Teen Health Series

Disease Management
SOURCEBOOK

First Edition

Health Reference Series

First Edition

Disease Management SOURCEBOOK

Basic Consumer Health Information about Coping with Chronic and Serious Illnesses, Navigating the Health Care System, Communicating with Health Care Providers, Assessing Health Care Quality, and Making Informed Health Care Decisions, Including Facts about Second Opinions, Hospitalization, Surgery, and Medications

Along with a Section about Children with Chronic Conditions, Information about Legal, Financial, and Insurance Issues, a Glossary of Related Terms, and Directories of Additional Resources

Edited by
Joyce Brennfleck Shannon

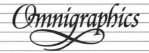

P.O. Box 31-1640, Detroit, MI 48231

Bibliographic Note

Because this page cannot legibly accommodate all the copyright notices, the Bibliographic Note portion of the Preface constitutes an extension of the copyright notice.

Edited by Joyce Brennfleck Shannon

Health Reference Series

Karen Bellenir, *Managing Editor*
David A. Cooke, M.D., *Medical Consultant*
Elizabeth Collins, *Research and Permissions Coordinator*
Cherry Stockdale, *Permissions Assistant*
EdIndex, Services for Publishers, *Indexers*

* * *

Omnigraphics, Inc.

Matthew P. Barbour, *Senior Vice President*
Kevin M. Hayes, *Operations Manager*

* * *

Peter E. Ruffner, *Publisher*

Copyright © 2008 Omnigraphics, Inc.

ISBN 978-0-7808-1002-0

Library of Congress Cataloging-in-Publication Data

Disease management sourcebook : basic consumer health information about coping with chronic and serious illnesses, navigating the health care system, communicating with health care providers, assessing health care quality, and making informed health care decisions, including facts about second opinions, hospitalization, surgery, and medications; along with a section about children with chronic conditions, information about legal, financial, and insurance issues, a glossary of related terms, and directories of additional resources / edited by Joyce Brennfleck Shannon.-- 1st ed.
    p. cm.
"Provides basic consumer health information about working with health care providers to manage serious and chronic illness, making decisions about care, understanding medications, and related financial and legal concerns. Includes index, glossary of related terms, and other resources"--Provided by publisher.
  Includes bibliographical references and index.
  ISBN-13: 978-0-7808-1002-0 (hardcover : alk. paper) 1. Chronic diseases--Treatment.
2. Consumer education. I. Shannon, Joyce Brennfleck.
  RC108.D58 2008
  616'.044--dc22
                                                                        2008004554

Table of Contents

Visit www.healthreferenceseries.com to view *A Contents Guide to the Health Reference Series*, a listing of more than 13,000 topics and the volumes in which they are covered.

Part III: Health Literacy and Making Informed Health Decisions

Part IV: Prescription (Rx) and Over-the-Counter (OTC) Medications

Part V: Managing Chronic Disease

Part VI: Children and Chronic Disease

Part VII: Legal, Financial, and Insurance Issues That Impact Disease Management

Part VIII: Additional Help and Information

Preface

About This Book

Making informed health care decisions requires the ability to obtain, process, and understand health information. Deficient health literacy skills are associated with lower rates of preventive service usage, higher rates of hospitalization, and higher health care costs. According to the U.S. Department of Health and Human Services' Office of Disease Prevention and Health Promotion, nearly nine out of ten adults in the U.S. lack the skills needed to manage their health and prevent disease. Health literacy skills are especially vital to the estimated 125 million Americans who are living with chronic illnesses, such as cardiovascular disease, diabetes, and cancer.

Disease Management Sourcebook addresses these concerns by providing facts about navigating the health care system, communicating with health care providers, and finding and evaluating health information. It discusses patient rights and responsibilities, privacy, medical errors, and health care fraud. It explains assistive technologies available to help people who have chronic illnesses and provides tips for dealing with legal, financial, and health insurance matters. Facts about medications—including prescription, generic, over-the-counter, and counterfeit drugs—are included. The book's end section features a glossary and directories of resources for patients and their families and caregivers.

How to Use This Book

This book is divided into parts and chapters. Parts focus on broad areas of interest. Chapters are devoted to single topics within a part.

Part I: Facts about Serious and Chronic Illnesses presents an overview of disease management in the United States. It includes information about risk factors for chronic disease and symptoms that may indicate serious health conditions or medical emergencies. It describes common screening and diagnostic tests and offers tips for finding support after receiving a diagnosis.

Part II: Working with Health Care Providers and the Health Care System provides information about effective communication in a doctor's office or hospital setting. Topics include second opinions, understanding medical specialties and alternative medicine, and clinical trials. Basic information is also provided about choosing a hospital and undergoing surgery, and issues related to health care quality are addressed.

Part III: Health Literacy and Making Informed Health Decisions discusses the skills that are essential for making knowledgeable health care choices. These include finding reliable health information, being aware of issues related to patient privacy rights, understanding informed consent, preventing medical errors, and recognizing fraud.

Part IV: Prescription (Rx) and Over-the-Counter (OTC) Medications provides information about what medications do and how to use them safely. It discusses purchasing and using prescription, generic, and over-the-counter drugs. Individual chapters provide details about common drug interactions, adverse drug reactions, drug name confusion, and counterfeit and misused drugs.

Part V: Managing Chronic Disease offers guidelines for self-management practices, including tips for dealing with pain, stress, and depression. Infection prevention, assistive technology, home modifications, and transitional and palliative care options are explained. A chapter offering tips for caregivers of individuals with chronic disease is also included.

Part VI: Children and Chronic Disease presents facts for parents and caregivers about serious illness in children, home health care, and the pediatric intensive care unit. It offers guidelines to help families and schools provide medical support for students with asthma, diabetes, and other chronic conditions, and it provides information about finding camps for children with special health needs.

Part VII: Legal, Financial, and Insurance Issues That Impact Disease Management includes information about health care benefit laws, the Americans with Disabilities Act, and the Family and Medical Leave Act. It describes advance directives and discusses hospital bills and access to free or reduced-cost health care. It also provides guidelines for purchasing health insurance and addresses such concerns as health savings accounts, medical discount plans and cards, the insurance needs of people with known medical risk factors, and the insurance claim process.

Part VIII: Additional Help and Information includes a glossary of related terms and directories of resources for information about disease management, health insurance, and financial assistance for medical treatments.

Bibliographic Note

This volume contains documents and excerpts from publications issued by the following U.S. government agencies: Administration on Aging; Agency for Healthcare Research and Quality (AHRQ); Centers for Disease Control and Prevention (CDC); Centers for Medicare and Medicaid Services (CMS); Federal Trade Commission (FTC); Health Care Financing Administration (HCFA); Health Resources and Services Administration (HRSA); National Cancer Institute (NCI); National Center for Complementary and Alternative Medicine (NCCAM); National Heart, Lung, and Blood Institute (NHLBI); National Human Genome Research Institute (NHGRI); National Institute on Aging (NIA); National Institute of Arthritis and Musculoskeletal and Skin Diseases (NIAMS); National Institute of Diabetes and Digestive and Kidney Diseases (NIDDK); National Institute of General Medical Sciences (NIGMS); National Institutes of Health (NIH); National Women's Health and Information Center (NWHIC); U.S. Department of Education (DOE); U.S. Department of Health and Human Services (HHS); U.S. Department of Justice (DOJ); U.S. Department of Labor (DOL); U.S. Department of the Treasury; U.S. Food and Drug Administration (FDA); and the U.S. Government Accountability Office (GAO).

In addition, this volume contains copyrighted documents from the following organizations: A.D.A.M., Inc.; American Academy of Family

Physicians; American Board of Medical Specialties; American College of Emergency Physicians; American Health Information Management Association; American Hospital Association; California Health Care Foundation; Cleveland Clinic; Families USA; Family Caregiver Alliance; Joint Commission; Lippincott Williams and Wilkins; National Association of Health Underwriters; National Family Caregivers Association (NFCA); National Health Care Anti-Fraud Association; National Pain Foundation; National Patient Safety Foundation; Nemours Foundation; Pharmaceutical Research and Manufacturers of America; and the Washington State Hospital Association.

Acknowledgements

In addition to the listed organizations, agencies, and individuals who have contributed to this *Sourcebook*, special thanks go to managing editor Karen Bellenir, research and permissions coordinator Liz Collins, and document engineer Bruce Bellenir for their help and support.

About the Health Reference Series

The *Health Reference Series* is designed to provide basic medical information for patients, families, caregivers, and the general public. Each volume takes a particular topic and provides comprehensive coverage. This is especially important for people who may be dealing with a newly diagnosed disease or a chronic disorder in themselves or in a family member. People looking for preventive guidance, information about disease warning signs, medical statistics, and risk factors for health problems will also find answers to their questions in the *Health Reference Series*. The *Series*, however, is not intended to serve as a tool for diagnosing illness, in prescribing treatments, or as a substitute for the physician/patient relationship. All people concerned about medical symptoms or the possibility of disease are encouraged to seek professional care from an appropriate health care provider.

A Note about Spelling and Style

Health Reference Series editors use *Stedman's Medical Dictionary* as an authority for questions related to the spelling of medical terms and the *Chicago Manual of Style* for questions related to grammatical structures, punctuation, and other editorial concerns. Consistent adherence is not always possible, however, because the individual volumes within the *Series* include many documents from a wide variety of different producers and copyright holders, and the editor's primary goal is to present material from each source as accurately as is possible following the terms specified by each document's producer. This sometimes means that information in different chapters or sections may follow other guidelines and alternate spelling authorities. For example, occasionally a copyright holder may require that eponymous terms be shown in possessive forms (Crohn's disease *vs.* Crohn disease) or that British spelling norms be retained (leukaemia *vs.* leukemia).

Locating Information within the Health Reference Series

The *Health Reference Series* contains a wealth of information about a wide variety of medical topics. Ensuring easy access to all the fact sheets, research reports, in-depth discussions, and other material contained within the individual books of the *Series* remains one of our highest priorities. As the *Series* continues to grow in size and scope, however, locating the precise information needed by a reader may become more challenging.

A *Contents Guide to the Health Reference Series* was developed to direct readers to the specific volumes that address their concerns. It presents an extensive list of diseases, treatments, and other topics of general interest compiled from the Tables of Contents and major index headings. To access A *Contents Guide to the Health Reference Series*, visit www.healthreferenceseries.com.

Medical Consultant

Medical consultation services are provided to the *Health Reference Series* editors by David A. Cooke, M.D. Dr. Cooke is a graduate of Brandeis University, and he received his M.D. degree from the University of Michigan. He completed residency training at the University of Wisconsin Hospital and Clinics. He is board-certified in Internal Medicine. Dr. Cooke currently works as part of the University of Michigan Health System and practices in Brighton, MI. In his free time, he enjoys writing, science fiction, and spending time with his family.

Our Advisory Board

We would like to thank the following board members for providing guidance to the development of this *Series*:

Health Reference Series *Update Policy*

The inaugural book in the *Health Reference Series* was the first edition of *Cancer Sourcebook* published in 1989. Since then, the *Series* has been enthusiastically received by librarians and in the medical community. In order to maintain the standard of providing high-quality health information for the layperson the editorial staff at Omnigraphics felt it was necessary to implement a policy of updating volumes when warranted.

Medical researchers have been making tremendous strides, and it is the purpose of the *Health Reference Series* to stay current with the most recent advances. Each decision to update a volume is made on an individual basis. Some of the considerations include how much new information is available and the feedback we receive from people who use the books. If there is a topic you would like to see added to the update list, or an area of medical concern you feel has not been adequately addressed, please write to:

Editor
Health Reference Series
Omnigraphics, Inc.
P.O. Box 31-1640
Detroit, MI 48231-1640
E-mail: editorial@omnigraphics.com

Part One

Facts about Serious and Chronic Illnesses

Chapter 1

Chronic Disease
in the United States

The Burden of Chronic Diseases

Chronic diseases such as heart disease, cancer, and diabetes are leading causes of disability and death in the United States. Every year, chronic diseases claim the lives of more than 1.7 million Americans. These diseases are responsible for seven of every ten deaths in the United States. Chronic diseases cause major limitations in daily living for more than one of every ten Americans or 25 million people. These diseases account for more than 70% of the $1 trillion spent on health care each year in the United States.

Although chronic diseases are among the most prevalent and costly health problems, they are also among the most preventable. Effective measures exist today to prevent or delay much of the chronic disease burden and curtail its devastating consequences.

Chronic diseases are not prevented by vaccines or generally cured by medication, nor do they just disappear. To a large degree, the major chronic disease killers—heart disease, cancer, stroke, chronic obstructive pulmonary disease, and diabetes—are an extension of what people do, or do not do, as they go about the business of daily living. Health-damaging behaviors—in particular tobacco use, lack of physical activity, and poor nutrition—are major contributors to heart disease

This chapter includes text from the following Centers for Disease Control and Prevention (CDC) documents: "Burden of Chronic Diseases 2004: Preface," reviewed April 4, 2006; "Chronic Disease Overview," November 18, 2005; and "Chronic Disease: Press Room Quick Facts," reviewed June 16, 2006.

3

and cancer, our nation's leading killers. A single behavior—tobacco use—is responsible for over 80% of deaths each year from chronic obstructive pulmonary disease, the nation's fourth leading cause of death. Clearly, promoting healthy behavior choices, through education and through community policies and practices, is essential to reducing the burden of chronic diseases.

In addition, we have the tools in hand to detect certain chronic diseases in their early stages, when treatment is most effective. Regular screening can detect cancers of the breast, cervix, colon, and rectum and is also critical for preventing the debilitating complications of diabetes, including blindness, kidney disease, and lower-extremity amputations. Screening and appropriate follow-up for high blood pressure and elevated cholesterol can save the lives of those at risk for cardiovascular disease. Access to high-quality, affordable prevention measures for all Americans is essential if we are to save lives and reduce medical care costs.

As the nation's prevention agency, the Centers for Disease Control and Prevention (CDC), in collaboration with its many partners (the states, voluntary and professional organizations, academic institutions, and other federal agencies), works to ensure that advances in basic scientific and behavioral research are put into practice to benefit all Americans. The framework for CDC efforts to prevent chronic diseases includes promoting healthy behaviors, expanding the use of early detection practices, reaching young people with important health messages, improving the health of communities, and supporting state-based public health interventions. Underpinning this framework is surveillance—the gathering of data to determine the extent of behavioral risks, to monitor the progress of prevention efforts, and ultimately, to make timely and effective public health decisions. The framework has been shown to be effective and, in many cases, cost-effective in reducing the chronic disease burden. Another generation of Americans need not suffer unnecessarily or die prematurely when so much is already known about how to prevent disability and death from chronic diseases.

Overview

The profile of diseases contributing most heavily to death, illness, and disability among Americans changed dramatically during the last century. Today, chronic diseases—such as cardiovascular disease (primarily heart disease and stroke), cancer, and diabetes—are among the most prevalent, costly, and preventable of all health problems. The prolonged course of illness and disability from such chronic diseases as diabetes and arthritis results in extended pain and suffering and decreases quality of life for millions of Americans.

Table 1.1. Causes of Death in the United States, 2004

Cause of Death	Percentage of All Deaths
Heart disease	27.2%
Cancer	23.1%
Cerebrovascular	6.3%
Chronic Lower Respiratory Disease	5.1%
Accidents	4.7%
Diabetes mellitus	3.1%
Alzheimer disease	2.8%
Pneumonia and influenza	2.5%
Other Causes	25.2%

Source: "Deaths: Final Data for 2004," National Center for Health Statistics (NCHS), January 11, 2007.

Costs of Chronic Disease

The United States cannot effectively address escalating health care costs without addressing the problem of chronic diseases:

- More than 90 million Americans live with chronic illnesses.

- Chronic diseases account for 70% of all deaths in the United States.

- The medical care costs of people with chronic diseases account for more than 75% of the nation's $1.4 trillion medical care costs.

- Chronic diseases account for one-third of the years of potential life lost before age 65.

- Hospitalizations for pregnancy-related complications occurring before delivery account for more than $1 billion annually.

- The direct and indirect costs of diabetes are nearly $132 billion a year.

- Each year, arthritis results in estimated medical care costs of more than $22 billion, and estimated total costs (medical care and lost productivity) of almost $82 billion.

- The estimated direct and indirect costs associated with smoking exceed $75 billion annually.

- In 2001, approximately $300 billion was spent on all cardiovascular diseases. Over $129 in lost productivity was due to cardiovascular disease.

- The direct medical cost associated with physical inactivity was nearly $76.6 billion in 2000.

- Nearly $68 billion is spent on dental services each year.

Cost-Effectiveness of Prevention

- For every $1 spent on water fluoridation, $38 is saved in dental restorative treatment costs.

- For a cost ranging from $1,108 to $4,542 for smoking cessation programs, one quality-adjusted year of life is saved. Smoking cessation interventions have been called the gold standard of cost-effective interventions.

- The direct medical cost associated with physical inactivity was $29 billion in 1987 and nearly $76.6 billion in 2000. Engaging in regular physical activity is associated with taking less medication and having fewer hospitalizations and physician visits.

- For each $1 spent on the Safer Choice Program (a school-based human immunodeficiency virus [HIV], other sexually transmitted disease [STD], and pregnancy prevention program), about $2.65 is saved on medical and social costs.

- For every $1 spent on preconception care programs for women with diabetes, $1.86 can be saved by preventing birth defects among their offspring.

- According to one Northern California study, for every $1 spent on the Arthritis Self-Help Program, $3.42 was saved in physician visits and hospital costs.

- A mammogram every two years for women aged 50–69 costs only about $9,000 per year of life saved. This cost compares favorably with other widely used clinical preventive services.

- For the cost of 100 Papanicolaou tests for low-income elderly women, about $5,907 and 3.7 years of life are saved.

- After controlling for physical limitation and major socioeconomic factors, more than 12% of annual medical costs of the inactive persons with arthritis is associated with physical inactivity. Physical activity interventions may be a cost-effective strategy for reducing the burden of arthritis.

Burden of Chronic Disease on Minority Racial Populations and Women

Breast and Cervical Cancer

African American women are more likely to die of breast cancer than are women of any other racial or ethnic group. The incidence of cervical cancer—a 100% preventable cancer—is more than five times greater among Vietnamese women in the United States than among white women.

Cardiovascular Disease

- More than half of persons who die each year of heart disease are women.

- Heart disease is the leading cause of death for all racial and ethnic groups in the United States. In 1998, rates of death from cardiovascular disease were about 30% higher among African American adults than among white adults.

Diabetes

- Diabetes affects more women than men.

- The prevalence of diabetes is 70% higher among African Americans and nearly 100% higher among Hispanics than among whites. The prevalence of diabetes among American Indians and Alaska Natives is more than twice that of the total population, and the Pimas of Arizona have the highest known prevalence of diabetes in the world.

Infant and Maternal Mortality

- African American, American Indian, and Puerto Rican infants have higher death rates than white infants. In 1998, the death rate among African American infants was 2.3 times greater than that among white infants.

- African American women are four times more likely to die of pregnancy-related complications than are white women, and American Indian and Alaska Native women are nearly twice as likely to die.

Table 1.2. Total Deaths and Deaths Due to Five Leading Chronic Disease Killers*, by State, 2001

State	Total Number of Deaths	Number of Deaths Due to Five Chronic Diseases*	Of all Deaths, Percentage Due to Five Chronic Diseases*
Alabama	45316	29554	65.2
Alaska	2974	1677	56.4
Arizona	41058	25768	62.8
Arkansas	27759	18735	67.5
California	234044	159606	68.2
Colorado	28294	16766	59.3
Connecticut	29827	19923	66.8
Delaware	7112	4726	66.5
District of Columbia	5951	3712	62.4
Florida	167269	113718	68.0
Georgia	64485	40180	62.3
Hawaii	8394	5553	66.2
Idaho	9753	6262	64.2
Illinois	105430	70866	67.2
Indiana	55198	37203	67.4
Iowa	27791	19133	68.8
Kansas	24647	16177	65.6
Kentucky	39861	27087	68.0
Louisiana	41757	27126	65.0
Maine	12421	8337	67.1
Maryland	43839	28879	65.9
Massachusetts	56754	36661	64.6
Michigan	86424	59089	68.4
Minnesota	37735	23576	62.5
Mississippi	28259	18937	67.0
Missouri	54982	37211	67.7
Montana	8265	5316	64.3
Nebraska	15174	9951	65.6

Table 1.2. (continued) Total Deaths and Deaths Due to Five Leading Chronic Disease Killers*, by State, 2001

State	Total Number of Deaths	Number of Deaths Due to Five Chronic Diseases*	Of all Deaths, Percentage Due to Five Chronic Diseases*
Nevada	16285	10579	65.0
New Hampshire	9815	6773	69.0
New Jersey	74710	50343	67.4
New Mexico	14129	8460	59.9
New York	159240	112074	70.4
North Carolina	70934	45953	64.8
North Dakota	6048	4102	67.8
Ohio	108027	73779	68.3
Oklahoma	34682	23622	68.1
Oregon	30158	19457	64.5
Pennsylvania	129729	87642	67.6
Rhode Island	10021	6864	68.5
South Carolina	36612	23394	63.9
South Dakota	6923	4639	67.0
Tennessee	55151	36641	66.4
Texas	152779	100494	65.8
Utah	12662	7113	56.2
Vermont	5201	3461	66.5
Virginia	56280	36744	65.3
Washington	44642	29885	66.9
West Virginia	20967	14357	68.5
Wisconsin	46628	31170	66.8
Wyoming	4029	2558	63.5
United States	2416425	1611833	66.7

* Diseases of the heart, all cancers, stroke, chronic lower respiratory disease, and diabetes.

Source: "Burden of Chronic Diseases 2004: Causes of Death," Centers for Disease Control and Prevention (CDC), reviewed October 2005.

Disability

Life expectancy is higher for women than for men, but women older than 70 years are more likely to be disabled.

Quick Facts: Economic and Health Burden of Chronic Disease

Heart Disease and Stroke

- More than 70 million Americans (over one-fourth of the population) live with a cardiovascular disease.
- Over 927,000 Americans die of cardiovascular disease or stroke each year, which amounts to one death every 34 seconds.

Cancer

- Cancer is the second leading cause of death in the United States. In 2005, approximately 570,280 Americans or more than 1,500 people a day, died of cancer.
- National Institutes of Health (NIH) estimates that the overall costs for cancer in the year 2004 were 189 billion—of this amount, $69 billion for direct medical costs and more than $120 billion for indirect costs such as lost productivity.

Tobacco

- An estimated 45.8 million adults in the United States smoke cigarettes even though this single behavior will result in death or disability for half of all regular users.
- Tobacco use is responsible for approximately 440,000 deaths each year. Additionally if current patterns of smoking continue, 6.4 million people currently younger than 18 will die prematurely from a tobacco-related disease.
- Smoking-related illnesses cost the nation more than $150 billion each year. The economic burden of tobacco use is enormous— more than $75 billion in medical expenditures and another $80 billion in indirect costs.

Diabetes

- Over 18.2 million Americans have diabetes, and about one-third of them don't know that they have the disease. By 2050, an estimated 29 million U.S. residents are expected to have diagnosed diabetes.

- Diabetes is the sixth leading cause of death. Over 200,000 people die each year of diabetes-related complications.

- The estimated economic cost of diabetes in 2002 was $132 billion. Of this amount, $92 billion was due to direct medical costs and $40 billion to indirect costs such as lost workdays, restricted activity, and disability due to diabetes.

Overweight/Obesity

- Between 1980 and 2000, obesity rates doubled among adults. About 60 million adults, or 30% of the adult population, are now obese. Since 1980, overweight rates have doubled among children and tripled among adolescents. About one in every six children (16.5%)—about 9 million young people—are considered overweight.

- The latest study from CDC scientists estimates that about 112,000 deaths are associated with obesity each year in the United States.

- Direct health costs attributable to obesity were estimated at $52 billion in 1995 and $75 billion in 2003. Among children and adolescents, annual hospital costs related to overweight and obesity more than tripled over the past two decades.

Additional Information

National Center for Chronic Disease Prevention and Health Promotion (NCCDPHP)
4770 Buford Hwy., N.E.
MS K–40
Atlanta, GA 30341-3717
Phone: 770-488-5131
Fax: 770-488-5962
Website: http://www.cdc.gov/nccdphp

Chapter 2

Family History Is Important to Your Health

Most of us know that we can reduce our risk of disease by eating a healthy diet, getting enough exercise, and not smoking. But did you know that your family history might be one of the strongest influences on your risk of developing heart disease, stroke, diabetes, or cancer? Even though you cannot change your genetic makeup, knowing your family history can help you reduce your risk of developing health problems.

Family History and Your Risk of Disease

Family members share their genes, as well as their environment, lifestyles, and habits. Everyone can recognize traits that run in their family, such as curly hair, dimples, leanness, or athletic ability. Risks for diseases such as asthma, diabetes, cancer, and heart disease also run in families. Everyone's family history of disease is different. The key features of a family history that may increase risk are:

- diseases that occur at an earlier age than expected (10 to 20 years before most people get the disease);

- disease in more than one close relative;

- disease that does not usually affect a certain gender (for example, breast cancer in a male); or

This chapter includes text from "Family History Is Important for Your Health," Centers for Disease Prevention (CDC), 2007; and excepts from "Family History: Frequently Asked Questions," CDC, April 19, 2007.

- certain combinations of diseases within a family (for example, breast and ovarian cancer, or heart disease and diabetes).

If your family has one or more of these features, your family history may hold important clues about your risk for disease.

Using Family History to Promote Your Health

People with a family history of disease may have the most to gain from lifestyle changes and screening tests. You can't change your genes, but you can change unhealthy behaviors, such as smoking, inactivity, and poor eating habits. In many cases, adopting a healthier lifestyle can reduce your risk for diseases that run in your family.

Screening tests (such as mammograms and colorectal cancer screening) can detect diseases like cancers at an early stage when they are most treatable. Screening tests can also detect disease risk factors like high cholesterol and high blood pressure, which can be treated to reduce the chances of getting disease.

Learning about Your Family History

To learn about your family history:

- ask questions,
- talk at family gatherings, and
- look at death certificates and family medical records, if possible.

Collect information about your grandparents, parents, aunts and uncles, nieces and nephews, siblings, and children. The type of information to collect includes:

- major medical conditions and causes of death,
- age of disease onset and age at death, and
- ethnic background.

Write down the information and share it with your doctor. Your doctor will:

- assess your disease risk based on your family history and other risk factors,
- recommend lifestyle changes to help prevent disease, and
- prescribe screening tests to detect disease early.

If your doctor notices a pattern of disease in your family, it may be a sign of an inherited form of disease that is passed on from generation to generation. Your doctor may refer you to a specialist who can help determine whether you have an inherited form of disease. Genetic testing may also help determine if you or your family members are at risk. Even with inherited forms of disease, steps can be taken to reduce your risk.

What If You Have No Family History?

Even if you don't have a history of a particular health problem in your family, you could still be at risk. This is because:

- your lifestyle, personal medical history, and other factors influence your chances of getting a disease;

- you may be unaware of disease in some family members;

- you could have family members who died young, before they had a chance to develop chronic conditions such as heart disease, stroke, diabetes, or cancer.

Being aware of your family health history is an important part of a lifelong wellness plan.

Frequently Asked Questions about Family Health History

What is family history?

Family history refers to health information about you and your close relatives. Family history is one of the most important risk factors for health problems like heart disease, stroke, diabetes, and cancer. (A risk factor is anything that increases your chance of getting a disease.)

Why is knowing my family history important?

Family members share their genes, as well as their environment, lifestyles, and habits. A family history helps identify people at increased risk for disease because it reflects both a person's genes and these other shared risk factors.

My mother had breast cancer. Does this mean I will get cancer, too?

Having a family member with a disease suggests that you may have a higher chance of developing that disease than someone without a similar family history. It does not mean that you will definitely develop the disease. Genes are only one of many factors that contribute to disease. Other factors to consider include lifestyle habits, such as diet and physical activity.

If you are at risk for breast cancer, consider following national guidelines for a healthy diet and regular exercise. It is also important to talk with your physician about your risk and follow recommendations for screening tests (such as mammograms) that may help to detect disease early, when it is most treatable.

Both of my parents had heart disease and I know I have bad genes. Is there anything I can do to protect myself?

First of all, there are no good or bad genes. Most human diseases, especially common diseases such as heart disease, result from the interaction of genes with environmental and behavioral risk factors that can be changed. The best disease prevention strategy for anyone, especially for someone with a family history, includes reducing risky behaviors (such as smoking) and increasing healthy behaviors (such as regular exercise).

How can knowing my family history help lower my risk of disease?

You can't change your genes, but you can change behaviors that affect your health, such as smoking, inactivity, and poor eating habits. People with a family history of chronic disease may have the most to gain from making lifestyle changes. In many cases, making these changes can reduce your risk of disease even if the disease runs in your family.

Another change you can make is to participate in screening tests, such as mammograms and colorectal cancer screening, for early detection of disease. People who have a family history of a chronic disease may benefit the most from screening tests that look for risk factors or early signs of disease. Finding disease early, before symptoms appear, can mean better health in the long run.

How do I learn about my family history if I'm adopted?

Learning about your family health history may be hard if you are adopted. Some adoption agencies collect medical information on birth relatives. This is becoming more common but is not routine. Laws concerning collection of information vary by state. Contact the health and social service agency in your state for information about how to access medical or legal records. The National Adoption Clearinghouse offers information on adoption and could be helpful if you decide to search for your birth parents. To learn more, visit http://www.childwelfare.gov/adoption/index.cfm.

What should I do with the information?

First, write down the information you collect about your family history and share it with your doctor. Second, remember to keep your information updated and share it with your siblings and children. Third, pass it on to your children, so that they too will have a family history record.

For More Information

CDC National Office of Public Health Genomics
4770 Buford Hwy.
Mail Stop K-89
Atlanta, GA 30341
Phone: 770-488-8510
Fax: 770-488-8355
Website: http://www.cdc.gov/genomics/public/famhist.htm
E-mail: genetics@cdc.gov

U.S. Surgeon General's Family History Initiative
Website: https://familyhistory.hhs.gov

This web-based tool helps users organize family health history information, print it out for presentation to the family doctor, save information to personal computers, and share that information with other family members.

Chapter 3

Assessing Risk Factors for Chronic Disease

Risk Factors for Chronic Disease and Use of Preventive Services by Adults in the United States

Poor Nutrition among Adults

Good nutrition, including a diet that is low in saturated fats and contains five or more servings of fruits and vegetables each day, plays a key role in maintaining good health. Improving the American diet could extend Americans' productive life span and reduce their risk for chronic diseases, including heart disease, stroke, some types of cancers, diabetes, and osteoporosis.

- Poor nutrition and lack of physical exercise are associated with at least 300,000 deaths each year in the United States.

- In 2002, more than three-fourths of U.S. adults reported not eating recommended amounts of fruits and vegetables daily.

- In 2002, the percentage of adults who did not eat the recommended amounts of fruits and vegetables ranged from 66% in the District of Columbia to 86% in Oklahoma.

Excerpts from "The Burden of Chronic Diseases and Their Risk Factors: National and State Perspectives 2004," Centers for Disease Control and Prevention (CDC), reviewed October 2005.

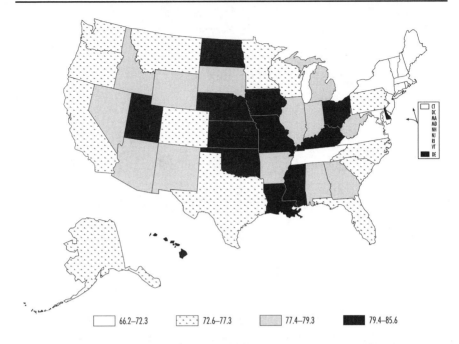

Figure 3.1. *Percentage of Adults Who Reported Eating Fewer Than Five Servings of Fruits and Vegetables per Day, 2002. Source: Centers for Disease Control and Prevention (CDC), Behavioral Risk Factor Surveillance System.*

No Leisure-Time Physical Activity among Adults

Regular physical activity reduces the risk for heart attack, colon cancer, diabetes, and high blood pressure, and may reduce the risk for stroke. It also helps to control weight; contributes to healthy bones, muscles, and joints; reduces falls among the elderly; helps to relieve the pain of arthritis; reduces symptoms of anxiety and depression; and can decrease the need for hospitalizations, physician visits, and medications. Moreover, physical activity need not be strenuous to be beneficial; people of all ages benefit from moderate physical activity, such as 30 minutes of brisk walking five or more times a week.

- In 2002, 25% of U.S. adults (28% of women and 22% of men) reported no leisure-time physical activity.

- No leisure time physical activity was more prevalent among Hispanics (37%) and blacks (33%) than among whites (22%).

- The percentage of adults reporting no leisure-time physical activity in 2002 ranged from 15% in Washington to 34% in Louisiana and Tennessee.

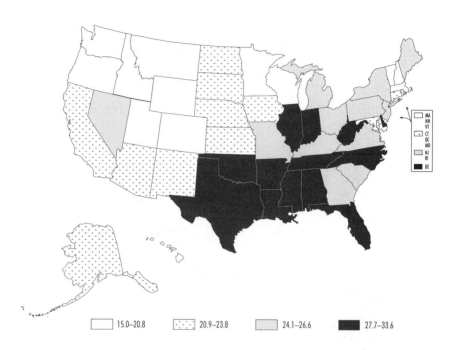

| | 15.0–20.8 | | 20.9–23.8 | | 24.1–26.6 | | 27.7–33.6 |

Figure 3.2. *Percentage of Adults Who Reported No Leisure-Time Physical Activity,˙ 2002. (˙No exercise, recreation, or physical activity (other than regular job duties) during the previous month.) Source: CDC, Behavioral Risk Factor Surveillance System.*

Cigarette Smoking among Adults

Tobacco use is the single most preventable cause of death and disease in the United States. Tobacco use increases the risk for lung and other cancers, cardiovascular disease, chronic lung disease, and adverse reproductive outcomes. Quitting smoking has major and immediate health benefits for men and women of all ages. Smokers who quit will, on average, live longer and have fewer years of disability.

- Cigarette smoking is responsible for more than 440,000 deaths each year, or one in every five deaths. Almost 10% of these deaths are a result of exposure to secondhand smoke.

- About 8.6 million people in the United States have at least one serious illness caused by smoking.

- The direct and indirect costs of smoking-related illnesses total more than $157 billion each year.

- The prevalence of cigarette smoking among adults in the United States in 2002 ranged from 13% in Utah to 33% in Kentucky.

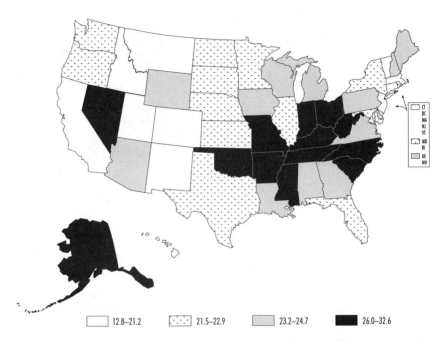

| | 12.8–21.2 | | 21.5–22.9 | | 23.2–24.7 | | 26.0–32.6 |

Figure 3.3. *Percentage of Adults Who Reported Cigarette Smoking,˙ 2002 (˙Ever smoked at least 100 cigarettes and now smoke every day or some days.) Source: CDC, Behavioral Risk Factor Surveillance System.*

Overweight and Obesity among Adults

Obesity has reached epidemic proportions in the United States, where it has more than doubled in the past two decades. People who are overweight (body mass index [BMI] over 25) or obese (BMI over 30) are at increased risk for heart disease, high blood pressure, diabetes, arthritis-related disabilities, and some cancers. In 2000, the direct and indirect cost attributable to obesity in the United States was $117 billion.

- In 2002, 59% of American adults were overweight on the basis of self-reported weight and height.

- In 2002, men were more likely than women to be overweight (67% versus 51%) on the basis of self-reported weight and height.

- The percentage of adults who reported being overweight on the basis of weight and height in 2002 ranged from 53% in Hawaii and the District of Columbia to 64% in West Virginia.

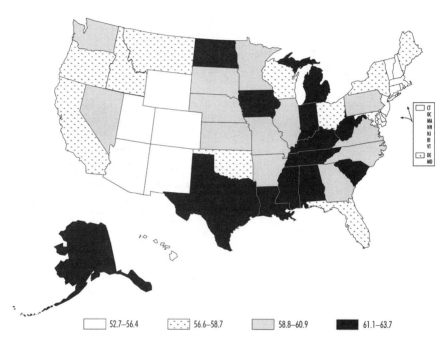

Figure 3.4. *Percentage of Adults Who Were Overweight or Obese, 2002. Source: CDC, Behavioral Risk Factor Surveillance System.*

High Blood Pressure

High blood pressure is a major modifiable risk factor for heart disease and stroke. All adults need to be aware that having their blood pressure checked regularly is an important first step in identifying and controlling high blood pressure. Medications to reduce blood pressure levels among people with high blood pressure can reduce their risk for heart disease, stroke, and other coronary events.

- A 12–13 point reduction in blood pressure among people with high blood pressure can reduce heart attacks by 21%, strokes by 37%, and total cardiovascular disease (CVD) deaths by 25%.

- Fifty million Americans have high blood pressure, and another 45 million are pre-hypertensive, or at high risk of developing high blood pressure.

- Seventy percent of people with high blood pressure do not have it under control.

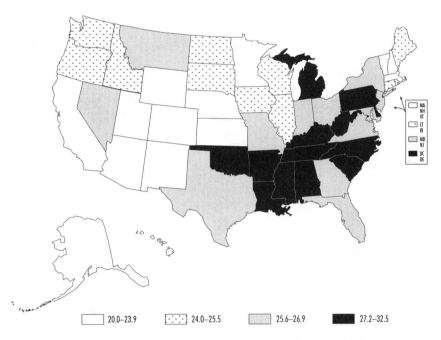

Figure 3.5. *Percentage of Adults Who Reported Having High Blood Pressure, 2001. Source: CDC, Behavioral Risk Factor Surveillance System.*

High Blood Cholesterol

High blood cholesterol is one of the major independent risk factors for heart disease and stroke. Educating the public and the health care community about the importance of prevention through controlling cholesterol levels is critical to reducing the health and economic burden of heart disease and stroke. Current guidelines recommend that all adults have their blood cholesterol levels checked every five years.

- An estimated 105 million Americans have a total cholesterol level of 200 milligrams (mg)/deciliter (dL) or higher, which is considered above optimal levels.

- Over 80% of those who have high blood cholesterol do not have it under control.

- A 10% decrease in total cholesterol levels may reduce the incidence of coronary heart disease by an estimated 30%.

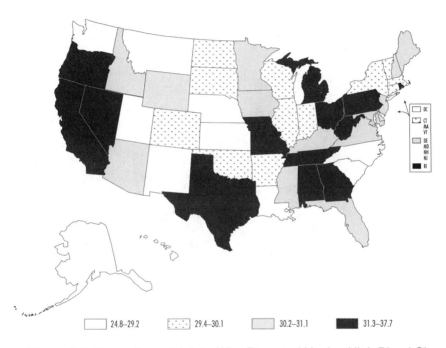

| | 24.8–29.2 | | 29.4–30.1 | | 30.2–31.1 | | 31.3–37.7 |

Figure 3.6. *Percentage of Adults Who Reported Having High Blood Cholesterol, 2001. Source: CDC, Behavioral Risk Factor Surveillance System.*

Lack of Mammography Screening

Mammography is the best available method to detect breast cancer in its earliest, most treatable stage, which on average is 1–3 years before a woman can feel a lump. Mammography also locates cancers too small to be felt during a clinical breast examination. Women aged 40 years and older should have a screening mammogram every 1–2 years.

- Timely mammography screening among women aged 40 or older can prevent approximately 16% of all deaths from breast cancer, and the risk reduction associated with screening increases as women get older.

- In 2002, 20% of American women aged 50 years or older reported that they had not had a mammogram in the previous two years.

- In 2002, the prevalence of not having had a mammogram during the previous two years among women aged 50 years or older ranged from 12% in Rhode Island to 31% in Arkansas.

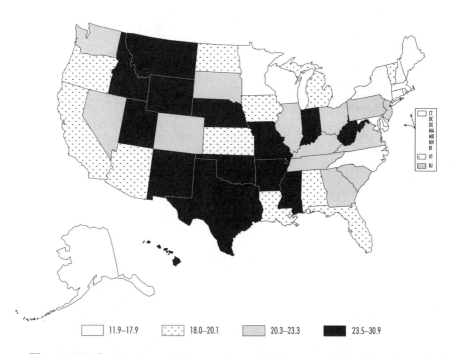

| | 11.9–17.9 | | 18.0–20.1 | | 20.3–23.3 | | 23.5–30.9 |

Figure 3.7. *Percentage of Women Aged 50 Years or Older Who Reported Not Having Had a Mammogram in the Previous Two Years, 2002. Source: CDC, Behavioral Risk Factor Surveillance System.*

Lack of Sigmoidoscopy or Colonoscopy

Colorectal cancer almost always develops from precancerous polyps (abnormal growths) in the colon or rectum. Sigmoidoscopy or colonoscopy can find polyps so they can be removed before they become cancerous. These screening tests can also find colorectal cancer early, when treatment works best. Sigmoidoscopy or colonoscopy is recommended every five years for people aged 50 years or older. Despite its proven effectiveness, colorectal cancer screening is used far less than screening for other cancers.

- Studies have found that people who had had a sigmoidoscopy had 59% fewer deaths from colorectal cancers within reach of a sigmoidoscope than people who had not had a sigmoidoscopy.

- In 2002, 60% of Americans aged 50 years or older reported not having had a sigmoidoscopy or colonoscopy within the previous five years.

- The prevalence of not having had a sigmoidoscopy or colonoscopy during the previous five years among Americans aged 50 years or older ranged from 45% in Minnesota to 70% in Oklahoma and Wyoming.

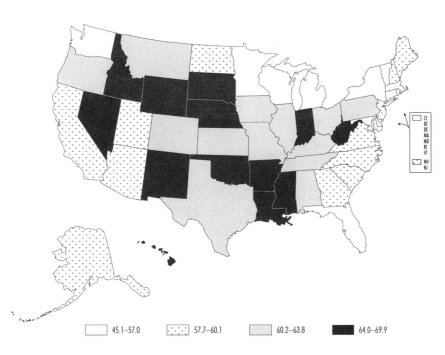

| | 45.1–57.0 | | 57.7–60.1 | | 60.2–63.8 | | 64.0–69.9 |

Figure 3.8. Percentage of Adults Aged 50 Years or Older Who Reported Not Having Had a Sigmoidoscopy or Coloscopy in the Previous Five Years, 2002. Source: CDC, Behavioral Risk Factor Surveillance System.

Lack of Fecal Occult Blood Test

The fecal occult blood test checks for occult (hidden) blood in the stool. Proven to be beneficial in screening for colorectal cancer, this test is recommended annually for people aged 50 years or older. Studies have shown that annual fecal occult blood tests can reduce the number of colorectal cancer deaths by one-third. Despite the availability of this effective screening test, it is widely underused.

- In 2002, 78% of Americans aged 50 years or older reported not having had a fecal occult blood test within the previous year.

- The prevalence of not having had a fecal occult blood test within the previous year among Americans aged 50 years or older ranged from 67% in Maine to 88% in Utah and Wyoming.

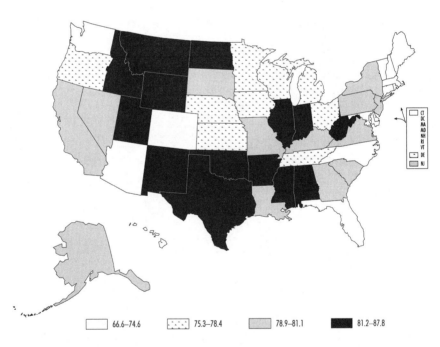

66.6–74.6   75.3–78.4   78.9–81.1   81.2–87.8

Figure 3.9. Percentage of Adults Aged 50 Years or Older Who Reported Not Having Had a Fecal Occult Blood Test within the Previous Year, 2002. Source: CDC, Behavioral Risk Factor Surveillance System.

No Health Care Coverage

Health care coverage includes health insurance, prepaid plans such as health maintenance organizations (HMO), and government plans such as Medicaid and Medicare. The U.S. health care system is rapidly changing. As this system evolves, health care plans need to ensure access to affordable, high-quality preventive services (for example, screening for early detection) for all Americans.

- In 2002, 18% of U.S. adults aged 18–64 years reported having no health care coverage.

- Hispanics were almost three times more likely than whites to report having no health care coverage.

- The prevalence of having no health care coverage among U.S. adults aged 18–64 years ranged from 8% in Minnesota to 31% in Texas.

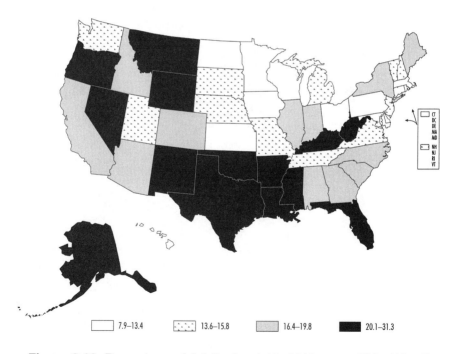

7.9–13.4   13.6–15.8   16.4–19.8   20.1–31.3

Figure 3.10. *Percentage of Adults Aged 18–64 Years or Older Who Reported Having No Health Care Coverage, 2002. Source: CDC, Behavioral Risk Factor Surveillance System.*

Risk Factors for Chronic Disease and Use of Preventive Services by High School Students in the United States

Cigarette Smoking among High School Students

Preventing tobacco use among young people is critical to the overall goal of reducing the prevalence of smoking. Almost all smokers begin smoking during their teenage years. Every year, nearly three-quarters of a million young people become regular smokers. If current patterns continue, more than six million young people who are regular smokers will eventually die from a tobacco-related disease. Factors associated with young people using tobacco include nicotine dependence, public attitudes about smoking, tobacco marketing, and peer and parental influences.

- According to a study by the Substance Abuse and Mental Health Services Administration (SAMHSA), every day 4,100 young people aged 12–17 try cigarettes for the first time.

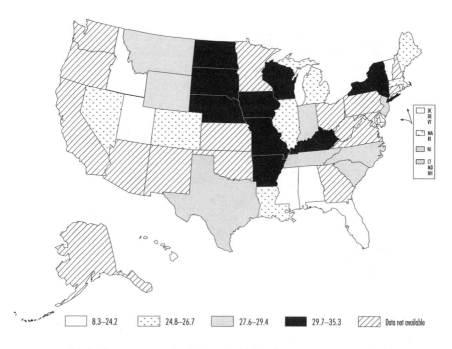

8.3–24.2   24.8–26.7   27.6–29.4   29.7–35.3   Data not available

Figure 3.11. *Percentage of High School Students Who Reported Cigarette Smoking,* 2001 (*Smoked cigarettes on one or more of the 30 days preceding the survey.) Source: CDC, Behavioral Risk Factor Surveillance System.*

30

- SAMHSA also reports that, among all people who ever smoked cigarettes, the average age at which they first smoked was 15.4 years.

- In 2001, 29% of U.S. high school students reported having smoked a cigarette in the last month.

- The percentage of high school students who reported having smoked a cigarette in the last month in the states that collected this information in 2001 ranged from 8% in Utah to 35% in Arkansas and North Dakota.

Overweight among High School Students

The obesity epidemic is not limited to adults. According to data from the National Health and Nutrition Examination Survey, the

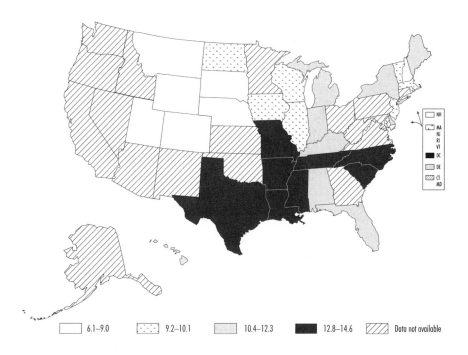

6.1–9.0   9.2–10.1   10.4–12.3   12.8–14.6   Data not available

Figure 3.12. Percentage of High School Students Who Reported Being Overweight, 2001. (*Body mass index greater than or equal to the 95th percentile by age and sex among participants in the First National Health and Nutrition Examination Survey, 1971–1975.) Source: CDC, Behavioral Risk Factor Surveillance System.*

31

percentage of adolescents who are overweight has more than doubled during the past two decades. Overweight or obesity that begins in childhood or adolescence may continue into adulthood and increase the risk later in life for heart disease, gallbladder disease, and some types of cancer.

- In 2001, 11% of U.S. high school students were overweight on the basis of self-reported weight and height, and 14% were at risk of becoming overweight.

- Being overweight was reported by a greater proportion of male students (14%) than female students (7%).

- In 2001, the percentage of high school students who reported being overweight in the states collecting this information ranged from 6% in Montana and Utah to 14% in Arkansas, Mississippi, and Texas.

Lack of Enrollment in Physical Education Class among High School Students

Regular physical activity in childhood and adolescence improves strength and endurance, helps build healthy bones and muscles, helps control weight, reduces anxiety and stress, increases self-esteem, and may improve blood pressure and cholesterol levels. High school physical education (PE) classes are important for ensuring that young people have a minimal, regular amount of physical activity and for establishing physical activity patterns that may be carried into adulthood.

- In 2001, 48% of U.S. high school students were not enrolled in a PE class.

- Among high school students in 2001, the percentage who attended PE class one or more days during an average school week declined with each successive grade, from 74% of 9th graders to 31% of 12th graders.

- The percentage of high school students who reported not being enrolled in a PE class in the states that collected this information in 2001 ranged from 6% in New York to 78% in South Dakota.

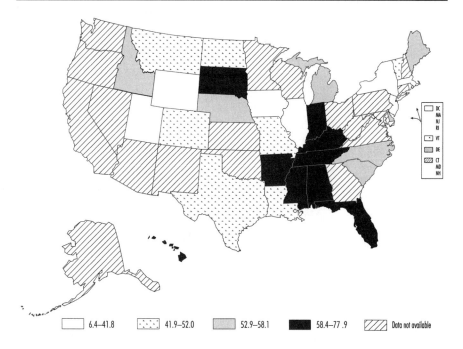

Figure 3.13. *Percentage of High School Students Who Reported Not Being Enrolled in Physical Education Class, 2001. Source: CDC, Behavioral Risk Factor Surveillance System.*

Chapter 4

When to See a Doctor: Symptoms of Serious Health Conditions

Some symptoms can be signs of serious health conditions and should be checked by a doctor or nurse. It is important to note that you might feel symptoms in one part of your body that could actually mean a problem in another part. Even if the symptoms do not seem related, they could be. Keep track of symptoms. If you have any of these symptoms, make an appointment to see your doctor. Listen to what your body is telling you, and be sure to describe every symptom in detail to your health care provider.

Signs of a Heart Attack

Some symptoms of a heart attack can happen a month or so before the heart attack. Before a heart attack, you may have one or more of these symptoms:

- unusual tiredness
- trouble sleeping
- problems breathing
- indigestion
- anxiety

"Tools to Help You Build a Healthier Life! Symptoms of Serious Health Conditions," National Women's Health Information Center, October 2006.

During a heart attack, you may have one or more of these symptoms:

- pain or discomfort in the center of the chest
- pain or discomfort in other areas of the upper body, including the arms, back, neck, jaw, or stomach
- other symptoms, such as shortness of breath, breaking out in a cold sweat, nausea, or light-headedness

If you have any of these symptoms, go to an emergency room right away or call 911.

Signs of a Stroke

Signs of a stroke happen suddenly and are different from signs of a heart attack.

- sudden or developing problems with speaking or understanding
- sudden or developing problems with sight
- sudden or developing problems with balance, coordination, walking, and dizziness
- sudden numbness or weakness in the face, arms, or legs
- sudden severe headache with no known cause

If you have any of these symptoms, go to an emergency room right away or call 911.

Symptoms of Reproductive Health Problems

- bleeding or spotting between periods
- itching, burning, or irritation (including bumps, blisters, or sores) of the vagina or genital area
- pain or discomfort during sex
- severe or painful bleeding with periods
- moderate to severe pelvic pain
- unusual (for you) vaginal discharge of any type or color or with strong odor

Symptoms of Breast Problems

- nipple discharge
- unusual breast tenderness or pain
- breast or nipple skin changes such as ridges, dimpling, pitting, swelling, redness, or scaling
- lump or thickening in or near breast or in underarm area, or tenderness

Symptoms of Lung Problems

- blood when you cough
- persistent cough that gets worse over time
- repeated bouts of bronchitis or pneumonia
- shortness of breath
- wheezing

Symptoms of Stomach or Digestive Problems

- bleeding from the rectum
- blood or mucus in the stool (including diarrhea) or black stools
- change in bowel habits or not being able to control bowels
- constipation, diarrhea, or both
- heartburn or acid reflux (feels like burning in throat or mouth)
- pain or feeling of fullness in stomach
- unusual abdominal swelling, bloating, or general discomfort
- vomiting of blood

Symptoms of Bladder Problems

- difficult or painful urination
- frequent urination or loss of bladder control
- blood in urine
- feeling the urge to urinate when bladder is empty

Symptoms of Skin Problems

- changes in the skin, such as changes in existing moles or new growths
- moles that are no longer round or have irregular borders
- moles that change colors or change in size (usually get bigger)
- frequent flushing (a sudden feeling of heat)
- jaundice (when the skin and whites of the eyes turn yellow)
- painful, crusting, scaling, or oozing sores that do not heal
- sensitivity to sun

Symptoms of Muscle or Joint Problems

- muscle pains and body aches that are persistent, or that come and go often
- numbness, tingling (pins and needles sensation), or discomfort in hands, feet, or limbs
- pain, stiffness, swelling, or redness in or around joints

Symptoms of Emotional Problems

These symptoms can have a physical cause and are usually treatable:

- anxiety and constant worry
- depression—feeling empty, sad all the time, or worthless
- extreme fatigue, even when rested
- extreme tension that cannot be explained
- flashbacks and nightmares about traumatic events
- no interest in getting out of bed or doing regular activities, including eating or sex
- thoughts about suicide and death
- seeing or hearing things that aren't there (hallucinations)
- seeing things differently from what they are (delusions)

- "baby blues" that haven't gone away two weeks after giving birth and seem to get worse over time

- thoughts about harming yourself, others, or your baby after giving birth

Symptoms of Headache Problems

- headaches between the eyes

- headaches that come on suddenly

- headaches that last longer than a couple of days

- seeing flashing lights or zigzag lines and temporary vision loss before a headache starts

- spreading pain in face that starts in one eye

- severe pain on one or both sides of head with upset stomach, nausea, or vision problems

Symptoms of Eating or Weight Problems

- extreme thirst or hunger

- losing weight without trying

- desire to binge on food excessively

- desire to vomit on purpose

- desire to starve (not eat at all)

Chapter 5

Is It a Medical Emergency?

When Should I Go to the Emergency Department?

More than 300,000 Americans on average are treated in our nation's emergency departments every day, according to the latest government statistics, and patients are treated for a wide variety of medical conditions.

How do you decide when a medical condition rises to the level of a medical "emergency?" The American College of Emergency Physicians (ACEP) offers a list of warning signs that indicate a medical emergency. These include:

- difficulty breathing, shortness of breath;

- chest or upper abdominal pain or pressure;

- fainting, sudden dizziness, weakness;

- changes in vision;

- confusion or changes in mental status;

- any sudden or severe pain;

- uncontrolled bleeding;

- severe or persistent vomiting or diarrhea;

- coughing or vomiting blood;

- suicidal feelings;

- difficulty speaking;

- shortness of breath; or

- unusual abdominal pain.

Children have unique medical problems and may display different symptoms than adults. Symptoms that are serious for a child may not be as serious for an adult. Children may also be unable to communicate their condition, which means an adult will have to interpret the behavior. Always get immediate medical attention if you think your child is having a medical emergency.

"If you or a loved one think you need emergency care, come to the emergency department and have a doctor examine you," said Dr. Frederick Blum, president of ACEP. "If you think the medical condition is life-threatening or the person's condition will worsen on the way to the hospital, then you need to call 9-1-1 and have your local emergency medical services provider come to you."

Emergency departments see patients based on the severity of their illnesses or injuries, not on a first-come, first-served basis. With that in mind, ACEP offers the following tips to patients when they come to an emergency department in order to get the best possible care as quickly as possible:

- Bring a list of medications and allergies: What's the name of the medication you are taking? How often do you take it and for how long? A list of allergies is important, especially if there are many of them. Be sure to include medications, foods, insects, or any other product that may cause an allergic reaction. Bring a medical history form with you.

- Know your immunizations: This will likely be a long list for children; mainly tetanus, flu and hepatitis B for adults.

- Remain calm: Obviously it is difficult to remain composed if you've been badly injured, but a calm attitude can help increase communication with the doctors and nurses who are caring for you.

Communication is important when you arrive at an emergency department," said Dr. Blum. "I want to know as much about the patient, as I can as quickly as I can, so the proper treatment can begin.

There can be long waits in the emergency department as doctors and nurses tend to those with the most severe conditions, but by all means tell them if you are in pain or there is any change in your condition while you are at the hospital."

What to Do in an Emergency

Main Points

- Emergency physicians are medical specialists who are trained to provide lifesaving care. They diagnose and treat every kind of medical condition that becomes an emergency.

- Emergency physicians provide lifesaving care 24 hours a day, 7 days a week, 365 days a year and care for everyone, regardless of their ability to pay.

- Emergency personnel educate the public to program their cell phones with an emergency contact name and phone number under the acronym ICE [in case of emergency].

- The initial minutes after an injury or medical crisis frequently are the most important. The key is knowing what to do, remaining calm and making a decision to act.

Preventing Medical Emergencies

- Preventing medical emergencies means getting yearly doctor's exams and regular exercise. Protect your health by determining whether you are at risk for any life-threatening conditions, and follow your doctor's suggestions to reduce any risk factors that can be dangerous to your health. For example, if you don't smoke, don't start. If you do smoke, quit.

- All medicines should be kept in childproof containers and well out of the reach of children.

- All poisonous materials should be stored out of reach of children in childproof containers.

- Drive carefully and appropriately to weather and traffic conditions. Children should be secured in child-safety seats. Your local police and fire department can help ensure you have installed the seat correctly.

- All passengers in motor vehicles should wear safety belts.

43

- Many states have regulations regarding the wearing of personal flotation devices (PFD) or lifejackets on watercraft. Even strong swimmers can become incapacitated in an accident.

- Never operate a vehicle if under the influence of alcohol or drugs. Read warning labels on all medications to see if they impair your ability to drive or operate machinery.

Preparing for Medical Emergencies

The initial minutes after an injury or medical crisis frequently are the most important. The key is knowing what to do, remaining calm and making a decision to act.

- Keep a list of emergency phone numbers by the phone. Include numbers for: police, fire, poison control, local hospital, ambulance service, and your family physician.

- Keep and maintain a well-stocked first-aid kit at home, at work, and in your vehicle. This will help you handle medical situations. ACEP offers information about what should be included in first-aid kits at www.acep.org.

- Keep a list of all your medications in your wallet, including drug names, strength, dosage form, and regimen. Also list all allergies, especially to medications.

- Also keep a list of emergency contacts such as family members.

- Wear your medical-alert bracelet or necklace.

- Take a first-aid class. This will not only help you stay calm and focused, but will also help you to help yourself and those around you in the event of an emergency.

Recognizing What Is and What Is Not an Emergency

- If the emergency is life threatening—call 9-1-1. This is a free call from any phone, including pay phones. Even non-activated cell phones, provided they have power, can be used to reach 911.

- If the emergency is not life threatening, do not call 911. It is more cost effective to drive or take a taxi to the hospital or doctor. Ask yourself the following questions:

- Could the victim's condition worsen and become life threatening on the way to the hospital?

- Could moving the victim need the skills or equipment of paramedics or emergency medical technicians?

- Would distance or traffic conditions cause a delay in getting the victim to the hospital?

- If you suspect a spinal injury, do not move the victim. Call 911 and wait for help to arrive. You may be asked to administer cardiopulmonary resuscitation (CPR) or the Heimlich maneuver in cases of stopped breathing or choking.

- The victims of any future attack; whether nuclear, chemical, biological or conventional; will be sent to emergency departments for treatment.

Responding Appropriately in Medical Emergencies

- Action can mean anything from calling paramedics, applying direct pressure to a wound, performing CPR, or splinting an injury. Never perform a medical procedure if you are unsure of how to do it.

- Calling 9-1-1 is the best thing to do in an emergency situation, even if you cannot speak. 911 operators can identify your location from the call. Do not hang up until instructed to do so by the operator.

- Emergency rooms provide services to any and all patients, regardless of their ability to pay, insurance coverage.

Additional Information

American College of Emergency Physicians
P.O. Box 619911
Dallas, TX 75261-9911
Toll-Free: 800-798-1822
Phone: 972-550-0911
Fax: 972-580-2816
Website: http://www.acep.org
E-mail: membership@acep.org

Chapter 6

Common Screening and Diagnostic Tests

Screening Tests: What You Need and When

Screening tests can find diseases early when they are easier to treat. Health experts from the U.S. Preventive Services Task Force have made recommendations, based on scientific evidence, about testing for the listed conditions. Talk to your doctor about which ones apply to you and when and how often you should be tested.

- **Obesity:** Have your body mass index (BMI) calculated to screen for obesity. (BMI is a measure of body fat based on height and weight.) You can also find your own BMI with the BMI calculator from the National Heart, Lung, and Blood Institute at http://www.nhlbisupport.com/bmi.

- **Breast cancer:** Have a mammogram every 1–2 years starting at age 40.

- **Cervical cancer:** Have a Pap smear every 1–3 years if you:

This chapter includes text from "Women: Stay Healthy at Any Age—Your Checklist for Health," Agency for Healthcare Research and Quality (AHRQ), Publication No. 07-IP005-A, February 2007, and excerpts from "Men: Stay Healthy at Any Age—Your Checklist for Health," AHRQ, Publication No. 07-IP006-A, February 2007. Text under the heading "Lab Tests" is from the U.S. Food and Drug Administration (FDA) February 2005. Text under the heading "Common Preventive and Diagnostic Tests" is from National Women's Health Information Center (NWHIC), October 2006.

- have ever been sexually active; or
- are between the ages of 21 and 65.

- **High cholesterol:** Have your cholesterol checked regularly starting at age 45. If you are younger than 45, talk to your doctor about whether to have your cholesterol checked if:
  - you have diabetes;
  - you have high blood pressure;
  - heart disease runs in your family; or
  - you smoke.

- **High blood pressure:** Have your blood pressure checked at least every two years. High blood pressure is 140/90 or higher.

- **Colorectal cancer:** Have a test for colorectal cancer starting at age 50. Your doctor can help you decide which test is right for you. If you have a family history of colorectal cancer, you may need to be screened earlier.

- **Diabetes:** Have a test for diabetes if you have high blood pressure or high cholesterol.

- **Depression:** Your emotional health is as important as your physical health. If you have felt down, sad, or hopeless over the last two weeks or have felt little interest or pleasure in doing things, you may be depressed. Talk to your doctor about being screened for depression.

- **Chlamydia and other sexually transmitted infections:** Have a test for chlamydia if you are 25 or younger and sexually active. If you are older, talk to your doctor about being tested. Also, ask whether you should be tested for other sexually transmitted diseases.

- **Human immunodeficiency virus (HIV):** Have a test to screen for HIV infection if you:
  - have had sex with men since 1975;
  - have had unprotected sex with multiple partners;
  - are pregnant;
  - have used or now use injection drugs;

- exchange sex for money or drugs or have sex partners who do;
- have past or present sex partners who are HIV-infected, are bisexual, or use injection drugs;
- are being treated for sexually transmitted diseases; or
- had a blood transfusion between 1978 and 1985.

- **Abdominal aortic aneurysm:** If you are between the ages of 65 and 75 and have ever smoked (100 or more cigarettes during your lifetime, you need to be screened once for abdominal aortic aneurysm—an abnormally large or swollen blood vessel in your abdomen.

- **Osteoporosis (thinning of the bones):** Have a bone density test beginning at age 65 to screen for osteoporosis. If you are between the ages of 60 and 64 and weigh 154 pounds or less, talk to your doctor about being tested.

Lab Tests

Laboratory tests are medical procedures that involve testing samples of blood, urine, or other tissues or substances in the body. Your doctor uses laboratory tests to help:

- identify changes in your health condition before any symptoms occur;
- diagnose a disease or condition before you have symptoms;
- plan your treatment for a disease or condition;
- evaluate your response to a treatment; or
- monitor the course of a disease over time.

How are lab tests analyzed?

After your doctor collects a sample from your body, it is sent to a laboratory. Laboratories perform tests on the sample to see if it reacts to different substances. Depending on the test, a reaction may mean you do have a particular condition, or it may mean that you do not have the particular condition. Sometimes laboratories compare your results to results obtained from previous tests to see if there has been a change in your condition.

What do lab tests show?

Lab tests show whether or not your results fall within normal ranges. Normal test values are usually given as a range, rather than as a specific number, because normal values vary from person to person. What is normal for one person may not be normal for another person.

Some laboratory tests are precise, reliable indicators of specific health problems, while others provide more general information that gives doctors clues to your possible health problems. Information obtained from laboratory tests may help doctors decide whether other tests or procedures are needed to make a diagnosis or to develop or revise a previous treatment plan. All laboratory test results must be interpreted within the context of your overall health and should be used along with other exams or tests.

What factors affect your lab test results?

Factors such as sex, age, and race can affect test results. Others factors include:

- medical history;
- general health;
- specific foods;
- drugs you are taking;
- how closely your follow preparatory instructions;
- variations in laboratory techniques; or
- variation from one laboratory to another.

Common Preventive and Diagnostic Tests

- **Angiogram:** Exam of your blood vessels using x-rays. The doctor inserts a small tube into the blood vessel and injects dye to see the vessels on the x-ray.

- **Barium enema:** A lubricated enema tube is gently inserted into your rectum. Barium flows into your colon. An x-ray is taken of the large intestine.

- **Biopsy:** A test that removes cells or tissues for examination by a pathologist to diagnose for disease. The tissue is examined under a microscope for cancer or other diseases.

- **Blood test:** Blood is taken from a vein in the inside elbow or back of the hand to test for a health problem.

- **Bone mineral density test (BMD):** Special x-rays of your bones are used to test if you have osteoporosis, or a weakening of the bones.

- **Bronchoscopy:** Exam of the lungs. A bronchoscope, or flexible tube, is put through the nose or mouth and into your windpipe (trachea).

- **Clinical breast exam (CBE):** A doctor, nurse, or other health professional uses his or her hands to examine your breasts and underarm areas to find lumps or other problems.

- **Chest x-ray:** An x-ray of the chest, lungs, heart, large arteries, ribs, and diaphragm.

- **Colonoscopy:** An examination of the inside of the colon using a colonoscope, inserted into the rectum. A colonoscope is a thin, tube-like instrument with a light and lens for viewing. It may also have a tool to remove tissue to be checked under a microscope for disease.

- **Computed tomographic (CT or CAT) scan:** The patient lies on a table and x-rays of the body are taken from different angles. Sometimes, a fluid is used to highlight parts of the body in the scan.

- **Echocardiogram:** An instrument (that looks like a microphone) is placed on the chest. It uses sound waves to create a moving picture of the heart. A picture appears on a monitor, and the heart can be seen in different ways.

- **Electroencephalogram (EEG):** Measures the electrical activity of the brain, using electrodes that are put on the patient's scalp. Sometimes patients sleep during the test.

- **Electrocardiogram (EKG or ECG):** Records the electrical activity of the heart, using electrodes placed on the arms, legs, and chest.

- **Exercise stress test:** Electrodes are placed on the chest, arms, and legs to record the heart's activity. A blood pressure cuff is placed around the arm and is inflated every few minutes. Heart rate and blood pressure are taken before exercise starts. The patient walks on a treadmill or pedals a stationary bicycle. The pace of the treadmill is increased. The response of the heart is monitored. The test continues until target heart rate is reached. Monitoring continues after exercise for 10–15 minutes or until the heart rate returns to normal.

- **Fecal occult blood test (FOBT):** Detects hidden blood in a bowel movement. There are two types: the smear test and flushable reagent pads.

- **Laparoscopy:** A small tube with a camera is inserted into the abdomen through a small cut in or just below the belly button to see inside the abdomen and pelvis. Other instruments can be inserted in the small cut as well. It is used for both diagnosing and treating problems inside the abdomen.

- **Magnetic resonance imaging (MRI):** A test that uses powerful magnets and radio waves to create a picture of the inside of your body without surgery. The patient lies on a table that slides onto a large tunnel-like tube, which is surrounded by a scanner. Small coils may be placed around your head, arm, leg, or other areas.

- **Mammogram:** X-rays of the breast taken by resting one breast at a time on a flat surface that contains an x-ray plate. A device presses firmly against the breast. An x-ray is taken to show a picture of the breast. Mammography is used to screen healthy women for signs of breast cancer. It can also be used to evaluate a woman who has symptoms of disease. It can, in some cases, detect breast cancers before you can feel them with your fingers.

- **Medical history:** The doctor or nurse talks to the patient about current and past illnesses, surgeries, pregnancies, medications, allergies, use of alternative therapies, vitamins and supplements, diet, alcohol and drug use, physical activity, and family history of diseases.

- **Pap test:** The nurse or doctor uses a small brush to take cells from the cervix (opening of the uterus) to look at under a microscope in a lab.

- **Pelvic exam:** A doctor or nurse asks about the patient's health and looks at the vaginal area. The doctor or nurse checks the fallopian tubes, ovaries, and uterus by putting two gloved fingers inside the vagina. With the other hand, the doctor or nurse will feel from the outside for any lumps or tenderness.

- **Physical exam:** The doctor or nurse will test for diseases, assess your risk of future medical problems, encourage a healthy lifestyle, and update your vaccinations.

- **Positron emission tomography (PET) scan:** The patient is injected with a radioactive substance, such as glucose. A scanner detects any cancerous areas in the body. Cancerous tissue absorbs more of the substance and looks brighter in images than normal tissue.

- **Sigmoidoscopy:** The sigmoidoscope is a small camera attached to a flexible tube. This tube, about 20 inches long, is gently inserted into the colon. As the tube is slowly removed, the lining of the bowel is examined.

- **Spirometry:** The patient breathes into a mouthpiece that is connected to an instrument called a spirometer. The spirometer records the amount and the rate of air that is breathed in and out over a specified time. It measures how well the lungs exhale.

- **Ultrasound:** A clear gel is put onto the skin over the area being examined. An instrument is then moved over that area. The machine sends out sound waves, which reflect off the body. A computer receives these waves and uses them to create pictures of the body.

Chapter 7

After Your Diagnosis: Finding Information and Support

This information is general advice for people with almost any disease or condition. And it has tips to help you learn more about your specific problem and how it can be treated. The online version at http://www.ahrq.gov/consumer/diaginfo.htm has many additional resources and their internet links.

Five Basic Steps

This chapter describes five basic steps to help you cope with your diagnosis, make decisions, and get on with your life.

Step 1: Take the time you need. Do not rush important decisions about your health. In most cases, you will have time to carefully examine your options and decide what is best for you.

Step 2: Get the support you need. Look for support from family and friends, people who are going through the same thing you are, and those who have been there. They can help you cope with your situation and make informed decisions.

Step 3: Talk with your doctor. Good communication with your doctor can help you feel more satisfied with the care you receive. Research shows it can even have a positive effect on things such as

"Next Steps After Your Diagnosis: Finding Information and Support," Agency for Healthcare Research and Quality (AHRQ), AHRQ Pub. No. 05-0049, July 2005.

symptoms and pain. Getting a second opinion may help you feel more confident about your care.

Step 4: Seek out information. When learning about your health problem and its treatment, look for information that is based on a careful review of the latest scientific findings published in medical journals.

Step 5: Decide on a treatment plan. Work with your doctor to decide on a treatment plan that best meets your needs.

As you take each step, remember this: Research shows that patients who are more involved in their health care tend to get better results and be more satisfied. Although most of the published research referred to in this publication focuses on cancer, it likely is relevant to people with other diseases and conditions as well.

Step 1: Take the Time You Need

A diagnosis can change your life in an instant. Like so many other people in your situation, you might be feeling one or more of the following emotions after getting your diagnosis:

- anger
- anxiety
- confusion
- denial
- depression
- fear
- helplessness
- numbness
- overwhelmed
- panicky
- powerless
- relieved (that you finally know what's wrong)
- sadness
- shame
- shock
- stress

It is perfectly normal to have these feelings. It is also normal, and very common, to have trouble taking in and understanding information after you receive the news—especially if the diagnosis was a surprise. And it can be even harder to make decisions about treating or managing your disease or condition.

Take time to make your decisions. No matter how the news of your diagnosis has affected you, do not rush into a decision. In most cases, you do not need to take action right away. Ask your doctor how much time you can safely take.

Taking the time you need to make decisions can help you:

- feel less anxious and stressed;

- avoid depression;

- cope with your condition;

- feel more in control of your situation; and

- play a key role in decisions about your treatment.

Step 2: Get the Support You Need

You do not have to go through it alone. Sometimes the emotional side of illness can be just as hard to deal with as the physical side. You may have fears or concerns. You may feel overwhelmed. No matter what your situation, having other people to turn to will help you know you are not alone.

Here are the kinds of support you might want to seek:

Family and friends: Talking to family and friends you feel close to can help you cope with your illness or condition. Just knowing that someone is there can be a comfort.

Sometimes it is hard to ask for help. And sometimes your family and friends want to help, but they do not want to intrude, or they do not know how to ask or what to offer. Think about specific ways people can help you. One idea is to ask someone to come with you to a doctor's appointment to help ask questions, take notes, and talk with you afterward.

If you do not have family or friends who can provide support, other people or groups can.

Support or self-help groups: Support groups are made up of people with the same disease or condition who get together to share information and concerns and to help one another. Support groups may or may not be led by experts. Self-help groups are similar to support groups but usually are led by the participants.

Research on support groups shows that participants feel less anxious, experience less depression, have a better quality of life, and have more success coping with their disease or condition. Similar findings have been reported for self-help groups.

Online support or self-help groups: The internet has support or self-help groups for people whose concerns and situations may be similar to yours. You can also find online message boards, where you can post questions and get answers. These communities can help you connect with people who can give you support and provide information, but be careful. Not every idea or treatment you come across in these groups will be scientifically proven to be safe and effective. If you read about something interesting and new, check it out with your doctor.

Counselor or therapist: A good counselor or therapist can help you cope with sadness, depression, and feelings of being overwhelmed. If you think this kind of help might be right for you, ask your doctor or other health care professional to recommend someone in your area.

People like you: You might want to meet and talk with someone in your own situation. Someone who has been there can talk about the real-life outcomes of their treatment choices as well as how they have learned to live with their disease or condition. Some advocacy or support groups can help you make this kind of contact.

Help is available: Take advantage of the support that is available to you.

Step 3: Talk with Your Doctor

Your doctor is your partner in health care. You probably have many questions about your disease or condition. The first person to ask is your doctor.

It is fine to seek more information from other sources; in fact, it is important to do so. But consider your doctor your partner in health care—someone who can discuss your situation with you, explain your options, and help you with the decisions that are right for you.

It is not always easy to feel comfortable around doctors. But research has shown that good communication with your doctor can actually be good for your health. It can help you to:

- feel more satisfied with the care you receive; and

- have better outcomes (end results), such as reduced pain and better recovery from symptoms.

Being an active member of your health care team also helps to reduce your chances of medical mistakes, and it helps you get high-quality care. Of course, good communication is a two-way street. Here are some ways to help make the most of the time you spend with your doctor.

Prepare for Your Visit

- Think about what you want to get out of your appointment. Write down all your questions and concerns.

- Prepare and bring to your doctor visit a list of all the medicines you take.

- Consider bringing along a trusted relative or friend. This person can help ask questions, take notes, and help you remember and understand everything once you leave the doctor's office.

Give Information to Your Doctor

- Do not wait to be asked.

- Tell your doctor everything he or she needs to know about your health—even the things that might make you feel embarrassed or uncomfortable.

- Tell your doctor how you are feeling—both physically and emotionally.

- Tell your doctor if you are feeling depressed or overwhelmed.

Get Information from Your Doctor

- Ask questions about anything that concerns you. Keep asking until you understand the answers. If you do not, your doctor may think you understand everything that is said.

- Ask your doctor to draw pictures if that will help you understand something.

- Take notes.

- Tape record your doctor visit, if that will be helpful to you. But first ask your doctor if this is okay.

- Ask your doctor to recommend resources such as websites, booklets, or tapes with more information about your disease or condition.

Do Not Hesitate to Seek a Second Opinion

A second opinion is when another doctor examines your medical records and gives his or her views about your condition and how it should be treated. You might want a second opinion to:

- be clear about what you have;

- know all of your treatment choices; or

- have another doctor look at your choices with you.

It is not pushy or rude to want a second opinion. Most doctors will understand that you need more information before making important decisions about your health. Check to see whether your health plan covers a second opinion. In some cases, health plans require second opinions.

Here are some ways to find a doctor for a second opinion:

- Ask your doctor. Request someone who does not work in the same office, because doctors who work together tend to share similar views.

- Contact your health plan or your local hospital, medical society, or medical school.

- Use the Doctor Finder online service of the American Medical Association at http://www.ama-assn.org.

Get Information about Next Steps

- Get the results of any tests or procedures. Discuss the meaning of these results with your doctor.

- Make sure you understand what will happen if you need surgery.

- Talk with your doctor about which hospital is best for your health care needs.

Finally, if you are not satisfied with your doctor, you can do two things: (1) talk with your doctor and try to work things out, or (2) switch doctors, if you are able to. It is very important to feel confident about your care.

Ten Important Questions to Ask Your Doctor after a Diagnosis

These ten basic questions can help you understand your disease or condition, how it might be treated, and what you need to know and do before making treatment decisions.

1. What is the technical name of my disease or condition, and what does it mean in plain English?

2. What is my prognosis (outlook for the future)?

3. How soon do I need to make a decision about treatment?

4. Will I need any additional tests, and if so what kind and when?

5. What are my treatment options?

6. What are the pros and cons of my treatment options?

7. Is there a clinical trial (research study) that is right for me?

8. Now that I have this diagnosis, what changes will I need to make in my daily life?

9. What organizations do you recommend for support and information?

10. What resources (for example, booklets, websites, audiotapes) do you recommend for further information?

Step 4: Seek Out Information

Now that you know your treatment options, you can learn which ones are backed up by the best scientific evidence. Evidence-based information—that is, information that is based on a careful review of the latest scientific findings in medical journals—can help you make decisions about the best possible treatments for you.

Evidence-based information comes from research on people like you. Evidence-based information about treatments generally comes from two major types of scientific studies:

- Clinical trials are research studies on human volunteers to test new drugs or other treatments. Participants are randomly assigned to different treatment groups. Some get the research treatment, and others get a standard treatment or may be given a placebo (a medicine that has no effect), or no treatment. The results are compared to learn whether the new treatment is safe and effective.

- Outcomes research looks at the impact of treatments and other health care on health outcomes (end results) for patients and populations. End results include effects that people care about, such as changes in their quality of life.

Take Advantage of the Available Evidence-Based Information

Health information is everywhere—in books, newspapers, and magazines, and on the internet, television, and radio. However, not all information is good information. Your best bets for sources of evidence-based information include the federal government, national nonprofit organizations, medical specialty groups, medical schools, and university medical centers.

Information about your disease or condition and its treatment is available from many sources. Some of the most reliable include:

- The healthfinder® site at http://www.healthfinder.gov/ organizations/OrgListing.asp is sponsored by the U.S. Department of Health and Human Services. It offers carefully selected health information websites from government agencies, clearinghouses, nonprofit groups, and universities.

- Health Information Resource Database available at http://www .health.gov/nhic/#Referrals is sponsored by the National Health Information Center. This database includes 1,400 organizations and government offices that provide health information upon request. Information is also available over the telephone at 800-336-4797.

- MEDLINEplus® available at http://www.nlm.nih.gov/medlineplus has extensive information from the National Institutes of Health and other trusted sources on over 650 diseases and conditions. The site includes many additional features.

- National nonprofit groups such as the American Heart Association, American Cancer Society, and American Diabetes Association can be valuable sources of reliable information. Many have chapters nationwide. Check your phone book for a local chapter in your community. The Health Information Resource Database can help you find national offices of nonprofit groups.

- Health or medical libraries run by government, hospitals, professional groups, and other reliable organizations often welcome consumers.

Current Medical Research

You can find the latest medical research in medical journals at your local health or medical library, and in some cases, on the internet. Here are two major online sources of medical articles:

- MEDLINE/PubMed® at http://www.ncbi.nlm.nih.gov/entrez/ query.fcgi: PubMed® is the National Library of Medicine's database of references to more than 14 million articles published in 4,800 medical and scientific journals. All of the listings have information to help you find the articles at a health or medical library. Many listings also have short summaries of the article (abstracts), and some have links to the full article. The article might be free, or it might require a fee charged by the publisher.

- PubMed® Central at http://www.pubmedcentral.nih.gov: PubMed® Central is the National Library of Medicine's database of journal articles that are available free of charge to users.

Clinical Trial

Perhaps you wonder whether there is a clinical trial that is right for you. Or you may want to learn about results from previous clinical trials that might be relevant to your situation. Here are two reliable resources:

- ClinicalTrials.gov at http://clinicaltrials.gov/ct/g/: ClinicalTrials .gov provides regularly updated information about federally and privately supported clinical research on people who volunteer to participate. The site has information about a trial's purpose, who may participate, locations, and phone numbers for more details. The site also describes the clinical trial process and includes news about recent clinical trial results.

- Cochrane Collaboration at http://www.cochrane.org: The Cochrane Collaboration writes summaries (reviews) about evidence from clinical trials to help people make informed decisions. You can

search and read the review abstracts free of charge at http://
www.cochrane.org/reviews/index.htm. Or you can read plain-
English consumer summaries of the reviews at http://www
.informedhealthonline.org. The full Cochrane reviews are available only by subscription. Check with your local medical or health
library to see whether you can access the full reviews there.

Outcomes Research

Outcomes research provides research about benefits, risks, and
outcomes (end results) of treatments so that patients and their doctors can make better informed decisions. The U.S. Agency for Healthcare
Research and Quality (AHRQ) supports improvements in health outcomes through research, and sponsors products that result from research such as:

- National Guideline Clearinghouse™ at http://www.guideline
  .gov: The National Guideline Clearinghouse™ is a database of
  evidence-based clinical practice guidelines and related documents.
  Clinical practice guidelines are documents designed to help doctors and patients make decisions about appropriate health care
  for specific diseases or conditions. The clearinghouse was originally created by AHRQ in partnership with the American Medical Association and America's Health Insurance Plans.

Step 5: Decide on a Treatment Plan

At this point, you have learned about your disease or condition and
how it can be treated or managed. Your information may have come
from the following sources:

- your doctor;

- second opinions from one or more other doctors;

- other people who are or were in the same situation as you; or

- information sources such as websites, health or medical libraries,
  and nonprofit groups.

Work with your doctor to make decisions. When you are ready to
make treatment decisions, you and your doctor can discuss:

- Which treatments have been found to work well, or not work
  well, for your particular condition.

- The pros and cons of each treatment option.

Make sure that your doctor knows your preferences and feelings about the different treatments—for example, whether you prefer medicine over surgery. Once you and your doctor decide on one or more treatments that are right for you, you can work together to develop a treatment plan. This plan will include everything that will be done to treat or manage your disease or condition—including what you need to do to make the plan work. Remember, being an active member of your health care team helps to reduce your chances of medical mistakes, and it helps you get high-quality care.

Summing It Up

You have taken important steps to cope with your diagnosis, make decisions, and get on with your life. Remember two things:

- Call on others for support as you need it.

- Make use of evidence-based information for any future health decisions.

For More Information

AARP Health Guide
Toll-Free: 888-687-2277
Website: http://www.aarp.org/health/healthguide

American Self-Help Group Clearinghouse
Website: http://mentalhelp.net/selfhelp

HON Code of Conduct (HONcode) for Medical and Health Web Sites
Health on the Net Foundation
Medical Informatics Division
University Hospital of Geneva
24 rue Micheli-du-Crest
1211 Geneva 14
Switzerland
Phone: +41-22-372-6250
Fax: +41-22-72-8885
Website: http://www.hon.ch/HONcode

National Institute of Mental Health–Locating Services
6001 Executive Blvd.
Room 8184, MSC 9663
Bethesda, MD 20892-9663
Toll-Free: 866-615-6464
Phone: 301-443-4513
TTY: 301-443-8431
Fax: 301-443-4279
Website: http://www.nimh.nih.gov/health/topics/
getting-help-locate-services/index.shtml
E-mail: nimhinfo@nih.gov

Toll-Free Number for Health Information

National Health Information Center
Website: http://www.health.gov/nhic/pubs/tollfree.htm.
Toll-Free: 800-336-4797

Part Two

Working with Health Care Providers and the Health Care System

Chapter 8

Talking with Your Health Care Provider

Ten Ways to Improve Communication with Your Doctor

Good health care begins with good communication. However, research indicates that as many as half of adults in this country have problems understanding health information. There are many reasons for this. Often, health care professionals use scientific terms that patients may not know. For example, you may use the word stomachache to describe how you feel, and your doctor may use the word gastroenteritis. Sometimes, the amount of information given in a medical appointment can be too much to take in. Other times patients report they cannot remember what their doctor has said after they leave.

Health literacy refers to understanding how to get and use health information to take care of yourself. Taking steps to make sure you understand health information you doctor has given you is important, as miscommunications and misunderstandings can lead to dangerous situations where people do not receive the medical treatment they need.

The following 10 steps can help improve communication between you and your doctor:

This chapter begins with "10 Ways to Improve Communication with Your Doctor," *Journal of Patient Safety*, Volume 1, Issue 4, p. 277, December 2005. © Lippincott Williams and Wilkins, Inc. Reprinted with permission. Text under the heading "How to Talk to Your Doctor or Nurse," is from the National Women's Health Information Center (NWHIC), October 2006. "Questions Are the Answer: Build Your Question List," is excerpted from a document of the same title by the Agency for Healthcare Research and Quality (AHRQ), June 20, 2003.

69

1. **Make a list.** Before you go to the doctor's office, write down any questions or concerns you have about your health. Take this list with you so you do not forget to ask all of your questions.

2. **Ask for definitions.** If your doctor uses a word you do not understand, ask him or her to re-explain using plain language. Many words sound alike or have different meanings when talked about in health care. For example, whereas the word negative has bad implications outside a doctor's office, when a test comes back negative, it is good news. It is okay to say you don't understand.

3. **Know your goals.** Ask your doctor to define your health care goals. For example, if your doctor tells you to check your blood pressure to make sure it is within normal range, you will need to know what normal means.

4. **Do the talking.** After your doctor has finished explaining something to you, explain it back to your doctor. This will help you remember it and help to make sure both you and your doctor understand the information in the same way.

5. **Picture it.** A picture can be worth a thousand words. Ask your doctor to draw a picture or give you an illustration of the concept he or she is talking about. For example, a doctor might suggest certain exercises for someone with low back pain. A drawing may be far easier to understand than a spoken description.

6. **Slow it down.** If your health care provider speaks quickly, ask him or her to speak slowly so that you do not miss information.

7. **Don't be shy.** If you have concerns regarding treatment, tell your health care provider. He or she may have information that will relieve your concerns, or there may be alternative treatments.

8. **Consider taking a partner.** Bringing a trusted family member or friend can be a big help when it comes to understanding information and remembering instructions once back at home.

9. **Ask for a recap.** At the end of your appointment, ask your doctor to repeat the main points and type or write down take-home instructions.

10. **Follow-up.** If you get home and cannot remember instructions, contact you doctor. If your physician offers communication via secure e-mail, you will have the added bonus of a written copy of the answer. (Regular e-mail does not provide complete privacy of your health information. If you have questions about whether your doctor uses secure e-mail, be sure to ask.)

Health care is a team effort. Make your doctor a partner in your health with open communication. This is your health, and it is important that you understand how to take care of it.

How to Talk to Your Doctor or Nurse

Waiting in your doctor's office can make you feel nervous, impatient, or even scared. You might worry about what's wrong with you. You might feel annoyed because you're not getting other things done. Then when you see your doctor or nurse, the visit seems to be so short. You might have only a few minutes to explain your symptoms and concerns. Later that day, you might remember something you forgot to ask. You wonder if your question and its answer matters. Knowing how to talk to your doctor, nurse, or other members of your health care team will help you get the information you need.

Tips: What to Do

- List your questions and concerns. Before your appointment, make a list of what you want to ask. When you're in the waiting room, review your list and organize your thoughts. You can share the list with your doctor or nurse.

- Describe your symptoms. Say when these problems started. Say how they make you feel. If you know, say what sets them off or triggers them. Say what you've done to feel better.

- Give your doctor a list of your medications. Tell what prescription drugs and over-the-counter medicines, vitamins, herbal products, and other supplements you're taking.

- Be honest about your diet, physical activity, smoking, alcohol or drug use, and sexual history. Not sharing information with your doctor or nurse can be harmful.

- Describe any allergies to drugs, foods, pollen, or other things. Don't forget to mention if you are being treated by other doctors, including mental health professionals.

- Talk about sensitive topics. Your doctor or nurse has probably heard it before. Don't leave something out because you're worried about taking up too much time. Be sure to talk about all of your concerns before you leave. If you don't understand the answers your doctor gives you, ask again.

- Ask questions about any tests and your test results. Get instructions on what you need to do to get ready for the test(s). Ask if there are any dangers or side effects. Ask how you can learn the test results. Ask how long it will take to get the results.

- Ask questions about your condition or illness. If you are diagnosed with a condition, ask your doctor how you can learn more about it. What caused it? Is it permanent? What can you do to help yourself feel better? How can it be treated?

- Tell your doctor or nurse if you are pregnant or intend to become pregnant. Some medicines may not be suitable for you. Other medicines should be used with caution if you are pregnant or about to become pregnant.

- Ask your doctor about any treatments he or she recommends. Be sure to ask about all of your options for treatment. Ask how long the treatment will last. Ask if it has any side effects. Ask how much it will cost. Ask if it is covered by your health insurance.

- Ask your doctor about any medicines he or she prescribes for you. Make sure you understand how to take your medicine. What should you do if you miss a dose? Are there any foods, drugs, or activities you should avoid when taking the medicine? Is there a generic brand of the drug you can use? You can also ask your pharmacist if a generic drug is available for your medication.

- Ask more questions if you don't understand something. If you're not clear about what your doctor or nurse is asking you to do or why, ask to have it explained again.

- Bring a family member or trusted friend with you. That person can take notes, offer moral support, and help you remember what was discussed. You can have that person ask questions, too.

- Call before your visit to tell them if you have special needs. If you don't speak or understand English well, the office may need to find an interpreter. If you have a disability, ask if they can accommodate you.

Build Your Question List

Are you visiting your health care clinician or pharmacist? It is important to be prepared. Create a personalized list of questions that you can take with you.

Did your clinician give you a prescription?

Questions to ask about prescriptions include:

- What is the name of the medicine?
- How do you spell the name?
- Can I take a generic version of this medicine?
- What is the medicine for?
- How am I supposed to take it?
- When should I take my medicine?
- How much medicine should I take?
- How long do I need to take the medicine?
- When will the medicine start working?
- Can I stop taking my medicine if I feel better?
- Can I get a refill?
- Are there any side effects?
- When should I tell someone about a side effect?
- Do I need to avoid any food, drinks, or activities?
- Does this new prescription mean I should stop taking any other medicines I'm taking now?
- Can I take vitamins with my prescription?
- What should I do if I forget to take my medicine?
- What should I do if I accidentally take more than the recommended dose?
- Is there any written information I can take home with me?
- Are there any tests I need to take while I'm on this medicine?

Are you scheduled to have medical tests?

Questions to ask about medical tests include:

- What is the test for?
- How is the test done?
- Will the test hurt?
- How accurate is the test?
- Is this test the only way to find out that information?
- What are the benefits and risks of having this test?
- What do I need to do to prepare for the test?
- How many times have you performed the test?
- When will I get the results?
- What will the results tell me?
- What's the next step after the test?

Did you recently receive a diagnosis?

Questions to ask about a diagnosis include:

- What is my diagnosis?
- What is the technical name of my disease or condition, and what does it mean in plain English?
- What is my prognosis (outlook for the future)?
- What changes will I need to make?
- Is there a chance that someone else in my family might get the same condition?
- Will I need special help at home for my condition?
- Is there any treatment?
- What are my treatment options?
- How soon do I need to make a decision about treatment?
- What are the benefits and risks associated with my treatment options?

- Is there a clinical trial (research study) that is right for me?

- Will I need any additional tests?

- What organizations and resources do you recommend for support and information?

Are you considering treatment for an illness or condition?

Questions to ask about treatment include:

- What are my treatment options?

- What do you recommend?

- Is the treatment painful?

- How can the pain be controlled?

- What are the benefits and risks of this treatment?

- How much does this treatment cost?

- Will my health insurance cover the treatment?

- What are the expected results?

- When will I see results from the treatment?

- What are the chances the treatment will work?

- Are there any side effects?

- What can be done about them?

- How soon do I need to make a decision about treatment?

- What happens if I choose to have no treatment at all?

Did your clinician recently recommend surgery?

Questions to ask about surgery include:

- Why do I need surgery?

- What kind of surgery do I need?

- What will you be doing?

- What are the benefits and risks of having this surgery?

- Have you done this surgery before?

- How successful is this surgery?
- Which hospital is best for this surgery?
- Will the surgery hurt?
- Will I need anesthesia?
- How long will the surgery take?
- How long will it take me to recover?
- How long will I be in the hospital?
- What will happen after the surgery?
- How much will the surgery cost?
- Will my health insurance cover the surgery?
- Is there some other way to treat my condition?
- What will happen if I wait or don't have this surgery?
- Where can I get a second opinion?

Are you choosing a clinician?

Questions to ask about clinician's include:

- Is this clinician part of my health plan?
- Does this clinician have the background and training I need?
- Is this clinician able to work at the hospital I like?
- Can I ask talk to this clinician and ask questions easily?
- Does this clinician listen to me?
- Does this clinician wash his or her hands between examining each patient?

Are you choosing a hospital?

Questions to ask about hospitals include:

- Which hospital has the best care for my condition?
- Is this hospital covered by my health insurance?
- Does the hospital meet national quality standards?

- How does the hospital compare with others in my area?

- Has the hospital had success with my condition?

- Does my clinician have privileges (is allowed to work) at this hospital?

- How well does the hospital check and improve on its own quality of care?

Chapter 9

Assessing Risks and Benefits in Medical Care

When it comes to making medical decisions, there are tradeoffs. Inasmuch as procedures and treatments can provide tremendous benefits, there are also risks. As an informed patient, it is important for you to have all information possible and to consider both the benefits and the risks before making a decision about medical care.

Some medical choices may provide more convenience. For example, some medications now come in extended-release formulas. Rather than taking a pill once a day, a patient may only need to take a pill once a week. For someone who has trouble swallowing, an extended-release formula may be a better option. However, this same choice may have unintended results, such as the medication not being taken because of a difficulty remembering a once-a-week pill. The convenience of each medical decision should be weighed against the potential downside of the same choice.

Another scenario may involve a family asking about a catheter (tube that drains liquid from the bladder) for their elderly mother who frequently struggles to use a restroom. Inasmuch as a catheter could improve certain aspects of this woman's day-to-day life, such as eliminating embarrassing accidents or having to wear underwear with padding, a catheter comes with risks, such as infections. In this case, the family and the physician would need to discuss if the convenience of a catheter is worth the risk of infection.

"Making Medical Decisions: A Patient's Guide," *Journal of Patient Safety*, Volume 2, Issue 2, June 2006. © Lippincott Williams and Wilkins, Inc. Reprinted with permission.

Even small decisions that may seem unimportant can lead to big safety risks. For example, if a patient decides to remove an identification bracelet during a hospital stay because he or she feels that it is a nuisance, this decision could lead to the wrong treatment being given. The consequences could be severe, even deadly.

Consider the following steps when making a medical decision:

- Choose health care providers with whom you feel comfortable. Have open and honest conversations. When decisions have to be made, ask about both risks and benefits.

- Remember the easiest solution may not always be the safest. In other situations, what is easiest may be the best choice for a particular person. Discuss both the pros and the cons of each option as they pertain to you.

- If you decide to undergo a treatment or procedure, learn how to lessen risks. For example, if a decision is made to use a catheter, learn how to prevent infections by taking steps such as regular catheter cleaning and frequent emptying of the reservoir.

- If you do not know why something is being done—ask. Once you understand the reason for something, it will be easier to avoid making decisions that may bring additional risks such as removing an identification bracelet.

- Know possible side effects of medical treatments and be on the lookout for symptoms. If you think there may be a problem, call your physician sooner rather than later.

Informed consent is the formal process of actually signing a document that says you understand the risks and benefits and have agreed that the procedure or treatment should be done in light of that understanding. It is very important not to assume that your physician would not go forward with a procedure if it was too risky. After all, risks are weighed in the eyes of the individual—what you consider too great a risk may be seen by someone else as an acceptable, or even minimal, risk. Thus, when asked to sign a consent form, it is reasonable to ask what risks there are, how likely they are to occur, what can be done to minimize the risks, and what alternatives there are to the proposed intervention.

Be an informed patient. Learn both sides of a medical decision before making a choice.

Chapter 10

Getting a Second Opinion

How to Get a Second Opinion

Even though doctors may get similar medical training, they can have their own opinions and thoughts about how to practice medicine. They can have different ideas about how to diagnose and treat conditions or diseases. Some doctors take a more conservative, or traditional, approach to treating their patients. Other doctors are more aggressive and use the newest tests and therapies. It seems like we learn about new advances in medicine almost every day.

Many doctors specialize in one area of medicine, such as cardiology or obstetrics or psychiatry. Not every doctor can be skilled in using all the latest technology. Getting a second opinion from a different doctor might give you a fresh perspective and new information. It could provide you with new options for treating your condition. Then you can make more informed choices. If you get similar opinions from two doctors, you can also talk with a third doctor.

Tips: What to Do

- Ask your doctor for a recommendation. Ask for the name of another doctor or specialist, so you can get a second opinion. Don't

This chapter includes text from "Tools to Help You Build a Healthier Life! How to Get a Second Opinion," National Women's Health Information Center (NWHIC), October 2006; and excerpts from "Getting a Second Opinion before Surgery," Centers for Medicare and Medicaid Services (CMS), CMS Publication No. 02173, revised July 2007.

worry about hurting your doctor's feelings. Most doctors welcome a second opinion, especially when surgery or long-term treatment is involved.

- Ask someone you trust for a recommendation. If you don't feel comfortable asking your doctor for a referral, then call another doctor you trust. You can also call university teaching hospitals and medical societies in your area for the names of doctors. Some of this information is also available on the internet.

- Check with your health insurance provider. Call your insurance company before you get a second opinion. Ask if they will pay for this office visit. Many health insurance providers do. Ask if there are any special procedures you or your primary care doctor need to follow.

- Ask to have medical records sent to the second doctor. Ask your primary care doctor to send your medical records to the new doctor. You need to give written permission to your current doctor to send any records or test results to a new doctor. You can also ask for a copy of your own medical records for your files. Your new doctor can then examine these records before your office visit.

- Learn as much as you can. Ask your doctor for information you can read. Go to a local library. Search the internet. Find a teaching hospital or university that has medical libraries open to the public. The information you find can be hard to understand, or just confusing. Make a list of your questions, and bring it with you when you see your new doctor.

- Do not rely on the internet or a telephone conversation. When you get a second opinion, you need to be seen by a doctor. That doctor will perform a physical examination and perhaps other tests. The doctor will also thoroughly review your medical records, ask you questions, and address your concerns.

Getting a Second Opinion before Surgery

A doctor might tell you that you need surgery for a health problem. Deciding what is best for you could mean getting a second opinion from another doctor. A second opinion is when another doctor gives his or her view about your health problem and how it should be treated. Medicare part B (medical insurance) helps pay for a second opinion before surgery.

When your doctor says you have a health problem or need surgery, you have the right to:

- know your treatment choices;

- have another doctor look at those choices with you; and

- participate in treatment decisions by making your wishes known.

Getting a second opinion can help you make a more informed decision.

When to Get a Second Opinion

- Don't wait for a second opinion if you need emergency surgery. Some types of emergencies that may require surgery right away include:

  - acute appendicitis,

  - blood clot or aneurysm, or

  - accidental injuries.

- If your doctor says you need surgery to diagnose or treat a health problem that is not an emergency, you should consider getting a second opinion. It is up to you to decide when and if you will have the surgery. You might also want a second opinion if your doctor tells you that you should have certain kinds of major non-surgical tests.

- Many insurance companies and Medicare do not pay for a second opinion for surgery or tests that are not medically necessary. For example, cosmetic surgery is not medically necessary and usually is not covered. So, private insurance and Medicare will not pay for a second opinion before this kind of surgery.

Finding a Doctor for a Second Opinion

Make sure the doctor giving the second opinion accepts your insurance. To find a doctor for a second opinion, you can do the following:

- Ask your doctor for the name of another doctor to see for a second opinion. Do not hesitate to ask; most doctors want you to get a second opinion. Or, you can ask another doctor you trust to recommend a doctor.

- Ask your local medical society for the names of doctors who treat your illness or injury. Your local library can help you identify these societies.

Getting a Second Opinion

Ask your doctor to send your medical records to the doctor giving the second opinion. That way, you may not have to repeat the tests you already had.

Before you visit the second doctor, call that office and make sure they have your records. During the visit, be sure that the doctor knows what tests you have had and what surgery you want to discuss.

It may help to write down a list of questions. Take the list of questions with you to the doctor who will be giving you a second opinion.

What if the first and second opinions are different?

If the second doctor does not agree with the first, you may feel confused about what to do. In that case, you may want to do the following:

- Talk more about your condition with your first doctor.

- Talk to a third doctor (insurance usually helps pay for a third opinion).

Getting a second opinion does not mean you have to change doctors. You decide which doctor you want to do your surgery.

How much does Medicare help pay for a second opinion before surgery?

Medicare part B helps pay for a second opinion just as it helps pay for other doctors' services that are medically necessary. If you have Medicare part B and are in the original Medicare plan:

- Medicare pays 80% of the Medicare-approved amount for a second opinion.

- Your share is usually 20% of the Medicare-approved amount after you have paid your $131 (in 2007) yearly part B deductible. The part B deductible may increase each year.

- If the second opinion does not agree with the first, Medicare pays 80% of the Medicare-approved amount for a third opinion.

- If you decide to have the surgery, Medicare part B covers the doctor's services, and Medicare part A (hospital insurance) covers other hospital services.

If you are in a Medicare health maintenance organization (HMO), you have the right to get a second opinion. Some HMO plans will only help pay for a second opinion if you first get a referral from your primary care doctor. (A referral is a written OK). After you get a referral, you must get the second opinion from the doctor named in the referral. If you want to get a second opinion from a doctor who does not belong to your plan, talk to your plan first. In some cases, HMO plans will help pay for this. If your plan will not pay, you could still get the second opinion from the doctor who does not belong to your plan, but you would have to pay the full cost. Call your plan for more information.

If you are in a Medicare preferred provider organization (PPO) or a Medicare private fee-for-service plan, your plan will help pay for a second opinion. You do not need a referral. If you are in a PPO, you may have to pay more if you get a second opinion from a doctor who does not belong to your plan.

If you belong to any of the Medicare plans, and the first two opinions are different, these plans will help pay for a third opinion. Call your plan for more information.

If you have Medicaid, it might also pay for second surgical opinions. To find out, call your state Medical Assistance (Medicaid) office.

Chapter 11

Medical Specialties Overview

Doctors are smart people, but these days we know more about the human body and keeping it healthy than any one person could possibly fit in their head, no matter how smart he or she might be. That's why we have specialists, doctors who focus on a particular aspect of patient care. For example, cardiologists focus on the heart and ways to treat heart disease, while endocrinologists focus on everything dealing with the endocrine glands and hormones.

Others concentrate on a specific area of the specialty and may focus on certain body systems, specific age groups or complex scientific techniques to diagnose or treat particular medical conditions.

Physician Specialties

Allergy and immunology: An allergist-immunologist is trained in evaluation, physical and laboratory diagnosis, and management of disorders involving the immune system.

Anesthesiology: An anesthesiologist is trained to provide pain relief and maintenance, or restoration, of a stable condition during and immediately following an operation or an obstetric or diagnostic procedure.

Colon and rectal surgery: A colon and rectal surgeon is trained to diagnose and treat various diseases of the intestinal tract, colon, rectum, anal canal, and perianal area by medical and surgical means.

Dermatology: A dermatologist is trained to diagnose and treat pediatric and adult patients with benign and malignant disorders of the skin, mouth, external genitalia, hair and nails, as well as a number of sexually transmitted diseases.

Emergency medicine: An emergency physician focuses on the immediate decision making and action necessary to prevent death or any further disability both in the pre-hospital setting by directing emergency medical technicians and in the emergency department.

Family medicine: A family physician is concerned with the total health care of the individual and the family, and is trained to diagnose and treat a wide variety of ailments in patients of all ages.

Internal medicine: A personal physician who provides long-term, comprehensive care in the office and the hospital, managing both common and complex illness of adolescents, adults, and the elderly.

Medical genetics: A specialist trained in diagnostic and therapeutic procedures for patients with genetically-linked diseases.

Neurological surgery: A neurological surgeon provides the operative and non-operative management (for example, prevention, diagnosis, evaluation, treatment, critical care, and rehabilitation) of disorders of the central, peripheral, and autonomic nervous systems.

Neurology and child neurology: A neurologist specializes in the diagnosis and treatment of all types of disease or impaired function of the brain, spinal cord, peripheral nerves, muscles, and autonomic nervous systems, as well as the blood vessels that relate to these structures.

Nuclear medicine: A nuclear medicine specialist employs the properties of radioactive atoms and molecules in the diagnosis and treatment of disease, and in research.

Obstetrics and gynecology: An obstetrician and gynecologist possesses special knowledge, skills, and professional capability in the medical and surgical care of the female reproductive system and associated disorders.

Ophthalmology: An ophthalmologist has the knowledge and professional skills needed to provide comprehensive eye and vision care.

Orthopaedic surgery: An orthopaedic surgeon is trained in the preservation, investigation, and restoration of the form and function of the extremities, spine, and associated structures by medical, surgical, and physical means.

Otolaryngology: An otolaryngologist—head and neck surgeon—provides comprehensive medical and surgical care for patients with diseases and disorders that affect the ears, nose, throat, the respiratory and upper alimentary systems, and related structures of the head and neck.

Pathology: A pathologist deals with the causes and nature of disease and contributes to diagnosis, prognosis, and treatment through knowledge gained by the laboratory application of the biologic, chemical, and physical sciences.

Pediatrics: A pediatrician is concerned with the physical, emotional, and social health of children from birth to young adulthood.

Physical medicine and rehabilitation: Physical medicine and rehabilitation, also referred to as rehabilitation medicine, is the medical specialty concerned with diagnosing, evaluating, and treating patients with physical disabilities.

Plastic surgery: A plastic surgeon deals with the repair, reconstruction, or replacement of physical defects of form or function involving the skin, musculoskeletal system, craniomaxillofacial structures, hand, extremities, breast and trunk, and external genitalia, or cosmetic enhancement of these areas of the body.

Preventive medicine: A preventive medicine specialist focuses on the health of individuals and defined populations in order to protect, promote, and maintain health and well-being, and to prevent disease, disability, and premature death.

Psychiatry: A psychiatrist specializes in the prevention, diagnosis, and treatment of mental, addictive, and emotional disorders.

Radiology: A radiologist uses radiologic methodologies to diagnose and treat disease.

Surgery: A surgeon manages a broad spectrum of surgical conditions affecting almost any area of the body; the surgeon establishes the diagnosis and provides the preoperative, operative, and postoperative care to surgical patients.

Thoracic surgery: A thoracic surgeon provides the operative, perioperative, and critical care of patients with pathologic conditions within the chest.

Urology: A urologist manages benign and malignant medical and surgical disorders of the genitourinary system and the adrenal gland.

Chapter 12

Selecting a Complementary and Alternative Medicine Practitioner

Selecting a health care practitioner—of conventional or complementary and alternative medicine (CAM)—is an important decision and can be key to ensuring that you are receiving the best health care.

Conventional medicine is medicine as practiced by holders of M.D. (medical doctor) or D.O. (doctor of osteopathy) degrees and by their allied health professionals, such as physical therapists, psychologists, and registered nurses. Some conventional medical practitioners are also practitioners of CAM.

What is CAM?

CAM is a group of diverse medical and health care systems, practices, and products that are not presently considered to be part of conventional medicine. Complementary medicine is used together with conventional medicine, and alternative medicine is used in place of conventional medicine. Some health care providers practice both CAM and conventional medicine. The list of what is considered to be CAM changes continually as those therapies that are proven to be safe and effective become adopted into conventional health care and as new approaches to health care emerge.

Excerpts from "Selecting a CAM Practitioner," National Center for Complementary and Alternative Medicine (NCCAM), February 12, 2007.

Defining Complementary, Alternative, and Integrative Medicine

The National Center for Complementary and Alternative Medicine (NCCAM) defines complementary, alternative, and integrative medicine as follows:

- Complementary medicine is used together with conventional medicine. An example of a complementary therapy is using aromatherapy—a therapy in which the scent of essential oils from flowers, herbs, and trees is inhaled to promote health and well-being. An example of a complementary therapy is using aromatherapy to help lessen a patient's discomfort following surgery.

- Alternative medicine is used in place of conventional medicine. An example of an alternative therapy is using a special diet to treat cancer instead of undergoing surgery, radiation, or chemotherapy that has been recommended by a conventional doctor.

- Integrative medicine, also called integrated medicine, combines treatments from conventional medicine and CAM for which there is some high-quality evidence of safety and effectiveness.

Source: "What Is CAM?" NCCAM, February 2007.

I am interested in a CAM therapy that involves treatment from a practitioner. How do I go about finding a practitioner?

Before selecting a CAM therapy or practitioner, talk with your primary health care provider(s). Tell them about the therapy you are considering and ask any questions you may have. They may know about the therapy and be able to advise you on its safety, use, and effectiveness, or possible interactions with medications. Here are some suggestions for finding a practitioner:

- Ask your doctor or other health professionals whether they have recommendations or are willing to make a referral.

- Contact a nearby hospital or a medical school and ask if they maintain a list of area CAM practitioners or could make a recommendation. Some regional medical centers may have CAM centers or CAM practitioners on staff.

- Ask if your therapy will be covered by insurance; for example, some insurers cover visits to a chiropractor. If the therapy will be covered, ask for a list of CAM practitioners who accept your insurance.

- Contact a professional organization for the type of practitioner you are seeking. Often, professional organizations have standards of practice, provide referrals to practitioners, have publications explaining the therapy (or therapies) that their members provide, and may offer information on the type of training needed and whether practitioners of a therapy must be licensed or certified in your state. Professional organizations can be located by searching the internet or directories in libraries (ask the librarian). One directory is the Directory of Information Resources Online (DIRLINE) compiled by the National Library of Medicine (dirline.nlm.nih .gov). It contains locations and descriptive information about a variety of health organizations, including CAM associations and organizations. You may find more than one member organization for some CAM professions; this may be because there are different "schools" of practice within the profession or for other reasons.

- Many states have regulatory agencies or licensing boards for certain types of practitioners. They may be able to provide you with information regarding practitioners in your area. Your state, county, or city health department may be able to refer you to such agencies or boards. Licensing, accreditation, and regulatory laws for CAM practices are becoming more common to help ensure that practitioners are competent and provide quality services.

Will insurance cover the cost of a CAM practitioner?

Few CAM therapies are covered by insurance, and the amount of coverage offered varies depending on the insurer. Before agreeing to a treatment that a CAM practitioner suggests, you should check with your insurer to see if they will cover any portion of the therapy's cost. If insurance does cover a portion of the cost, you will want to ask if the practitioner accepts your insurance or participates in your insurer's network. Even with insurance, you may be responsible for a percentage of the cost of therapy.

I have located the names of several practitioners. How do I select one?

Begin by contacting the practitioners on your list and gathering information.

- Ask what training or other qualifications the practitioners have. Ask about their education, additional training, licenses, and certifications. If you have contacted a professional organization, see if the practitioners' qualifications meet the standards for training and licensing for that profession.

- Ask if it is possible to have a brief consultation in person or by phone with the practitioners. This will give you a chance to speak with them directly. The consultation may or may not involve a charge.

- Ask if there are diseases or health conditions in which the practitioners specialize and how frequently they treat patients with problems similar to yours.

- Ask if the practitioners believe the therapy can effectively address your complaint and if there is any scientific research supporting the treatment's use for your condition.

- Ask how many patients the practitioners typically see in a day and how much time they spend with each patient.

- Ask whether there is a brochure or website to tell you more about the practice.

- Ask about charges and payment options. How much do treatments cost? If you have insurance, do the practitioners accept your insurance or participate in your insurer's network? Even with insurance, you may be responsible for a percentage of the cost.

- Ask about the hours appointments are offered. How long is the wait for an appointment? Consider whether this will be convenient for your schedule.

- Ask about office location. If you need a building with an elevator or a wheelchair ramp, ask about it.

- Ask what will be involved in the first visit or assessment.

- Observe how comfortable you feel during these first interactions.

Once you have gathered the information, assess the answers and determine which practitioner was best able to respond to your questions and best suits your needs.

I have selected a practitioner. What questions should I ask at my first visit?

The first visit is very important. Come prepared to answer questions about your health history, such as surgeries, injuries, and major illnesses, as well as prescriptions, vitamins, and other supplements you take. Not only will the practitioner wish to gather information from you, but you will want to ask questions, too. Write down ahead of time the questions you want to ask, or take a family member or friend with you to help you remember the questions and answers. Some people bring a tape recorder to record the appointment. (Ask the practitioner for permission to do this in advance.) Here are some questions you may want to ask:

- What benefits can I expect from this therapy?
- What are the risks associated with this therapy?
- Do the benefits outweigh the risks for my disease or condition?
- What side effects can be expected?
- Will the therapy interfere with any of my daily activities?
- How long will I need to undergo treatment? How often will my progress or plan of treatment be assessed?
- Will I need to buy any equipment or supplies?
- Do you have scientific articles or references about using the treatment for my condition?
- Could the therapy interact with conventional treatments?
- Are there any conditions for which this treatment should not be used?

How do I know if the practitioner I have selected is right for me?

After your first visit with a practitioner, evaluate the visit. Ask yourself:

- Was the practitioner easy to talk to? Did the practitioner make me feel comfortable?
- Was I comfortable asking questions? Did the practitioner appear willing to answer them, and were they answered to my satisfaction?
- Was the practitioner open to how both CAM therapy and conventional medicine might work together for my benefit?
- Did the practitioner get to know me and ask me about my condition?

- Did the practitioner seem knowledgeable about my specific health condition?

- Does the treatment recommended seem reasonable and acceptable to me?

- Was the practitioner clear about the time and costs associated with treatment?

Can I change my mind about the treatment or the practitioner?

Yes, if you are not satisfied or comfortable, you can look for a different practitioner or stop treatment. However, as with any conventional treatment, talk with your practitioner before stopping to make sure that it is safe to simply stop treatment—it may not be advisable to stop some therapies midway through a course of treatment.

Discuss with your practitioner the reasons you are not satisfied or comfortable with treatment. If you decide to stop a therapy or seek another practitioner, make sure that you share this information with any other health care practitioners you may have, as this will help them make decisions about your care. Communicating with your practitioner(s) can be key to ensuring the best possible health care.

Can I receive CAM treatment through a clinical trial?

NCCAM supports clinical trials (research studies in people) on CAM therapies. Clinical trials on CAM are taking place in many locations worldwide, and study participants are needed. To find out more about clinical trials on CAM, go to the website http://nccam.nih.gov/clinicaltrials. You can search this site by the type of therapy being studied or by disease or condition.

For More Information

National Center for Complementary and Alternative Medicine (NCCAM) Clearinghouse
P.O. Box 7923
Gaithersburg, MD 20898-7923
Toll-Free: 888-644-6226, Phone: 301-519-3153
TTY: 866-464-3615, Fax: 866-464-3616
Website: http://nccam.nih.gov
E-mail: info@nccam.nih.gov

Chapter 13

An Introduction to Clinical Trials

Choosing to participate in a clinical trial is an important personal decision. The following frequently asked questions provide detailed information about clinical trials. In addition, it is often helpful to talk to a physician, family members, or friends about deciding to join a trial. After identifying some trial options, the next step is to contact the study research staff and ask questions about specific trials.

What is a clinical trial?

Although there are many definitions of clinical trials, they are generally considered to be biomedical or health-related research studies in human beings that follow a predefined protocol. ClinicalTrials.gov includes both interventional and observational types of studies. Interventional studies are those in which the research subjects are assigned by the investigator to a treatment or other intervention, and their outcomes are measured. Observational studies are those in which individuals are observed and their outcomes are measured by the investigators.

Why participate in a clinical trial?

Participants in clinical trials can play a more active role in their own health care, gain access to new research treatments before they are widely available, and help others by contributing to medical research.

National Institutes of Health (NIH), May 8, 2007.

Who can participate in a clinical trial?

All clinical trials have guidelines about who can participate. Using inclusion and exclusion criteria is an important principle of medical research that helps to produce reliable results. The factors that allow someone to participate in a clinical trial are called inclusion criteria and those that disallow someone from participating are called exclusion criteria. These criteria are based on such factors as age, gender, the type and stage of a disease, previous treatment history, and other medical conditions. Before joining a clinical trial, a participant must qualify for the study. Some research studies seek participants with illnesses or conditions to be studied in the clinical trial, while others need healthy participants. It is important to note that inclusion and exclusion criteria are not used to reject people personally. Instead, the criteria are used to identify appropriate participants and keep them safe. The criteria help ensure that researchers will be able to answer the questions they plan to study.

What happens during a clinical trial?

The clinical trial process depends on the kind of trial being conducted. The clinical trial team includes doctors and nurses as well as social workers and other health care professionals. They check the health of the participant at the beginning of the trial, give specific instructions for participating in the trial, monitor the participant carefully during the trial, and stay in touch after the trial is completed.

Some clinical trials involve more tests and doctor visits than the participant would normally have for an illness or condition. For all types of trials, the participant works with a research team. Clinical trial participation is most successful when the protocol is carefully followed and there is frequent contact with the research staff.

What is informed consent?

Informed consent is the process of learning the key facts about a clinical trial before deciding whether or not to participate. It is also a continuing process throughout the study to provide information for participants. To help someone decide whether or not to participate, the doctors and nurses involved in the trial explain the details of the study. If the participant's native language is not English, translation assistance can be provided. Then the research team provides an informed consent document that includes details about the study, such as its purpose, duration, required procedures, and key contacts. Risks and potential benefits are explained in the informed consent document. The participant then decides whether or not to sign the document. Informed consent is not a contract, and the participant may withdraw from the trial at any time.

What are the benefits and risks of participating in a clinical trial?

Benefits: Clinical trials that are well-designed and well-executed are the best approach for eligible participants to:

- play an active role in their own health care;
- gain access to new research treatments before they are widely available;
- obtain expert medical care at leading health care facilities during the trial; and
- help others by contributing to medical research.

Risks: There are risks to clinical trials.

- There may be unpleasant, serious or even life-threatening side effects to experimental treatment.
- The experimental treatment may not be effective for the participant.
- The protocol may require more of their time and attention than would a non-protocol treatment, including trips to the study site, more treatments, hospital stays or complex dosage requirements.

What are side effects and adverse reactions?

Side effects are any undesired actions or effects of the experimental drug or treatment. Negative or adverse effects may include headache, nausea, hair loss, skin irritation, or other physical problems. Experimental treatments must be evaluated for both immediate and long-term side effects.

How is the safety of the participant protected?

The ethical and legal codes that govern medical practice also apply to clinical trials. In addition, most clinical research is federally regulated with built-in safeguards to protect the participants. The trial follows a carefully controlled protocol, a study plan which details what researchers will do in the study. As a clinical trial progresses, researchers report the results of the trial at scientific meetings, to medical journals, and to various government agencies. Individual participants' names will remain secret and will not be mentioned in these reports.

What should people consider before participating in a trial?

People should know as much as possible about the clinical trial and feel comfortable asking the members of the health care team questions about it, the care expected while in a trial, and the cost of the trial. The following questions might be helpful for the participant to discuss with the health care team. Some of the answers to these questions are found in the informed consent document.

- What is the purpose of the study?
- Who is going to be in the study?
- Why do researchers believe the experimental treatment being tested may be effective? Has it been tested before?
- What kinds of tests and experimental treatments are involved?
- How do the possible risks, side effects, and benefits in the study compare with my current treatment?
- How might this trial affect my daily life?
- How long will the trial last?
- Will hospitalization be required?
- Who will pay for the experimental treatment?
- Will I be reimbursed for other expenses?
- What type of long-term follow-up care is part of this study?
- How will I know that the experimental treatment is working? Will results of the trials be provided to me?
- Who will be in charge of my care?

What kind of preparation should a potential participant make for the meeting with the research coordinator or doctor?

- Plan ahead and write down possible questions to ask.

- Ask a friend or relative to come along for support and to hear the responses to the questions.

- Bring a tape recorder to record the discussion to replay later.

Every clinical trial in the U.S. must be approved and monitored by an Institutional Review Board (IRB) to make sure the risks are as low as possible and are worth any potential benefits. An IRB is an independent committee of physicians, statisticians, community advocates, and others that ensures that a clinical trial is ethical and the rights of study participants are protected. All institutions that conduct or support biomedical research involving people must, by federal regulation, have an IRB that initially approves and periodically reviews the research.

Does a participant continue to work with a primary health care provider while in a trial?

Yes. Most clinical trials provide short-term treatments related to a designated illness or condition, but do not provide extended or complete primary health care. In addition, by having the health care provider work with the research team, the participant can ensure that other medications or treatments will not conflict with the protocol.

Can a participant leave a clinical trial after it has begun?

Yes. A participant can leave a clinical trial, at any time. When withdrawing from the trial, the participant should let the research team know about it, and the reasons for leaving the study.

Where do the ideas for trials come from?

Ideas for clinical trials usually come from researchers. After researchers test new therapies or procedures in the laboratory and in animal studies, the experimental treatments with the most promising laboratory results are moved into clinical trials. During a trial, more and more information is gained about an experimental treatment, its risks, and how well it may or may not work.

Who sponsors clinical trials?

Clinical trials are sponsored or funded by a variety of organizations or individuals such as physicians, medical institutions, foundations, voluntary groups, and pharmaceutical companies, in addition to federal agencies such as the National Institutes of Health (NIH), the Department of Defense (DOD), and the Department of Veteran's Affairs (VA). Trials can take place in a variety of locations, such as hospitals, universities, doctors' offices, or community clinics.

What is a protocol?

A protocol is a study plan on which all clinical trials are based. The plan is carefully designed to safeguard the health of the participants as well as answer specific research questions. A protocol describes what types of people may participate in the trial; the schedule of tests, procedures, medications, and dosages; and the length of the study. While in a clinical trial, participants following a protocol are seen regularly by the research staff to monitor their health and to determine the safety and effectiveness of their treatment.

What is a placebo?

A placebo is an inactive pill, liquid, or powder that has no treatment value. In clinical trials, experimental treatments are often compared with placebos to assess the experimental treatment's effectiveness. In some studies, the participants in the control group will receive a placebo instead of an active drug or experimental treatment.

What is a control or control group?

A control is the standard by which experimental observations are evaluated. In many clinical trials, one group of patients will be given an experimental drug or treatment, while the control group is given either a standard treatment for the illness or a placebo.

What are the different types of clinical trials?

Treatment trials test experimental treatments, new combinations of drugs, or new approaches to surgery or radiation therapy.

Prevention trials look for better ways to prevent disease in people who have never had the disease or to prevent a disease from returning. These approaches may include medicines, vitamins, vaccines, minerals, or lifestyle changes.

Diagnostic trials are conducted to find better tests or procedures for diagnosing a particular disease or condition.

Screening trials test the best way to detect certain diseases or health conditions.

Quality of life trials (or supportive care trials) explore ways to improve comfort and the quality of life for individuals with a chronic illness.

What are the phases of clinical trials?

Clinical trials are conducted in phases. The trials at each phase have a different purpose and help scientists answer different questions:

- In Phase I trials, researchers test an experimental drug or treatment in a small group of people (20–80) for the first time to evaluate its safety, determine a safe dosage range, and identify side effects.

- In Phase II trials, the experimental study drug or treatment is given to a larger group of people (100–300) to see if it is effective and to further evaluate its safety.

- In Phase III trials, the experimental study drug or treatment is given to large groups of people (1,000–3,000) to confirm its effectiveness, monitor side effects, compare it to commonly used treatments, and collect information that will allow the experimental drug or treatment to be used safely.

- In Phase IV trials, post-marketing studies delineate additional information including the drug's risks, benefits, and optimal use.

What is an expanded access protocol?

Most human use of investigational new drugs takes place in controlled clinical trials conducted to assess safety and efficacy of new drugs. Data from the trials can serve as the basis for the drug marketing application. Sometimes, patients do not qualify for these carefully controlled trials because of other health problems, age, or other factors. For patients who may benefit from the drug use but don't qualify for the trials, FDA regulations enable manufacturers of investigational new drugs to provide for expanded access use of the drug. For example, a treatment investigational new drug application (IND) or treatment protocol is a relatively unrestricted study. The primary intent of a treatment IND or protocol is to provide for access to the new drug for people with a life-threatening or serious disease for which there is no good alternative treatment. A secondary purpose for a treatment IND or protocol is to generate additional information about the drug, especially its safety. Expanded access protocols can be undertaken only if clinical investigators are actively studying the experimental treatment in well-controlled studies, or all studies have been completed. There must be evidence that the drug may be an effective treatment in patients like those to be treated under the protocol. The drug cannot expose patients to unreasonable risks given the severity of the disease to be treated.

Some investigational drugs are available from pharmaceutical manufacturers through expanded access programs listed in ClinicalTrials.gov. Expanded access protocols are generally managed by the manufacturer, with the investigational treatment administered by researchers or doctors in office-based practice. If you or a loved one is interested in treatment with an investigational drug under an expanded access protocol listed in ClinicalTrials.gov, review the protocol eligibility criteria and location information and inquire at the Contact Information number.

Additional Information

ClinicalTrials.gov
Website: http://clinicaltrials.gov

Chapter 14

Patient-Reported Outcomes: A Tool for Clinical Trials and Clinical Practice

A patient-reported outcome (PRO) is a measurement of any aspect of a patient's health status that comes directly from the patient, without the interpretation of the patient's responses by a physician or anyone else.

How Do Patient-Reported Outcomes Differ from Other Measurements?

A visit to the doctor often means being poked and prodded with various instruments, such as a thermometer stuck in the mouth, a stethoscope placed on the chest, or a blood pressure cuff wrapped around an arm. All of these instruments give the physician measurements—blood pressure, temperature, heart rate—that help in diagnosing or treating an illness. But none of these instruments measure how much pain patients feel, how depressed they are, how well they sleep at night, or whether they have enough energy to walk up a flight of stairs. That information must come directly from the patients.

Along with getting a physical examination and lab tests, patients are routinely asked how they are feeling or how well they are functioning, says Robert Temple, M.D., director of the Food and Drug Administration's Office of Medical Policy, but the information they provide

Excerpted from "The Importance of Patient-Reported Outcomes—It's All about the Patients," by Linda Bren, *FDA Consumer magazine*, November–December 2006, U.S. Food and Drug Administration (FDA).

is filtered through a knowledgeable interpreter—the physician. For example, a person with heart failure will be examined for large amounts of fluid in the body tissues (edema), for fluid in the lungs, and for abnormal heart sounds. He or she might get a chest x-ray or echocardiogram, and would be asked about his or her ability to exercise. The patient would be given a heart failure classification, a widely recognized four-category description of the severity of exercise limitations that makes use of non-standardized questions and has considerable room for judgment. In these evaluations, the patients' own assessment of their well-being has not been ignored, but their reports have been interpreted by the physician.

Increasingly, however, information about symptoms and performance is being obtained directly from patients using structured questionnaires that are shown to give reproducible, meaningful, quantitative assessments of how patients feel and how they function—measures that are called patient-reported outcomes (PRO). The questionnaires used to collect this information are called PRO instruments.

What is really new, says Temple, is that these instruments are being used to assess symptoms without the physician's interpretation. "The use of PRO instruments is part of a general movement toward the idea that the patient, properly queried, is the best source of information about how he or she feels," says Temple.

Why Is the FDA Interested in PRO?

The FDA is encouraging the medical research community to use PRO in clinical trials to help tell whether a new drug or medical device is working, and how well it is working. If PRO is collected, measured, and assessed properly, the information can be used by drug or device developers to support the approval of a new medical product and claims about that product. Beyond clinical trials, researchers also are investigating how PRO can be used in clinical practice to enhance the treatment of patients.

The goal of using PRO measures is to provide better information to doctors and patients so that the best treatment for patients can be determined, says Laurie Burke, R.Ph., M.P.H., director of the FDA's study endpoints and label development team in the Office of New Drugs. "It's all about the patients. Just like a doctor may ask, 'How are you feeling today?' but then probes with further questions, a PRO instrument probes in a structured, formal way," Burke says.

Getting information directly from patients about their symptoms and about how they feel or function is not new. More recently, many researchers have developed their own PRO measuring instruments, says Burke. "But the problem is that although those measures are familiar to the people who developed them, we often can't interpret the measures."

The FDA is working with the research community, the pharmaceutical and medical device industry, and other government agencies to ensure that the PRO instruments used are reliable, interpretable, and valid—in other words, that they measure what they are intended to measure and that they are backed up by solid, scientific rationale.

Why Use PRO Instruments?

PRO instruments offer a structured interview technique that minimizes measurement error and ensures consistency, ultimately providing a more reliable measurement than one that can be obtained by informal interviews.

PRO is useful because some treatment effects are known only to the patient, says Bob Rappaport, M.D., director of the FDA's Division of Anesthesia, Analgesia, and Rheumatology Products, and it is helpful to standardize the questions asked of patients. For example, pain intensity and pain relief have always been measured with PRO instruments. "In most cases, the only way to know if someone is feeling better is to ask how much pain they are in," he says.

PRO and Quality of Life

PRO measurements are sometimes confused with quality of life measurements. Quality of life is a broad concept referring to all aspects of a person's well-being. PRO instruments are used to measure quality of life, but they also can focus much more narrowly—for example, on a single symptom, such as pain.

Some manufacturers of drugs or medical devices are interested in showing, and claiming, that a treatment improves patients' quality of life. Such a claim would imply an evaluation of the impact of a treatment on all aspects of a person's well-being. Quality of life measurements assess not just the physical consequences of disease, such as symptoms and decreased function, but also the effect of disease on a person's emotional state, feelings, coping behaviors, self-identity (psychological functioning), and on a person's ability to interact well with others (social functioning).

Despite the interest in examining effects of drugs on quality of life, the FDA has rarely allowed a claim that a product improves quality of life because it has been very difficult to show such broad effects from drugs that are directed at specific symptoms. But a health-related quality of life (HRQOL) claim would be considered by the FDA if the PRO instrument reliably captured the impact of treatment on the most important aspects of HRQOL. HRQOL represents an individual's perceptions of how an illness and its treatment affect, at a minimum, the physical, mental, and social aspects of his or her life.

HRQOL PRO instruments have been developed for specific diseases, and the FDA has permitted HRQOL claims on the label of certain drugs. For example, the label of the asthma drug Advair, an FDA-approved inhaled bronchodilator, is allowed to carry an HRQOL claim because, says Burke, "the drug sponsor successfully measured an impact of Advair on not only the symptoms of asthma but also on physical, social, and psychological functioning in asthma patients." The Advair label states, in part:

> "The subjective impact of asthma on patients' perception of health was evaluated through use of an instrument called the Asthma Quality of Life Questionnaire (AQLQ). Patients receiving Advair ... had clinically meaningful improvements in overall asthma-specific quality of life."

Drug Approvals Based on PRO

From 1997–2002, 30 percent of the new drugs approved by the FDA contained PRO in their labels. Many drugs approved more recently also have shown effectiveness based on PRO. In the past decade, the FDA has approved six cancer drugs based, at least in part, on PRO instruments which showed that the drugs improved functioning or relieved symptoms, such as pain, difficulty swallowing, or dry mouth. Five of these drugs also showed evidence of attacking the cancer itself. The sixth, Novantrone (mitoxantrone), was approved based primarily on pain relief using a PRO instrument called a pain intensity scale, says Edwin Rock, M.D., Ph.D., a cancer specialist in the FDA's Office of Oncology Drug Products.

Types of PRO Instruments

Many different types of PRO instruments are used. One of the most common instruments for measuring pain requires the patient to verbally rate the level of perceived pain intensity using, for example, adjectives such as none, mild, moderate, and severe, or numbers from

0–10, with zero representing no pain and with ten representing the worst possible pain.

PRO can also be used in children, says Rappaport, but different scales are used, such as pictures of faces. "The series of faces start on the left with smiley and happy faces, there's a bland expression on the face in the middle, and on the right side are frowns and sad faces."

FDA Guidance

The FDA published draft guidance in February 2006 that tells researchers how the agency intends to evaluate PRO instruments. The guidance, called "PRO Measures: Use in Medical Product Development to Support Claims," also describes how sponsors of new drugs or devices can use study results measured by PRO instruments to support claims in the labels or the advertising of approved products.

Beyond Clinical Trials

The phone rings, and a patient picks it up and hears a voice say, "It's time for your health check. Would you like to take a few minutes now to answer some questions, or shall we remind you later?" The patient speaks into the phone when prompted, hangs up when done, and doesn't think much more about it—until a call comes in from a medical clinic. "I see your pain is more severe than it was last week," says a nurse, "and the doctor would like to adjust your medication."

This scenario may already be playing out in some clinics, says Bryce Reeve, Ph.D., program director for outcomes research at the National Cancer Institute, but he envisions that in the future, PRO instruments will be used more with interactive systems to monitor health and to guide treatment recommendations, especially in people who require long-term care, such as cancer patients.

"Reminders can be sent by e-mail or phone," says Reeve. Or when patients go in for a medical appointment, they can be given a laptop computer to respond to a brief questionnaire while they're waiting to see the doctor, he adds. "Or they can answer the questions from home before going to the doctor's office and the information could be available by the time they arrive at their appointment."

The responses would be sent to the doctor's office electronically and linked to a person's electronic medical record. The computer would generate a one-page status report for the physician that summarizes the patient-reported data, flagging any significant symptom changes, such as worsening of pain, says Reeve.

Reeve sees these technological advances as a way to enhance doctor-patient communications and decision-making. "Doctors obviously are very short on time," he says. "Combining PRO with technology will help them perform a comprehensive assessment of their patient. It also empowers the patient to be actively involved in their treatment and well-being."

Chapter 15

Health Care Quality Issues

Chapter Contents

Section 15.1

Understanding Health Care Quality

Excerpted from "Guide to Health Care Quality," Agency for
Healthcare Research and Quality (AHRQ), September 2005.

You Deserve Quality Health Care

Getting quality health care can help you stay healthy and recover
faster when you become sick. However, we know that often, people do
not get high-quality care. A 2004 study of 12 large U.S. communities
found that just over half (54.9 percent) of people were receiving the
care they needed.

What exactly is health care quality? We know that quality means
different things to different people. Some people think that getting
quality health care means seeing the doctor right away, being treated
courteously by the doctor's staff, or having the doctor spend a lot of
time with them.

While these things are important to all of us, clinical quality of care
is even more important. Think of it like this: getting quality health
care is like taking your car to a mechanic. The people in the shop can
be friendly and listen to your complaints, but the most important thing
is whether they fix the problem with your car.

Health care providers, the government, and many other groups are
working hard to improve health care quality. You also have a role to
play to make sure you and your family members receive the best quality care possible.

Be Active: Take Charge of Your Health Care

The single, most important thing you can do to ensure you get high
quality health care is to find and use health information and take an
active role in making decisions about your care. Here are some steps
you can take to improve your care:

- Work together with your doctor and other members of the
  health care team to make decisions about your care.

- Be sure to ask questions.

- Ask your doctor what the scientific evidence has to say about your condition.

- Do your homework; go online or to the library to find out more information about your condition.

- Find and use quality information in making health care choices. Be sure the information comes from a reliable source.

Talking with Your Doctor

Here are some examples of questions to ask your doctor. It is not a complete list. You will probably have many other questions. You should keep asking questions until you understand what is wrong with you and what you need to do to get better.

Understand Your Diagnosis

- What is wrong with me?
- What do I need to do to get better?
- Where can I get more information about my condition?

If You Need Tests, Ask Your Doctor

- How will the test be done?
- How accurate will the results be?
- What are the benefits and risks of the test?
- When and how will I receive the results?
- What should I do if I don't receive the results?

Questions about New Prescriptions

- What is the name of the medicine?
- What is it supposed to do?
- When should I take the medicine, and how much should I take?
- Does the medicine have any side effects?

If You Need Surgery

- What kind of operation do I need?

- Why do I need an operation?
- What are the benefits and risks of the operation?
- How long will it take to recover?
- What will happen if I don't have the operation?
- Are there any other treatments I could have instead of an operation?
- Where can I get a second opinion?

Understanding Health Care Quality

Research has shown that science-based measures can be used to assess quality for various conditions and for specific types of care. For example, quality health care is:

- doing the right thing (getting the health care services you need);
- at the right time (when you need them);
- in the right way (using the appropriate test or procedure);
- to achieve the best possible results.

Providing quality health care also means striking the right balance of services by:

- avoiding underuse (for example, not screening a person for high blood pressure);
- avoiding overuse (for example, performing tests that a patient doesn't need); and
- eliminating misuse (for example, providing medications that may have dangerous interactions).

We would like to think that every doctor, nurse, pharmacist, hospital, and other provider gives high-quality care, but we know this is not always the case. Quality varies depending on where you live. Quality can vary from one state to another, and it can vary from one doctor's office across the street to another. Health care quality varies widely and for many reasons. For example, timely receipt of clot-busting drugs can save lives for patients suffering heart attacks. The national standard for providing clot-busting drugs is within 30 minutes of a patient's arrival at the hospital. But we know that this varies widely across states, from a low of 20 minutes in one state to a high of 140 minutes in another.

Efforts to Improve Health Care Quality

Improving health care quality is a team effort, and it is ongoing on many levels. To succeed, every part of the health care system must become involved, including government and private organizations, doctors, nurses, pharmacists, hospitals, other providers, and you—the patient.

One way to assess and track quality of care is by using measures that are based on the latest scientific evidence. A health care measure clearly defines which health care services should be provided to patients who have or are at risk for certain conditions. Measures also set standards for screening, immunizations, and other preventive care.

There are two types of measures: clinical measures and consumer ratings. Because measures are intended to set general standards for a broad population, they may or may not apply to you. Always check with your doctor about your level of risk for a particular condition and which types of screening and tests you should have.

Clinical Measures

Clinical measures can be used to assess quality of care and patient satisfaction. Examples are provided here of measures that can be used to assess care quality for three of the most common conditions: diabetes, heart disease, and cancer.

Diabetes

More than six percent of all Americans have diabetes. Diabetes is the leading cause of blindness, leg amputation not resulting from trauma, and kidney disease. Diabetes increases the risk of complications in pregnant women, and it is a risk factor for heart disease and stroke. People who have diabetes are two to four times as likely to die from heart disease or stroke as those without diabetes. The following five measures can be used to assess quality of care for diabetes. If you have diabetes, you should receive the following tests and exams:

- regular hemoglobin A1c (blood glucose) testing,
- regular cholesterol testing,
- annual retinal eye exam,

- annual foot exam, and
- a flu shot each year.

Heart Disease

Heart disease—or cardiovascular disease—is a collection of diseases of the heart and blood vessels that includes heart attack, stroke, and heart failure. About 64 million Americans are living with heart disease. Heart disease is the number one cause of death in the United States. Maintaining control of blood pressure and cholesterol can help you prevent heart attack and stroke. The following are examples of measures that can be used to assess care for heart disease.

For adults age 18 and older:

- blood pressure measurement, and
- cholesterol testing.

More than 60 million men and women are living with heart disease. Everyone should know what constitutes good quality care for heart disease. In general,

- if you smoke, being advised to stop smoking; and
- if you suffer a heart attack, receiving aspirin within 24 hours of hospital admission and being prescribed beta-blocker therapy at hospital discharge.

Cancer

Cancer is the nation's second leading cause of death, after heart disease. Each year, more than one million new cases of cancer are diagnosed. Four cancers account for over half of the new cases reported each year. The four cancers are lung, colorectal, breast, and prostate. Screening to permit early detection holds the most promise for successful cancer treatment.

Talk to your doctor about screening tests for all of these cancers, especially if other members of your family have had these cancers or if you smoke. The following are examples of quality measures for several types of cancer screening.

Breast and Cervical Cancer

- mammography exam for women age 40 and older

- Pap smear testing for women age 18 and older

Colorectal Cancer

Men and women age 50 and older should receive the following tests:

- fecal occult blood testing (a test to detect blood in the stool)
- flexible sigmoidoscopy/colonoscopy exam (Check with your doctor about how often you should have this screening.)

Finding Quality Information

Today, you can find a great deal of information about health care quality, both online and in print. New tools and resources for assessing and improving health care quality are being developed and will be available soon. Meanwhile, here is a brief look at what is available now.

Report Cards

Reports cards and other quality reports include consumer ratings, clinical performance measures, or both. They can help you select the right treatment and the right health care provider based on what is most important to you. You may be able to get quality reports from:

- your employer—ask your personnel office for information on health plans;
- health plans—ask the plan's customer service office about quality reports; or
- other health care providers—hospitals, nursing homes, and community health clinics may have quality reports.

Several government agencies publish quality reports and other types of quality information.

- U.S. Department of Health and Human Services (HHS) has a quality tool that helps you compare the care provided by hospitals in your area. This tool is available online at http://www .hospitalcompare.hhs.gov.
- Another website (http://www.medicare.gov/NHCompare/home .asp) provided by the Centers for Medicare and Medicaid Services has detailed information on the past performance of every Medicare and Medicaid certified nursing home in the country.

Accreditation

Accreditation is another indicator that can be used to judge quality. Accreditation is a seal of approval given by a private, independent group. Health care organizations—such as hospitals—must meet national standards, including clinical performance measures, in order to be accredited.

Accreditation reports present quality information on hospitals, nursing homes, and other health care facilities. For example, the Joint Commission (formerly Joint Commission on Accreditation of Healthcare Organizations) prepares a performance report on each hospital that it surveys. Another group, the National Committee for Quality Assurance (NCQA), rates health plans like HMOs. The NCQA Health Plan Report Card presents accreditation results for hundreds of health plans across the country.

If you need help in finding quality reports, accreditation reports, or other types of quality information, check with your local library or your local or state health department. You can find your state health department listed in the blue pages of your phone book.

Consumer Ratings

Consumer ratings tell you what other people like you think about their health care. Some consumer ratings focus on health plans. For example, a survey called Consumer Assessment of Healthcare Providers and Systems (CAHPS®) asks people about the quality of care in their own health plans. Their answers can help you decide whether you want to join one of those plans. Hospital CAHPS (HCAHPS®) will be released for the first time in 2006. It will ask patients about their experiences with hospital care.

Choosing Quality Health Care

Here are some tips for making quality a key factor in the health care decisions you make about health plans, doctors, treatments, hospitals, and long-term care. Look for a health plan that:

- has been given high ratings by its members on the things that are important to you;
- has the doctors and hospitals you want or need;
- provides the benefits (covered services) you need;
- provides services where and when you need them; and

- has a documented history of doing a good job of preventing and treating illness.

Look for a doctor who:

- has received high ratings for quality of care;
- has the training and experience to meet your needs; and
- will work with you to make decisions about your health care.

If you become ill, make sure you understand:

- your diagnosis;
- how soon you need to be treated;
- your treatment choices, including the benefits and risks of each treatment; and
- how much experience your doctor has in treating your condition.

Look for a hospital that:

- is accredited by the Joint Commission;
- is rated highly by the state and by consumer groups or other organizations;
- has a lot of experience and success in treating your condition; and
- monitors quality of care and works to improve quality.

In choosing a nursing home or other long-term care facility, look for one that:

- has been found by state agencies and other groups to provide quality care; and
- provides a level of care, including staff and services, that will meet your needs.

Resources for More Information

Accreditation Association for Ambulatory Health Care
5250 Old Orchard Rd., Suite 200
Skokie, IL 60077
Phone: 847-853-6060

Fax: 847-853-9028
Website: http://www.aaahc.org
E-mail: info@aaahc.org

Agency for Healthcare Research and Quality (AHRQ)
P.O. Box 8547
Silver Spring MD 20907-8547
Toll-Free: 800-358-9295
Websites: http://www.guideline.gov; or,
http://www.qualitytools.ahrq.gov
E-mail: info@ahrq.gov

The Joint Commission
(Formerly Joint Commission on Accreditation of Healthcare
Organizations)
One Renaissance Blvd.
Oakbrook Terrace, IL 60181-4294
Phone: 630-792-5000
Fax: 630-792-5005
Website: http://www.jcaho.org

National Committee for Quality Assurance
1100 13th St., N.W., Suite 1000
Washington, DC 20005
Toll-Free: 888-275-7585
Phone: 202-955-3500
Fax: 202-955-3599
Website: http://www.ncqa.org
E-mail: customersupport@ncqa.org

Section 15.2

Identifying Quality Laboratory Services

"Helping You Identify Quality Laboratory Services,"
© 2007 The Joint Commission. Reprinted with permission.

Selecting quality health care services for yourself, a relative, or friend requires special thought and attention. The Joint Commission has prepared this information to help you make your selection. Knowing what to look for and what to ask will help you choose a laboratory that provides quality care and best meets your needs.

Although you may not always have the opportunity to choose the laboratory where your tests are processed, you can obtain some important information about the laboratory. By doing so, you'll have confidence that your tests will be performed properly. Begin by asking your doctor why he or she selected the laboratory and then discuss specifics about the quality improvement processes the laboratory has in place.

General Questions

- What is the name and location of the laboratory?

- What criteria did your doctor use to choose the laboratory?

- Does the doctor have confidence in the accuracy of the test results?

- Does the laboratory notify the doctor if a specimen is incorrectly collected? What is the follow-up procedure?

- Has the doctor ever received an incorrect result from the laboratory? How did the doctor handle the situation?

- How are complaints about inaccurate test results handled?

Questions about Sample Collection

- Are you given instructions about how to prepare for the lab test (for example, no eating or drinking)?

- Does the laboratory give your doctor clear instructions about how to properly collect specimens? Is this information included in the office staff's orientation and training materials? Is it periodically updated?

- If you are collecting the specimen yourself, did you receive clear instructions?

- When the specimen was collected, did the technician use two identifiers to label the sample collection containers in your presence?

Questions about the Test Results

- How soon can you expect to learn the test results?

- How will you be informed of test results? Will you receive a personal phone call if there was an abnormal test result?

- Is there a number you can call if you have questions?

Quality Oversight

- Is the laboratory accredited by a nationally recognized accrediting body such as The Joint Commission? Joint Commission accreditation means the organization voluntarily sought accreditation and met national health and safety standards.

Additional questions and considerations are included in another Joint Commission consumer brochure called "Speak Up: Prevent Errors in Your Care."

To find out if the laboratory you are considering is accredited by The Joint Commission, see Quality Check® on their website (www.jointcommission.org). Quality Check is a search engine for health care organizations. Joint Commission-accredited organizations are identified by the Gold Seal of Approval on Quality Check.

Quality Check provides Quality Reports that include information on the organization's overall performance level and how it compares to other organizations nationwide and statewide in specific performance areas. If a report is not available on Quality Check, or if you would like a printed copy, please call the Customer Service Center at 630-792-5800.

To report information or concerns about accredited organizations:

- Call or e-mail the Office of Quality Monitoring at 800-994-6610 or complaint@jointcommission.org.

- You can also fill out a Quality Incident Report form online.

Section 15.3

Choosing Quality Ambulatory Care

"Helping You Choose Quality Ambulatory Care,"
© 2007 The Joint Commission. Reprinted with permission.

Choosing quality health care services for yourself, a family member, or a close friend is one of the most important decisions you will ever make. Knowing what to look for and what to ask will help you choose an ambulatory care organization that provides quality care and best meets your needs—or those of a loved one.

Ambulatory care services include those provided by community health centers, medical practices, outpatient clinics, student health services, urgent and emergency care centers, and specialty services such as cardiac catheterization centers, imaging centers, and surgery centers.

Begin by asking your doctor or insurance case manager to recommend several conveniently located ambulatory care organizations. Visit or call each one and talk with the manager or other staff members about the organization's services, policies, history, and staff credentials. Then use the following questions to determine whether the organization meets your needs.

General Questions

- Does the organization explain your rights and responsibilities as a patient? Ask to see a copy of the organization's patient rights and responsibilities.

- Do you know the organization's policy regarding visitors? Are family members allowed in the recovery area?

- Does the organization maintain the confidentiality of patient files?

- How is confidentiality maintained and under what circumstances is specific patient information released?

- Does the organization have a written description of its services and fees? Is the organization able to help you find financial assistance if you need it? Will your insurance company reimburse you for the procedure?

- Is the organization licensed or certified by an appropriate state agency? Is the organization certified by Medicare?

- Is the organization accredited by a nationally recognized accrediting body such as The Joint Commission? Joint Commission accreditation means the organization voluntarily seeks accreditation and meets national health and safety standards.

Questions about Staff Qualifications

- Are the professionals qualified to offer the services and procedures you need? Are the doctors certified by appropriate medical specialty boards? Do the doctors practice at nearby hospitals? Are staff nurses and other personnel trained in emergency services such as cardiopulmonary resuscitation?

- If anesthesia or sedation is necessary for your procedure, are those who will administer it trained or certified?

- If high-tech equipment such as a laser is used in procedures, is staff properly trained to use and care for the equipment?

Questions about Emergency Care

- Does the organization have a 24-hour telephone number you can call if a complication arises after the procedure? Who will answer the phone, and what is the procedure for dealing with such emergencies after hours?

- Does the organization have an emergency patient care plan in case of a power failure or a natural disaster? In case of an emergency, will the organization still provide its services?

- Is the organization affiliated with any area hospitals? What is its transfer plan in case of an emergency?

Questions about Your Specific Care

- What is the organization's success record for the specific medical procedure you need? What is the specific training of the doctor who will be performing the procedure? How often is the procedure performed?

- Does the doctor provide you with information about the procedure and its risks? Are the doctor and staff receptive to your questions?

To find out if the ambulatory care organization you are considering is accredited by The Joint Commission, see Quality Check® on their website (www.jointcommission.org). Quality Check is a search engine for health care organizations. Joint Commission-accredited organizations are identified by the Gold Seal of Approval on Quality Check.

Quality Check® also provides Quality Reports that include information on a Joint Commission-accredited organization's performance and how it compares to other organizations nationwide and statewide. If a report is not available on Quality Check® or you would like a printed copy, call the Customer Service Center, 630-792-5800.

To report information or concerns about accredited organizations:

- Call or e-mail the Office of Quality Monitoring at 800-994-6610 or complaint@jointcommission.org.

- You can also fill out a Quality Incident Report form.

Chapter 16

Hospitalization

Chapter Contents

Section 16.1

Choosing a Hospital

Excerpted from "Choosing a Hospital," Health
Care Financing Administration (HCFA), May 2006.

Why Choose a Hospital?

In a medical emergency—when every second counts—you may not
be able to choose the hospital you go to. But often going into the hospital is not an emergency. You have time to think about it and to choose
the hospital you think will give you the best care.

Your choice of a hospital may depend on your doctor. It may also
depend on how you get your insurance or Medicare health care. In
most cases, you must use hospitals that belong to your plan. Some
managed care plans let you pay extra to use a hospital not on the
plan's list. Look at your plan's membership materials. Call your plan
to find out if you can do this and how much it would cost.

Questions to Ask when Choosing a Hospital

Is this a hospital where my doctor can treat patients?

The first thing to find out is if your doctor can treat you while you
are in this hospital. (Doctors usually have privileges in only a few
hospitals.) If not, you may want to choose a hospital where your doctor can treat you. Or you may choose to go to this hospital, knowing
that you will need to be under another doctor's care while you are
there.

Do staff at this hospital treat a lot of people with my health problem?

Your choice of hospital may depend on the kind of health problem
you have. Sometimes a hospital is known for treating a certain kind
of problem, like heart disease. If you need that kind of treatment, you
may want to choose that hospital. If you have a rare or serious health

128

problem, you may want to go to a hospital that treats a lot of people who have that problem. It may be helpful to talk with your doctor about which hospital you should choose.

How well do staff at this hospital treat people with my health problem?

Research shows that hospital staff have better success when they do a procedure often. You may want to ask your doctor:

- How often is this procedure done at this hospital?
- How often does the doctor do this procedure?
- How well do patients do after they have the procedure?

What is done to make sure patients get the best quality care?

Many hospitals are trying to make their quality of care better. One way to do this is to keep track of how well patients do. For example, if a lot of patients get infections while they are in the hospital, the hospital tries to find out what might be causing the problem. Then it makes changes and tries to do better so that fewer patients get infections.

Your Rights as a Patient in the Hospital

No matter which hospital you choose, as a patient you have certain rights while you are in the hospital. You have the right to get all the care you need while you are in the hospital and after you leave. If you feel you are being asked to leave the hospital before you are ready to go, you have a right to ask for a review of that decision.

Things to Remember

- If being cared for by your own doctor is important to you, you will want to choose a hospital where your doctor can treat patients.
- In most managed care plans, you must use hospitals that belong to your plan. Some plans let you pay extra to use hospitals not on the plan's list.
- In a private fee-for-service plan, you may use any hospital that accepts the plan's payment terms.

- Research shows that patients do better when a hospital does the same procedure often.

- No matter which hospital you choose, as a patient you have certain rights while you are in the hospital.

Section 16.2

Basics of a Hospital Stay

"When You Are in the Hospital: A Guide for Patients," *Journal of Patient Safety*, Volume 2, Issue 1, March 2006, p. 55. © Lippincott Williams and Wilkins, Inc. Reprinted with permission. Also, excerpts from "Hospital Hints," National Institute on Aging (NIA), December 2005.

When You Are in the Hospital: A Guide for Patients

Hospital stays can be a stressful time for both patient and family. Whether you are hospitalized for a scheduled procedure or unexpected illness, there are several steps you can take to help ensure that you receive the best care possible.

As a first step, make sure your health care team has all the information they need. The more details you provide about your medical history, the better care they can provide you.

When You Are Admitted

1. **Medications:** If you are taking medications or have recently taken medications, bring an updated list, including both name and dosage. This list should include herbal supplements, vitamins, and over-the-counter medications. If you are having surgery, it is particularly important that your health care team knows of any herbal supplement use. There are services that allow you to keep such a list, as well as a personal medical record. Options include www.ihealthrecord.org and www.medicalert .org. Such services can be particularly helpful in an emergency.

2. **Your doctor:** During an emergency visit, ask the hospital to contact your primary care doctor. Because your doctor knows

your health history, his or her involvement can be a tremendous help during an unplanned hospital stay.

3. **Allergies:** If you have a known allergy, make sure it is noted in your record and then remind each health care team member of this allergy before medications are administered or procedures are started.

4. **Chronic Conditions:** Make sure your record includes any chronic conditions you have, such as asthma, arthritis, diabetes, or high blood pressure. Tell each health care team member about these conditions and be sure to alert someone if symptoms flare. If this is a scheduled visit to the hospital, ask for directions in advance about whether you should take regular medications on the day before and day of your procedure. If you have chronic conditions or medication allergies, wearing a medical alert bracelet or pendant can provide key information to an emergency care team.

5. **Substance use:** You may be asked questions about your lifestyle, such as how much alcohol you drink, if you smoke, and whether you use street drugs. Sometimes, patients are embarrassed or fear they are being judged, so they do not answer honestly. These questions are being asked for your safety. For example, if you drink alcohol regularly, your liver may process certain medications differently; if you smoke, you are at higher risk of an infection after surgery. It is very important that you answer these questions honestly.

During Your Stay

There are several safety checks and measures you can take to lessen the chance of mistakes or complications while you are in the hospital.

- Check identification information to make sure it is correct. Your name, weight, and age are particularly important. Once in the hospital room, make sure the information in the hospital registry matches yours, not the patient who stayed in the room previously.

- To prevent infections, wash your hands with soap every time you use the restroom. All visitors and family members, as well as doctors and health care staff, should have clean hands before touching you. Do not be afraid to remind those around you to use soap and water. If visitors are not feeling well, ask them to visit with a phone call rather than in person.

- Monitors are used to make sure that vital systems in your body are working right. They track information such as your breathing and heart rate. Although beeps and other noises from monitors may seem disruptive, do not remove attachments or change settings on these machines. Monitors can be life saving.

Share this information with family and friends. You may want to appoint a person to act as your health advocate during your stay to make sure you are being taken care of as you wish. Your voice or that of your advocate is one of the most important safety measures you can use. Ask questions and raise concerns if you have them.

Hospital Hints

The following information is for people who plan to enter the hospital by choice rather than for those who go to the hospital because of an emergency. Relatives and friends of patients who are admitted to the hospital also may find this information useful.

What to Bring

It's best to pack as little as you can. However, be sure to bring the following items:

- nightclothes, bathrobe, and sturdy slippers (label all personal items)
- comfortable clothes to wear home
- a toothbrush, toothpaste, shampoo, comb and brush, deodorant, and razor
- a list of your medicines, including prescription and over-the-counter drugs
- details of past illnesses, surgeries, and allergies
- your insurance card
- a list of the names and telephone numbers (home and business) of family members to contact in an emergency
- $10 or less for newspapers, magazines, or other items you may wish to buy in the hospital gift shop

What to Leave Home

Leave cash, jewelry (including wedding rings, earrings, and watches), credit cards, and checkbooks at home or have a family member or friend keep them for you. If you must bring valuables, ask if they can be kept in the hospital safe during your stay. In addition, leave electric razors, hair dryers, and curling irons at home.

Safety Tips

Because you may feel weak or tired, please take a few extra safety steps while in the hospital:

- Use the call bell or button when you need help.
- Use the controls to lower your bed before getting in or out.
- Be careful not to trip over the wires and tubes that may be around the bed.
- Try to keep the things you need within easy reach.
- Take only prescribed medicines. If you bring your own medicines with you, tell your nurse or doctor. Do not take other drugs without your doctor's permission.
- Hold on to grab bars for support when getting in and out of the bathtub or shower.
- Use handrails on stairways and in hallways.

Patient Rights

You can decide in advance what medical treatments you want or do not want in the hospital in case you lose your ability to speak for yourself. You can do this by preparing an advance directive. In an advance directive, you tell people how to make medical decisions for you when you cannot make them for yourself. You also can name someone else to make medical decisions for you. Two common advance directives are a living will and a durable power of attorney for health care.

Discharge Planning

Before going home, you'll need discharge orders from your doctor and a release form from the hospital business office. Discharge planning before leaving the hospital can help you prepare for your health and home care needs after you go home. The discharge planner can help you arrange for a visiting nurse, hospital equipment, meals-on-wheels, or other services. The discharge planner also knows about senior centers, rehabilitation centers, nursing homes, and other long-term care services.

Section 16.3

Communicating Effectively in the Hospital Setting

Caregivers know all too well the feelings of helplessness that often accompany their role of caring for a loved one with a chronic illness. When a hospitalization is involved, it is not uncommon to feel as though you have lost all control. There are steps you can take to ease the stress of a hospitalization and to ensure that you remain a part of the health care team should a hospital stay take place.

Most patients enter the hospital today as the result of a serious complication of a chronic illness or a life-threatening acute event. Because your loved one is likely to be seriously ill, there may be a great deal of uncertainty involved with his or her prognosis. Your loved one may experience a significant decline in function, and you may be forced to make crucial decisions without his or her input. By being proactive now, prior to any hospitalization, you will ensure that you and your loved one have a voice when it counts the most.

The Papers You Need

Having the proper legal documents in place is critical if you want to ensure that your loved one will receive the type of care he or she wants and needs. The following list outlines the basic documents we all should have.

- **Durable power of attorney for health care:** A durable power of attorney for health care, also known as a health care agent or proxy, is an individual you have appointed to make decisions about your medical care if you become unconscious or can no longer speak for yourself. A health care agent can be assigned as part of the advance directive form.

- **Advance medical directive:** An advance directive informs your physician and family members what kind of care you wish to receive in the event that you can no longer make your own medical decisions.

- **Living will:** A living will is a type of advance directive that outlines what kind of medical treatment you want in certain situations. It only comes into effect if you are diagnosed with a terminal illness and have less than six months to live, or if you are in a persistent vegetative state. A living will does not, however, allow you to name someone to make decisions on your behalf.

- **Do-not-resuscitate (DNR) order:** Another conversation that should take place prior to any hospitalization involves your loved one's wishes regarding resuscitation (efforts to restart the heart after it has stopped). Does he/she want resuscitation to occur regardless of circumstances? What are his or her feelings about ventilators and other life-sustaining equipment? If the decision is made that cardiopulmonary resuscitation is not what your loved one desires, then a do-not-resuscitate order must be written by your physician. A DNR can be part of your advance directive.

If your loved one does not already have a living will or an advance directive, now is the time to discuss his or her wishes for end-of-life treatment. A durable health care power of attorney should be appointed before a crisis develops. In the event your loved one is incapable of making decisions, this individual will have the legal authority to act on his or her behalf. Advance directives, living wills, and durable power of attorney forms are all simple documents to complete. Samples may be obtained through your local hospital, your attorney, or your state's attorney general's office. Your physician may also have copies of some of these documents. Signed copies should be given to your family physician. The documents must also be placed in the hospital chart each time your loved one is hospitalized.

Information You Need to Provide to Hospital Personnel

In addition to having the vital documents mentioned above, you can facilitate your loved one's transition to the hospital by providing the health care team with the following information:

- the patient's medical history, in writing
- a list of the patient's allergies
- a list of current medications and dosages
- a list of all physicians and consultants who are caring for your loved one, along with phone numbers

Providing this information immediately upon admission to the hospital can save crucial hours and improve communication. Often the hospitalization begins in the emergency room. The information will ensure that in the busy emergency room setting, your loved one's care is facilitated and physicians familiar with his or her case are involved from the start.

The Health Care Team

As a family caregiver, you are a part of the health care team, which also includes the attending physician, the hospital nurses, and a hospital social worker or case manager. Each of these individuals, including you, has a role in the hospitalization. Stand up for your role on the team. The other members of the health care team need your input in order to evaluate, educate, prognosticate, advise, and treat your loved one. Here are four things you should do upon arrival at the hospital.

1. **Find out the name of the attending physician of record for your loved one.** This is the individual who will be coordinating the care throughout his or her hospital stay. This physician will be the primary doctor on the case. The attending physician will be in communication with the other consulting physicians and know their recommendations. Sometimes it is necessary to talk to a consultant about a specific issue, but often the attending physician can summarize the entire treatment plan. Make sure you understand and agree with that plan. Don't hesitate to continue to ask questions until you feel comfortable with the answers. You may find it helpful to keep a running

list of questions that you wish to discuss each time you see the physician.

2. **The first time you speak with the attending physician, make sure to find out the best way to get in touch with him or her.** Who will initiate the phone contact? At what number can the physician be reached and what times are best to call? Make sure the fact sheet in your loved one's hospital chart contains your name and your correct phone numbers.

3. **Get to know the nurses who are caring for your loved one.** They can answer your day-to-day questions and are an excellent source of information and support. Don't be afraid to ask the nurses about any new procedures or changes in your loved one's course of treatment. They are the natural starting point for questions and will direct you to the attending physician when necessary. This will cut down on any frustration you might feel at not being able to reach your attending physician every time you have a new issue to discuss. Realize that the change of shifts is a very busy time for the nurses, so find out when the shifts occur and try to hold your questions until the nurse coming on duty has received his or her report.

    *   **Note:** Many elderly patients, upon admission to a hospital, will experience disorientation in their new environment and may become uncooperative. They may sleep poorly and may be found wandering the halls in the evening. You may notice deterioration in their concentration and memory. Don't panic. These reactions are common and the health care team is experienced in dealing with these challenges.

4. **As soon as you are able, speak to a hospital social worker or case manager, who will help you with any discharge planning issues.** This includes what follow-up is necessary after you leave the hospital; who will be providing home health care, if necessary; what home health equipment you might need; and who will be paying for these additional expenses. Make sure you obtain the numbers of all home health companies providing goods and services and the names and numbers of companies that will deliver the equipment. A hospitalization may be the transition to a nursing home or hospice setting. The hospital social worker or case manager can help you make a smooth transition and can provide support for you, the caregiver, as well as for the patient.

137

Maintaining Some Control

Medicine is full of "lesser of the evils" choices, and at no time is this truer than when a chronically ill patient is hospitalized. The goal of hospitalization in these cases is often symptom management, with the understanding that the underlying problem cannot be fixed. The focus in the hospital will be on palliation and management rather than cure. It is important for you, as the primary caregiver, to keep this in mind, and to strive to understand the risks and benefits of any proposed course of treatment. It is also your role to make clear to everyone on the health care team what your loved one's wishes are regarding short- and long-term treatment. By being more proactive in your communication, you will not only simplify everyone's job, you will maintain some degree of control. At no time is your role as caregiver more important than when you speak on behalf of the person you love.

—by Patricia L. Tomsko, M.D., and Sandy Padwo Rogers

Patricia L. Tomsko, M.D., is board certified in family practice, geriatrics, and hospice and palliative medicine. Sandy Padwo Rogers is a freelance writer and editor.

Chapter 17

Surgery

Chapter Contents

Section 17.1

What You Need to Know about Surgery

Excerpted from "Having Surgery? What You Need to Know,"
Agency for Healthcare Research and Quality (AHRQ), AHRQ
Pub No. 05(06)–0074–A, October 2005.

Are you facing surgery? You are not alone. Every year, more than 15 million Americans have surgery. Most operations are not emergencies and are considered elective surgery. This means that you have time to learn about your operation to be sure it is the best treatment for you. You also have time to work with your surgeon to make the surgery as safe as possible. Be active in your health care to have quality care.

Your regular doctor is your primary care doctor. He or she may be the doctor who suggests that you have surgery and may refer you to a surgeon. You may also want to find another surgeon to get a second opinion, to confirm if surgery is the right treatment for you. You might want to ask friends or coworkers for the names of surgeons they have used.

This chapter gives you some questions to ask your primary care doctor and surgeon before you have surgery. Your doctors should welcome questions. If you do not understand the answers, ask the doctor to explain them clearly. Bring a friend or relative along to help you talk with the doctor. Research shows that patients who are well informed about their treatment are more satisfied with their results.

Get the Basic Facts

Why do I need an operation?

There are many reasons to have surgery. Some operations can relieve or prevent pain. Others can reduce a symptom of a problem or improve some body function. Some surgeries are done to find a problem. Surgery can also save your life. Your doctor will tell you the purpose of the procedure. Make sure you understand how the proposed operation will help fix your medical problem. For example, if something is going to be repaired or removed, find out why it needs to be done.

140

What operation are you recommending?

Ask your surgeon to explain the surgery and how it is done. Your surgeon can draw a picture or a diagram and explain the steps in the surgery.

Is there more than one way of doing the operation? One way may require more extensive surgery than another. Some operations that once needed large incisions (cuts in the body) can now be done using much smaller incisions (for example, laparoscopic surgery). Some surgeries require that you stay in the hospital for one or more days. Others let you come in and go home on the same day. Ask why your surgeon wants to do the operation one way over another.

Laparoscopic surgery: Some surgeries that used to need a large incision can now be done using a few small cuts. Instead of a large scar, you will have only a few small scars. Usually, you will recover from laparoscopic surgery more quickly. The incisions let doctors insert a thin tube with a camera (a laparoscope) into the body to help them see. Then they use small tools to do the surgery. Removing the gallbladder, for example, is now mostly done with this type of surgery.

Are there alternatives to surgery?

Sometimes, surgery is not the only answer to a medical problem. Medicines or treatments other than surgery, such as a change in diet or special exercises, might help you just as well—or more. Ask your surgeon or primary care doctor about the benefits and risks of these other choices. You need to know as much as possible about these benefits and risks to make the best decision.

One alternative to surgery may be watchful waiting. During a watchful wait, your doctor and you check to see if your problem gets better or worse over time. If it gets worse, you may need surgery right away. If it gets better, you may be able to wait to have surgery or not have it at all.

How much will the operation cost?

Even if you have health insurance, there may be some costs for you to pay. This may depend on your choice of surgeon or hospital. Ask what your surgeon's fee is and what it covers. Surgical fees often also include some visits after the operation. You also will get a bill from the hospital for your care and from the other doctors who gave you care during your surgery.

141

Before you have the operation, call your insurance company. They can tell you how much of the costs your insurance will pay and what share you will have to pay. If you are covered by Medicare, call 800-MEDICARE (800-633-4227) to find out your share of surgery costs.

Learn about the Benefits and Risks

What are the benefits of having the operation?

Ask your surgeon what you will gain by having the operation. For example, a hip replacement may mean that you can walk again with ease.

Ask how long the benefits will last. For some procedures, it is not unusual for the benefits to last for a short time only. You may need a second operation at a later date. For other procedures, the benefits may last a lifetime.

When finding out about the benefits of the operation, be realistic. Sometimes patients expect too much and are disappointed with the outcome or results. Ask your doctor if there is anything you can read to help you understand the procedure and its likely results.

What are the risks of having the operation?

All operations have some risk. This is why you need to weigh the benefits of the operation against the risks of complications or side effects.

Complications are unplanned events linked to the operation. Typical complications are infection, too much bleeding, reaction to anesthesia, or accidental injury. Some people have a greater risk of complications because of other medical conditions. There also may be side effects after the operation. Often, your surgeon can tell you what side effects to expect. For example, there may be swelling and some soreness around the incision.

There is almost always some pain with surgery. Ask your surgeon how much pain there will be and what the doctors and nurses will do to help stop the pain. Controlling the pain will help you to be more comfortable while you heal. Controlling the pain will also help you get well faster and improve the results of your operation.

What if I don't have this operation?

Based on what you learn about the benefits and risks of the operation, you might decide not to have it. Ask your surgeon what you will gain—or lose—by not having the operation now. Could you be in more pain? Could your condition get worse? Could the problem go away?

Learn How to Get More Information

Where can I get a second opinion?

Getting a second opinion from another doctor is a very good way to make sure that having the operation is the best choice for you. You can ask your primary care doctor for the name of another surgeon who could review your medical file. If you consult another doctor, make sure to get your records from the first doctor so that your tests do not have to be repeated.

Many health insurance plans ask patients to get a second opinion before they have certain operations that are not for an emergency. If your plan does not require a second opinion, you may still ask to have one. Check with your insurance company to see if they will pay for a second opinion. You should discuss your insurance questions with your health insurance company or your employee benefits office. If you are eligible for Medicare, they will pay for a second opinion.

Find Out More about Your Operation

What kind of anesthesia will I need?

Anesthesia is used so that surgery can be performed without unnecessary pain. Your surgeon can tell you whether the operation calls for local, regional, or general anesthesia and why this form of anesthesia is best for your procedure. Section 17.2, "Anesthesia Basics," provides further detailed information about anesthesia.

How long will it take me to recover?

Your surgeon can tell you how you might feel and what you will be able to do—or not do—the first few days, weeks, or months after surgery. Ask how long you will be in the hospital. Find out what kind of supplies, equipment, and help you will need when you go home. Knowing what to expect can help you get better faster.

Ask how long it will be before you can go back to work or start regular exercise again. You do not want to do anything that will slow your recovery. For example, lifting a 10-pound bag of potatoes may not seem to be too much a week after your operation, but it could be. You should follow your surgeon's advice to make sure you recover fully as soon as possible.

Making Sure Your Surgery Is Safe

Check with your insurance company to find out if you may choose a surgeon or hospital or if you must use ones selected by the insurer. Ask your doctor about which hospital has the best care and results for your condition if you have more than one hospital to choose from. Studies show that for some types of surgery, numbers count—using a surgeon or hospital that does more of a particular type of surgery can improve your chance of a good result.

If you do have a choice of surgeon or hospital, ask the surgeon the following questions.

What are your qualifications?

You will want to know that your surgeon is experienced and qualified to perform the operation. Many surgeons have taken special training and passed exams given by a national board of surgeons. Ask if your surgeon is board certified in surgery. Some surgeons also have the letters F.A.C.S. after their name. This means they are Fellows of the American College of Surgeons and have passed another review by surgeons of their surgical skills.

How much experience do you have doing this operation?

One way to reduce the risks of surgery is to choose a surgeon who has been well trained to do the surgery and has plenty of experience doing it. You can ask your surgeon about his or her recent record of successes and complications with this surgery. If it is easier for you, you can discuss the surgeon's qualifications with your primary care doctor.

At which hospital will the operation be done?

Most surgeons work at one or two local hospitals. Find out where your surgery will be done and how often the same operation is done there. Research shows that patients often do better when they have surgery in hospitals with more experience in the operation. Ask your doctor about the success rate at the hospitals you can choose between. The success rate is the number of patients who improve divided by all patients having that operation at a hospital. If your surgeon suggests using a hospital with a lower success rate for your surgery, find out why.

How long you will be in the hospital?

Until recently, most patients who had surgery stayed in the hospital overnight for one or more days. Today, many patients have surgery done as an outpatient in a doctor's office, a special surgical center, or a day surgery unit of a hospital. These patients have an operation and go home the same day. Outpatient surgery is less expensive because you do not have to pay for staying in a hospital room.

Ask whether your operation will be done in the hospital or in an outpatient setting, and ask which of these is the usual way the surgery is done. If your doctor recommends that you stay overnight in the hospital (inpatient surgery) for an operation that is usually done as outpatient surgery—or recommends outpatient surgery that is usually done as inpatient surgery—ask why. You want to be in the right place for your operation.

Have the Surgeon Mark the Surgery Site

Rarely, surgeons will make a mistake and operate on the wrong part of the body. A number of groups of surgeons now urge their members to use a marking pen to show the place that they will operate on. The surgeons do this by writing directly on the patient's skin on the day of surgery. Don't be afraid to ask your surgeon to do this to make your surgery safer.

Section 17.2

Anesthesia Basics

This information was provided by TeensHealth, one of the largest resources online for medically reviewed health information written for teens, kids, and parents. For more articles like this one, visit www.TeensHealth.org, or www.KidsHealth.org. © 2006 The Nemours Foundation.

No doubt about it, getting an operation can be stressful. If you're scheduled for surgery, you may have questions or concerns about anesthesia. The thought of being unconscious or temporarily losing sensation can be downright unnerving.

From a minor procedure with a shot to numb the area to a more serious surgery in which you will be "asleep," knowing the basics about anesthesia may help answer your questions and ease some concerns.

What is anesthesia?

Basically, anesthesia is the use of medicine to prevent the feeling of pain or another sensation during surgery or other procedures that might be painful (such as getting stitches or having a wart removed). Given as an injection or through inhaled gases or vapors, different types of anesthesia affect the nervous system in various ways by blocking nerve impulses and, therefore, pain.

In today's hospitals and surgery centers, highly trained professionals use a wide variety of safe, modern medications and extremely capable monitoring technology. An anesthesiologist is a doctor who specializes in giving and managing anesthetics—the medications that numb an area of the body or help you fall and stay asleep.

In addition to administering anesthesia medications before the surgery, the anesthesiologist will:

- monitor your major bodily functions (such as breathing, heart rate and rhythm, body temperature, blood pressure, and blood oxygen levels) during surgery;

- address any problems that might arise during surgery;

- manage any pain you may have after surgery; and

146

- keep you as comfortable as possible before, during, and after surgery.

A specially trained nurse anesthetist or resident physician, who works with the anesthesiologist and surgeon, may also give you anesthesia (although the anesthesiologist will be the one to manage the anesthesia during the operation).

What are the types of anesthesia?

Anesthesia is broken down into three main categories: general, regional, and local, all of which can be administered using various methods and different medications that affect the nervous system in some way. The American Society of Anesthesiologists (ASA) compares the nervous system to an office's telephone system—with the brain as the switchboard, the nerves as the cables, and the body parts feeling pain as the phones.

- **General anesthesia:** The goal is to make and keep the person completely unconscious (or asleep) during the operation, with no sensations, feeling of pain, awareness, movement, or memory of the surgery. General anesthesia can be given through an intravenous (IV)—which requires a needle stick into a vein, usually in the arm—or by inhaling gases or vapors.

- **Regional anesthesia:** An anesthetic drug is injected near a cluster of nerves, numbing a larger area of the body (such as below the waist). A person who receives regional anesthesia is usually asleep before the procedure is done. However, older children or those who would be at unacceptable risk by being asleep may be awake or sedated during the procedure. For example, if a person is overweight, it may be difficult for the anesthesiologist to feels the bones that help guide correct placement of the needle. To avoid nerve damage, getting feedback from an awake person would be a safer option. This type of anesthesia includes things like epidurals, caudal blocks (which are similar to epidurals, but are placed in the tailbone), and spinal blocks (which further numb the lower body).

- **Local anesthesia:** An anesthetic drug numbs only a small, specific part of the body (for example, a hand or patch of skin). Depending on the size of the area, local anesthesia can be given as a shot, spray, or ointment. With local anesthesia, a person may be awake or sedated. Local anesthesia lasts for a short period of time and is often used for minor surgeries and outpatient procedures (when patients come in for an operation and can go home that same day). If you are having surgery in a clinic or doctor's office (such as the dentist or dermatologist), this is probably the type of anesthetic that will be used.

The type and amount of anesthesia will be specifically tailored to your needs and will depend on various factors, including your age and weight, the type and area of the surgery, any allergies you may have, and your current medical condition.

What are the common side effects?

You will most likely feel disoriented, groggy, and a little confused when waking up after surgery. Some other common side effects, which should go away fairly quickly, include:

- nausea or vomiting which can usually be alleviated with anti-nausea medication;
- chills;
- shakiness; or
- sore throat (if a tube was used to administer the anesthesia or help with breathing).

What are the risks?

Anesthesia today is very safe. In very rare cases, anesthesia can cause complications (such as strange heart rhythms, breathing problems, allergic reactions to medications, and even death). However, rare complications usually involve patients with other medical problems. The risks depend on the kind of procedure, the condition of the patient, and the type of anesthesia used. Be sure to talk to your doctor, surgeon, and/or anesthesiologist about any concerns.

Most complications can usually be prevented by simply providing the anesthesiologist with complete information before the surgery about things like:

- your current and past health (including diseases or conditions such as recent or current colds, or other issues such as snoring or depression);
- any medications (prescription and over-the-counter), supplements, or herbal remedies you are taking;

- any allergies (especially to foods, medications, or latex) you may have;

- whether you smoke, drink alcohol, or take any recreational drugs; or

- any previous reactions you or any family member has had to anesthesia

To ensure your safety during the surgery or procedure, it's extremely important to answer all of the anesthesiologist's questions as honestly and thoroughly as possible. Things that may seem harmless could interact with or affect the anesthesia and cause you to react to it.

It's also important that you follow the doctor's recommendations about what not to do before the surgery. You probably won't be able to eat or drink (usually nothing after midnight the day before) and may need to stop taking herbal supplements for a certain period of time before surgery.

You can rest assured that the safety of anesthetic procedures has improved a lot in the past 25 years, thanks to advances in technology and the extensive training anesthesiologists receive. The more informed, calm, and reassured you are about the surgery and the safety of anesthesia, the easier the experience will probably be.

For More Information

The American College of Surgeons (ACS)
Office of Public Information
633 N. St. Clair St.
Chicago, IL 60611-3211
Toll-Free: 800-621-4111
Phone: 312-202-5000
Website: http://www.facs.org/public_info/ppserv.html

American Society of Anesthesiologists (ASA)
520 North Northwest Highway
Park Ridge, IL 60068-2573
Phone: 847-825-5586
Fax: 847-825-1692
Website: http://www.asahq.org
E-mail: mail@asahq.org

Part Three

Health Literacy and Making Informed Health Decisions

Chapter 18

Health Literacy Defined

You may not have considered it, but every time you read health information, from food labels to medical forms, you're exercising your health literacy skills. Health literacy is the ability to obtain, process, and understand health information needed to make informed health decisions. Health literacy affects your ability to:

- use the health care system, including filling out complex forms and locating health care providers and services;

- share personal information, such as your health history, with providers;

- care for yourself and manage any chronic disease;

- interpret nutrition labels and understand what you're putting in your body;

- understand how to correctly use over-the-counter and prescription medicines to get the most benefit and avoid risks; and

- understand math concepts such as probability and risk.

In addition to basic literacy skills, health literacy requires knowledge of health topics and math. For example, you use math skills to

---

"Health Literacy: Hints for a Healthier You," *FDA and You*, Winter 2007, U.S. Food and Drug Administration (FDA).

calculate cholesterol and blood sugar levels, measure medications, and understand nutrition labels.

If you have limited health literacy, you may lack knowledge or have misinformation about the body as well as the nature and causes of disease. Without this knowledge, you may not understand the relationship between lifestyle factors such as diet and exercise and various health outcomes.

Why is health literacy important?

According to the Institute of Medicine, a nonprofit organization that offers advice on science matters, approximately one-half of the adult population may lack the needed literacy skills to use the U.S. health care system. Low literacy has been linked to poor health outcomes such as higher rates of hospitalization, less frequent use of preventive services, and higher health care costs.

What do research studies say about the relationship between health literacy and health outcomes?

Use of preventive services: People with limited health literacy skills are more likely to skip important preventive measures such as Pap smears and flu shots. When compared to those with adequate health literacy skills, studies have shown that patients with limited health literacy skills enter the health care system when they are sicker.

Knowledge about medical conditions and treatment: People with limited health literacy skills are more likely to have chronic conditions and are less able to manage them effectively. Studies have found that patients with high blood pressure, diabetes, asthma, or human immunodeficiency virus (HIV)/acquired immunodeficiency syndrome (AIDS) who have limited health literacy skills have less knowledge of their illness and its management.

Rates of hospitalization: Limited health literacy skills are associated with an increase in preventable hospital visits and admissions. Studies have shown a higher rate of hospitalization and use of emergency services among patients with limited literacy skills.

Health status: Studies show that people with limited health literacy skills are significantly more likely than people with adequate health literacy skills to report their health as poor.

Health care costs: Those with limited health literacy skills use more services designed to treat complications of disease and less services designed to prevent complications. Higher rates of hospitalization and use of emergency services among patients with limited health literacy skills is associated with higher health care costs.

Stigma and shame: Low health literacy may also have negative psychological effects. One study found that those with limited health literacy skills reported a sense of shame about their skill level. As a result, they may hide reading or vocabulary difficulties to maintain their dignity.

How can I become more health literate?

Study: While you're in school, many of the classes you're taking will help raise your health literacy. Reading, English, science, math, and health classes are all important for raising health literacy skills.

Research: If you do have a health problem, be an informed consumer by researching your condition. A good place to start your research is http://www.healthfinder.gov, a federal website developed for consumers, by the U.S. Department of Health and Human Services and other federal agencies. The FDA website (http://www.fda.gov) can also help you find health information about topics such as drugs, medical devices, and food.

Ask: Your health care provider can answer questions you have about your health. Advice from your health care provider can keep you safe while improving your health literacy.

What is FDA doing to improve health literacy skills?

FDA participates in a workgroup to improve health literacy skills by raising awareness, building support, and improving practices around health literacy.

Chapter 19

Consumers in Health Care: How Do People Make Health Care Decisions?

Changes in the health care environment are forcing consumers to make more—and more complex—decisions than ever before. The rise of consumer-directed health plans requires consumers to shop for and evaluate health care services; individuals selecting hospitals or providers lack comprehensive data on quality and outcomes; and those looking for coherent information on treatment options are often stymied by the sheer volume of resources available to help them make decisions about their care. Providing support to consumers as they navigate the health care system can have positive results not only for individuals but for the health care system as a whole, since informed and knowledgeable consumers can encourage better system performance and quality through the decisions they make.

The Changing Environment for Decision Making

Fundamental changes taking place in the health care system underscore the importance of helping consumers understand and evaluate the complex choices they face. These changes include:

- The rapid growth in the availability and use of health care information, fueled largely by the internet.

Excerpts from "Consumers in Health Care: The Burden of Choice," reprinted with permission from the California HealthCare Foundation © 2007.

- A growing desire by many American consumers to be more active and involved in the management of their health care.

- A movement to shift more responsibility for the cost of health insurance benefits and the purchase of health services to individuals through consumer-directed health plans.

- The growing customization of products and services, including health benefit plans that offer consumers opportunities to choose among levels of premiums, deductibles, and coinsurance, as well as offering a degree of choice within hospital and doctor networks.

- Increasing advertising "clutter" that makes it difficult to attract and hold people's attention, even if the goal of doing so is to help them make good decisions.

- Declining levels of consumer trust in key institutions, including insurance companies, physicians, and health care organizations, such as managed care companies.

These trends point to the growing need for and challenge of providing effective decision-support information that consumers can understand and use to make better health care choices.

Key Findings from Decision Research

Research on how people make choices and the cognitive steps they go through in processing and using information reveals important insights for the developers of decision-support information for health care consumers. These findings include:

- Contrary to popular notions that more information is better, decision-making research shows that more information does not always improve decision making, and frequently may actually undermine it.

- In the face of complex choices, people focus on familiar terms or concepts, or take mental short cuts that reduce the cognitive effort required to make decisions. They often wind up sacrificing thoroughness in favor of greater ease in making the decision.

- Consumer preferences shift during the decision-making process, suggesting that the content and presentation of information can influence people's perceptions about that information and their willingness to act on it.

- Individuals use different modes of thinking—some analytical and some experiential—to make decisions; designers of decision-support information should take this into account to increase the likelihood of a good decision.

Lessons from Advertising and Social Marketing

Commercial advertising capitalizes on the power of emotions to influence consumer decisions. Building brand awareness is one of the principal strategies for using emotion to capture and retain customers for a given product or service. Branding is the central means by which marketers cut through the clutter of advertising to present a message that stands out and builds consumer awareness and loyalty. To be most effective, the specific segment of the consumer audience or market with the needs, values, motivations, and behaviors most likely to be receptive to the brand's message must be identified and targeted.

Social marketing is a field of social research and practice that uses the principles of marketing to motivate changes in behavior that are beneficial to the society at large. By identifying the barriers to desired behavior, social marketers are able to offer the target audience incentives to move toward the desired behavior by helping them perceive the benefits of doing so. The social marketing model has been successful in a variety of areas, including recycling, smoking cessation, improved diet and nutrition, and teen pregnancy reduction.

What are the lessons of branding, audience segmentation, and social marketing strategies for developers of decision-support information? If decision-support and comparative information tools are to get noticed and used, promoters will need to develop and market a successful brand image in the face of multiple competing messages. They will need to understand who their target audience is, what specific behaviors they want to encourage, and what benefits can be offered to motivate such behavior change.

Implications of Findings for Supporting Consumer Health Care Decisions

Taken together, the findings from consumer decision research and the lessons from advertising and social marketing suggest a number of implications for developers of health care decision support information:

- Make decision-support information relevant and appropriate to the specific type of health care decisions. Those interested in

159

helping consumers make good choices need to understand the context in which choices are being made and to make decision-support information relevant and appropriate to the specific type of decision being made. For example, information to support choice of health plan may be needed only once a year during open enrollment, but information for managing the treatment of a chronic disease may be required frequently. The most appropriate content and structure of any particular set of decision-support information will depend on the frequency and complexity of the decision, the degree of choice, and the factors that are most important to consumers who make these choices, like cost, convenience, and quality.

- Help decision makers simplify their choices systematically. Recognizing that consumers cannot and will not deal with large amounts of information and manifold sources, developers of decision-support information must give them ways to simplify the decision process. This can be done through a range of methods, from "low-tech" design strategies, such as a simple health plan comparison chart with visual cues that help people navigate and understand the core implications of information, to more sophisticated online approaches that enable users to "customize" information to their specific preferences and circumstances.

- Focus on those most receptive to the information. Decision-support information must be targeted to the audience segment(s) most likely to be receptive to it. To be effective, segmentation strategies should go beyond basic demographics to understand underlying cultural differences and the values, attitudes, motivations, and behaviors of those most likely to benefit from and use the information. Successful marketing to these groups may help identify strategies for eventually reaching nonusers, by identifying precisely what users respond to and finding ways to market these features and benefits to others.

- Work through trusted advisors. Because many consumers (especially the elderly and certain ethnic groups) tend to make their health care decisions based wholly or in part on the guidance of trusted advisers, sponsors of report cards, and other decision-support information should consider these advisors to be a key target for their marketing and distribution efforts. In addition, they should engage consumers in the development of these materials through focus groups and other methods. Trusted advisors

160

include friends and family, physicians, senior centers, civic organizations, and consumer advocates. Developers of consumer information should consider training these "information intermediaries" on the importance and use of these materials and providing them with technical assistance on an ongoing basis.

- Cultivate an image as a trusted source. In order to create credibility and recognition, developers of decision-support information should determine whether they are known by their target audience of health care consumers, what their reputation is with those consumers, whether they have the resources to build a brand on their own, or whether it might make sense to partner with an already recognized brand identity. Focus groups with current and prospective users of information support provide one way to investigate perceptions and to test out new ideas for creating a trusted brand image.

- Integrate multiple types of information. As consumers are forced to take on more responsibility and risk for the cost of their decisions, they will likely need resources that integrate information on all of the factors they need to consider, such as quality, cost, the degree of choice among providers, and convenience. Increasingly, such one-stop service may be required to accommodate the growing complexity of decisions that consumers face.

- Promote information by emphasizing benefits, not features. Marketing theory and practice suggest that it is more effective to emphasize benefits than to describe features. The most appealing benefits for consumers are usually immediate and tangible, and tap into emotion-laden core values, like a desire for control or independence, or the desire to care for one's family. Making the appeal emotional rather than intellectual may help cut through the defenses of consumers inundated with demands for their time, and open them up to the idea of integrating "cold" analytical information into some of the most personal—and daunting—decisions that individuals may make.

Chapter 20

How to Find
Medical Information

Searching for medical information can be confusing, especially for first-timers. However, if you are patient and stick to it, you can find a wealth of information. Today's computer technology is making it easier than ever for people to track down medical and health information. Other good sources of information include textbooks, journal articles, reference books, and health care organizations. This chapter explains how to locate these important sources of information.

Start with Your Community Library

Most people have a library in or near their community, and it's a good place to start to look for medical information. Before going to the library, you may find it helpful to make a list of topics you want information about and questions you have. Your topic list will make it easier for the librarian to direct you to the best resources.

The following are some types of resources you are likely to find at, or access through, your local library.

Basic Medical References

Many community libraries have a collection of basic medical references. These references may include medical dictionaries or encyclopedias, drug information handbooks, basic medical and nursing

National Institute of Arthritis and Musculoskeletal and Skin Diseases (NIAMS), NIH Publication No. 05–4745, January 2005.

163

textbooks, and directories of physicians and medical specialists (listings of doctors). You may also wish to find magazine articles on a certain topic. Look in the *Reader's Guide to Periodical Literature* for articles on health and medicine that were published in consumer magazines.

Computer Databases

Infotrac, a CD-ROM computer database available at libraries or on the web, indexes hundreds of popular magazines and newspapers, as well as some medical journals such as the *Journal of the American Medical Association* and *New England Journal of Medicine.*

Your library may also carry searchable computer databases of medical journal articles, including MEDLINE®/PubMed® (http://pubmed .gov) or the Cumulative Index to Nursing and Allied Health Literature. Many of the databases or indexes have abstracts that provide a summary of each journal article. Although most community libraries don't have a large collection of medical and nursing journals, your librarian may be able to get copies of the articles you want. Interlibrary loans allow your librarian to request a copy of an article from a library that carries that particular medical journal. Your library may charge a fee for this service.

Articles published in medical journals can be technical, but they may be the most current source of information on medical topics.

Medical and Health Directories

You may find many useful medical and health information directories at your library. Ask your librarian about the following resources:*

- *Directory of Physicians in the United States.* Chicago, IL: American Medical Association (AMA). Updated yearly. Provides information such as address, medical school attended, year of license, specialty, and certifications for physicians who are members of the AMA.

- *Health Hotlines.* A booklet of toll-free numbers of health information hotlines available from the National Library of Medicine (NLM) or on the internet at http://healthhotlines.nlm.nih.gov/.

- *Medical and Health Information Directory.* Detroit, MI: Gale Research. Updated yearly. Includes publications, organizations, libraries, and health services (three volumes).

- The *Official ABMS Directory of Board Certified Medical Specialists*. New Providence, NJ: Marquis Who's Who. Updated yearly. Provides information on physicians certified in various specialties by the American Board of Medical Specialists.

- Rees, A., editor. *The Consumer Health Information Sourcebook*. *7th edition*. Phoenix, AZ: Oryx Press, 2003. Lists information clearinghouses, books, and other resources.

- White, B.J., and Madone, E., editors. *The Self-Help Sourcebook: The Comprehensive Reference of Self-Help Group Resources*. *7th edition*. American Self-Help Group Clearinghouse, 2003. Lists over 1,000 organizations that offer support groups.

*Names of resources and organizations included in this chapter are provided as examples only, and their inclusion does not mean that they are endorsed by the National Institutes of Health or any other Government agency. Also, if a particular resource or organization is not mentioned, this does not mean or imply that it is unsatisfactory.

MedlinePlus.gov also has a number of directories available freely to search for health facilities, health providers, and services at: http://www.nlm.nih.gov/medlineplus/directories.html.

If you find a particularly useful book at the library, you can buy a copy at your local bookstore. If the book isn't in stock, your bookstore can probably order a copy for you.

Some medical references have been converted from book form to a CD-ROM or disk for use on a personal computer. If you have a computer with a CD-ROM drive, color monitor, and sound card, you can use compact disks to locate medical information. Check with your local bookstore or computer store for software programs that contain health information. Many other medical references or databases are available online through the internet.

Take Advantage of Services Provided by the Federal Government and Other Organizations

The federal government as well as many medical societies and nonprofit health organizations are also good sources of information.

The federal government operates a number of clearinghouses and information centers. Services vary but may include publications, referrals, and answers to consumer inquiries. To obtain a free list of federal information clearinghouses contact:

National Health Information Center
P.O. Box 1133
Washington, DC 20013-1133
Toll-Free: 800-336-4797
Phone: 301-984-4167
Fax: 301-984-4256
Website: http://www.health.gov/nhic
E-mail: nhicinfo@health.org

Many voluntary health organizations are devoted to specific diseases or conditions (for example, the Scleroderma Foundation, National Alopecia Areata Foundation, National Psoriasis Foundation, Arthritis Foundation, Lupus Foundation of America). Other organizations, such as the American Association of Retired Persons, serve a particular population group and provide information on a variety of topics, including health-related ones.

Many of these organizations offer referrals, publications, newsletters, educational programs, and local support groups. Your doctor may be able to tell you about support groups in your community as well.

Look for a Medical Library

Medical libraries can usually be found at medical, nursing, and dental schools; large medical centers; and community hospitals. Not all hospital or academic libraries are open to the public, but a librarian at your community library may be able to give you information about the closest medical library open to the public. Medical libraries may also be listed in your telephone book under hospitals, schools, or universities. In addition, you can call the National Network of Libraries of Medicine (http://nnlm.gov) of the National Library of Medicine (NLM), National Institutes of Health (NIH), at 800-338-7657 to find the location of the nearest medical library open to the public.

A medical library has a large collection of resources, including many medical and nursing textbooks and a comprehensive collection of medical and health-related journals. Although you may not be allowed to check out materials, most libraries have photocopiers you can use to copy material you want to take home.

Investigate Other Options for Finding Information

People who are unable to get to a community or medical library have several options for finding additional medical information. Some community libraries provide access to online databases that can be searched from a home computer via a modem. In addition, your doctor, nurse, pharmacist, dietitian, or the patient education department at your local hospital may be able to provide you with pamphlets, brochures, and journal articles or direct you to classes, seminars, and health screenings.

Use Telephone and Fax Services

Some communities have a telephone medical service that allows callers to listen to audiotapes on certain disease topics. Also, your health insurance company or health maintenance organization may have a nurse available to answer health-related questions over the telephone.

If you have access to a fax machine, you can get health information from some organizations in just a few minutes. If a faxback system is available, use the telephone on your fax machine to call the faxback number of the organization and listen to the instructions. In most cases, you can request a list or menu of information to be sent to you first.

The Centers for Disease Control and Prevention at 888-232-3299 (toll-free) is an example of an organization that has information available by fax. Your librarian can help you locate other fax services.

Explore Computer Databases

The computer has become an important tool for helping people locate medical and health information quickly and easily. Most software and information services are user friendly and allow people with no formal training in computer searching to use databases to obtain information. Using a computer at home or in the library, you can find health information by searching CD-ROM databases, searching online on the internet, or using a health-related software program.

As mentioned earlier, many public libraries have Infotrac, a database that includes consumer health information. It indexes popular magazines and newspapers and 2–4 years of medical publications. Medical libraries have more extensive medical databases. Just ask your librarian to help you find the most appropriate CD-ROM or online databases for your needs. Many medical databases can also be accessed from your own home or work computer or wherever you have internet access.

Some Major Databases Worth Searching

- MEDLINE®/PubMed®. This database contains citations and often abstracts for over 15 million articles in over 4,800 biomedical journals on all aspects of biomedicine and allied health fields. Online at http://pubmed.gov, it now covers the literature from 1951 to the present and is available free of charge through the NLM website at http://www.nlm.nih.gov. Some free full-text articles are available through publishers and PubMed Central™ at http://pubmedcentral.nih.gov.

- DIRLINE®. This database contains location and description information about a wide variety of resources, including organizations, research resources, projects, databases, and electronic bulletin boards concerned with health and biomedicine. The database is available online through the NLM at no fee at http://dirline.nlm .nih.gov.

Search the Internet

The internet is a worldwide network of computers that can exchange information almost instantaneously. The worldwide web (abbreviated www in computer addresses), or more simply, the web, is a system of electronic documents linked together and available on the internet for anyone with a computer, a modem, and an internet provider account. While the terms internet and worldwide web are often used interchangeably, the web is actually the part of the internet that supports the use of graphics, pictures, sound, and even video.

In addition to the aforementioned databases, you can find a wealth of information on the web—everything from the latest medical research to facts about particular conditions. The internet also offers other resources such as bulletin boards, online publications, forums for discussion of current medical issues, and online support groups.

Help with Searching on the Internet

Searching for health information on the internet can be confusing and difficult. The sheer volume of information can be overwhelming, and people often find it difficult to narrow down search topics or find specific websites. Although an internet search engine such as Google® or YAHOO!® is meant to help you find information, search results on specific topics often reveal thousands of websites, many of which may be unrelated to the information you want. You may want to get a copy of a reference book that provides tips on how to find health information on the internet.

Some Health Resources to Check Out on the WWW

- National Institute of Arthritis and Musculoskeletal and Skin Diseases at http://www.niams.nih.gov

- National Institutes of Health at http://www.nih.gov

- Combined Health Information Database at http://chid.nih.gov

- MedlinePlus® at http://medlineplus.gov

- healthfinder® at http://www.healthfinder.gov

- National Library of Medicine at http://www.nlm.nih.gov

- Agency for Healthcare Research and Quality at http://www.ahrq.gov

- Arthritis Foundation at http://www.arthritis.org

- American Academy of Dermatology at http://www.aad.org

Don't Believe Everything You Read

As you make purchases for your home library or search the internet, keep in mind that not all information is written by qualified medical experts. Your doctor or a health organization may be able to recommend some good books or helpful internet sites. When looking for health information on the internet, don't believe everything you see. Articles published in peer-reviewed medical journals are checked for accuracy, but anyone can put information on the internet, so there's no guarantee that the information you find is accurate or up-to-date. In addition, many companies set up websites primarily to sell their products. It may be helpful to ask a health professional about the information you find on the internet, particularly before you buy any products. If you search and shop with care, you can add some medically sound reference materials to your home library and find accurate information on the internet.

Use Information Wisely

It can be hard to judge the accuracy and credibility of medical information you read in books or magazines, see on television, or find on the internet. Even people with medical backgrounds sometimes find this task challenging. The following are some important tips to help you decide what information is believable and accurate.

Books, Articles, and Television Reports

- Compare several different resources on the same topic. Check two or three other articles or books to see whether the information or advice is similar.

- Check the author's credentials by looking up his or her affiliations, such as university and medical school attended, associations, and lists of other publications. For doctors, this information can be found in one of the physician directories at your library or on the American Medical Association's (AMA) website at http://www .ama-assn.org (click on AMA Physician Select). You can also call the American Board of Medical Specialists at 866-275-2267 to see whether a physician is board certified in his or her specialty. Your librarian can help you find other resources to check the credentials of non-physicians.

- Ask yourself if the information or advice rings true. That is, is it feasible, plausible, and common sense, or is it wishful thinking or sensationalism?

- Look for a list of references at the end of the article or book. Information that is backed up by other medical professionals and researchers is more likely to be accurate.

- Check out your information source. Was the article published in a peer-reviewed journal? Look for a list of editorial or review board members at the beginning of a journal. In a peer-reviewed journal, articles are reviewed by other qualified members of the profession for accuracy and reliability.

- Look very carefully at information published in newspapers and magazines or reported on television. Most reporters are journalists rather than medical experts. In addition, newspapers and television reporters may use sensationalism to attract more readers or viewers. Medical facts and statistics can be misrepresented or incomplete. Check to see whether the newspaper or magazine cites a source for its information and includes the credentials of the persons cited.

- Examine a magazine's list of editors. Do medical experts serve as editors and review articles? Be especially wary of personal testimonials of miracle cures. There's often no way of judging whether the story is true. Furthermore, don't trust medical product advertisements claiming miracle cures or spectacular results.

The Internet

- Compare the information you find on the internet with other resources. Check two or three articles in the medical literature or medical textbooks to see whether the information or advice is similar.

- Check the author's or organization's credentials. They should be clearly displayed on the website. If the credentials are missing, consider this a red flag. Unfortunately, there are many so-called doctors and other health professionals making false claims on the internet.

- Find out if the website is maintained by a reputable health organization. Remember that no one regulates information on the internet. Anyone can set up a home page and claim anything. Some reliable websites providing health information include those of government agencies, health foundations and associations, and medical colleges. In general, sites ending in ".gov" (government), ".edu" (education) and ".org" (organization) are more likely to provide more reputable medical information than those ending in ".com" (commercial; that is, a site designed to sell a product or products).

- Be wary of websites advertising and selling products that claim to improve your health. More important, be very careful about giving out credit card information on the internet. Further, even if nothing is being sold on a website, ask yourself if the site host has an interest in promoting a particular product or service.

- Ask yourself whether the information or advice seems to contradict what you've learned from your doctor. If so, talk to your doctor to clarify the differences in the information.

- Be cautious when using information found on bulletin boards or during chat sessions with others. Testimonials and personal stories are based on one person's experience rather than on objective facts or proven medical research.

To Make Informed Decisions about Your Health Care, You Need to Understand Your Health Problem

Medical information, especially material written for health care providers, can be hard to understand, confusing, and sometimes frightening. As you read through your materials, write down any words or information you don't understand or find confusing. Make a list of your questions and concerns. During your next office visit, ask your doctor, nurse, or other health professional to review the information with you so that you understand clearly how it might be helpful to you.

If the medical information you gathered is for a personal health problem, you may want to share what you found with your spouse, other family members, or a close friend. Family members and friends who understand your health problem are better able to provide needed support and care. Finally, you might want to consider joining a support group in your community. You may find it helpful to be able to talk with others who have the same health problem and share your feelings or concerns.

Ultimately, the information you gather from print and electronic resources can help you approach issues about your health care: how to prevent illness, maintain optimal health, and address your specific health problems. Armed with this knowledge, you can more actively work in partnership with your doctor and other health care professionals to explore treatment options and make health care decisions. Health care experts predict that today's computer and telecommunication systems will result in a new era—the health care system information age—built around health-savvy, health-responsible consumers who are the primary managers of their own health and medical care.

Chapter 21

Consumer e-Health Tools Offer Solutions but Pose Problems, Too

The economic pressures of ever-increasing health care costs and suboptimal health outcomes are driving the search for new approaches to health management. Policy makers and the President now speak of the National Health Information Network and interoperable electronic health records as important and necessary instruments of health care for the entire population. The President has also called for universal, affordable access to broadband technology.

Consumer-controlled electronic health records, or personal health records, are an element, likely a cornerstone, of evolving personal health record systems. These emerging systems signify the growing momentum of the consumer e-health phenomenon, in which consumer engagement, decision making, and tools come together to support and enhance health. The internet, in particular, facilitates the spread of consumer e-health and has become a popular public channel for finding health and health care information and communicating with peers and health experts.

The idea behind much of the current policy interest in e-health is what is commonly called personal health management. This term is used by an increasing number of organizations and policy documents to describe individuals' responsibility for their own health. Although many, if not most, consumers already do much of their own coordination to cope with a fragmented health care system, the underlying

Excerpts from "Expanding the Reach and Impact of Consumer e-Health Tools," U.S. Department of Health and Human Services (HHS), January 2007.

assumption of personal health management is that individuals both want and will have to take even more responsibility for and control of their own health and health care.

The concept of personal health management refers to individuals' orientation toward their health, information, and health care services as well as their capacity to engage in tasks that require ongoing attention. Personal health management implies that everyone has at least some capacity, no matter how limited, that can be applied to decisions and actions about health. For example, highly activated, capable consumers would regularly seek out health information, maintain or cultivate a healthy lifestyle, participate in shared decision making with providers, monitor health conditions, maintain personal health records, and compare health care cost and quality. Less activated persons might perform these tasks less frequently, less systematically, or with less precision; or they might ask someone else to do it on their behalf.

Electronic Tools

Electronic tools offer many consumers a broad range of integrated, interactive functions to enable personal health management. For those consumers who are least able to cope with the volume of health information, decisions, and care coordination, these tools—if designed and disseminated appropriately—could potentially ease the burden. The functions include the following:

- **Health information:** Virtually all e-health tools provide access to health information, either a spectrum of searchable information or more narrowly defined content. Providing information is the main or sole purpose of some tools.

- **Behavior change and prevention:** Some e-health tools are designed to support a specific behavior change, such as stopping smoking or binge drinking, starting regular exercise, or getting a mammogram. Most prevention-related tools are developed through research with defined target audiences under controlled conditions.

- **Health self-management:** Consumers use health self-management tools to achieve and maintain healthy behavior in various lifestyle areas such as diet and fitness. Some are marketed online directly to consumers; others are distributed by employers, health plans, and insurance companies.

174

- **Online communities:** Internet-based communities facilitate interaction around common health concerns among consumers, patients, or informal caregivers. Many online communities have multiple capabilities—not only providing social support, but also exchanging health information and facilitating decision-making. Many disease management tools and some with other functions offer users an online community option.

- **Decision support:** The tools in this category provide structured support to consumers. Some tools support treatment decisions, such as weighing the tradeoffs between different cancer treatments. Demand management tools help consumers choose and evaluate insurance programs or health care providers. Managing health care benefits is a related e-health tool function. Demand and benefits management tools are growing in prominence as a function of prevailing consumer-driven strategies, such as health savings accounts.

- **Disease management:** These tools provide monitoring, record keeping, and communication devices to help consumers manage a specific disease, such as diabetes or cancer, typically in close interaction with health care providers.

- **Health care tools:** These e-health tools facilitate interaction between patients and clinical professionals and health care organizations. Some tools may be free-standing, such as personal health records (PHR) provided by a non-health care entity, or they may be available to patients or members, who have considerable control over their use. The most common forms of health care tools are PHR, patient portals, and secure doctor-patient e-mail. PHR and portals are a gateway to many other e-health functions and may become the way that most Americans are introduced to e-health tools.

Most e-health tools support several of the listed functions, generally structured around a primary purpose such as disease management. The linking of functions makes it possible, for example, for Medicare enrollees who log on to the Beneficiary Portal not only to view their claims history but also to search the National Library of Medicine's MedlinePlus for information on a health condition or to use a search engine to find a commercial e-health product to help with smoking cessation. Migrant farm workers who keep family health records online with the MiVIA program could also use that service to e-mail the doctor, download nutritional information, or participate in a Spanish-language online community.

e-Health Tools' Potential

Today, more and more decision makers are interested in e-health tools as critical components of personal health management and health care reform strategies. Decision makers are seeking viable approaches to reduce health care costs, improve the quality of care, and increase consumers' ability to manage their own health. Conditions are favorable for a greater investment in consumer-oriented e-health tools. The technology marketplace is dynamic; the public is increasingly turning to information and communication technologies for a better life; health care organizations are adopting and offering health information technology; and government policy is placing great emphasis on both health information technology and personal health management for consumers. Such activities are now part of everyday news.

E-health practices have the potential to be part of the solution to health disparities and other health policy challenges if appropriate and useful e-health resources are made available to a larger proportion of the U.S. population than is now the case. So far, market forces and fragmented public-sector efforts have failed to harness technological innovation to improve population health. Some observers worry that an uneven distribution of high-quality e-health tools or consumers' varying ability to use such tools could worsen health disparities. Extending the benefits of these technologies to diverse users requires public leadership, robust public-private partnerships, and consumer-centric research, analysis, and strategies.

Chapter 22

Evaluating Internet Health Information

The growing popularity of the internet has made it easier and faster to find health information. Much of this information is valuable; however, the internet also allows rapid and widespread distribution of false and misleading information. It is important for people to carefully consider the source of information and to discuss the information they find with their health care provider. This chapter can help people decide whether the health information they find on the internet or receive via e-mail from a website is likely to be reliable.

Who runs the website?

Any website should make it easy for people to learn who is responsible for the site and its information. On the National Cancer Institute's (NCI) website, for example, the NCI is clearly noted on every major page, along with a link to the site's home page.

Who pays for the website?

It costs money to run a website. The source of a website's funding should be clearly stated or readily apparent. For example, internet addresses ending in ".gov" are federal government-sponsored sites,

---

The chapter includes text from "How to Evaluate Health Information on the Internet: Questions and Answers," National Cancer Institute (NCI), September 1, 2005; and excerpts from "Finding Reliable Health Information Online," National Human Genome Research Institute, October 3, 2007.

".edu" indicates educational institutions, ".org" is often used by non-commercial organizations, and ".com" denotes commercial organizations. The source of funding can affect what content is presented, how the content is presented, and what the owners want to accomplish on the site.

What is the purpose of the website?

The purpose of the website is related to who runs and pays for it. Many websites have a link to information about the site. The link, which is often called "About This Site," should clearly state the purpose of the site and help users evaluate the trustworthiness of the information on the site.

What is the original source of the information on the website?

Many health and medical websites post information collected from other websites or sources. If the person or organization in charge of the site did not write the material, the original source should be clearly identified.

How is the information on the website documented?

In addition to identifying the original source of the material, the site should identify the evidence on which the material is based. Medical facts and figures should have references (such as citations of articles in medical journals). Also, opinions or advice should be clearly set apart from information that is "evidence-based" (that is, based on research results).

How is information reviewed before it is posted on the website?

Health-related websites should give information about the medical credentials of the people who prepare or review the material on the website. For example, the NCI's website contains cancer information summaries from the Institute's PDQ® database. All PDQ cancer information summaries are peer-reviewed and updated regularly by six editorial boards of cancer specialists in adult treatment, pediatric (childhood) treatment, supportive care, screening and prevention, genetics, and complementary and alternative medicine. The editorial boards review current literature from more than 70 biomedical journals, then evaluate its relevance, and synthesize it to write the PDQ summaries.

How current is the information on the website?

Websites should be reviewed and updated on a regular basis. It is particularly important that medical information be current, and that the most recent update or review date be clearly posted. Even if the information has not changed, it is helpful to know that the site owners have reviewed it recently to ensure that the information is still valid.

How does the website choose links to other sites?

Reliable websites usually have a policy about how they establish links to other sites. Some medical websites take a conservative approach and do not link to any other sites; some link to any site that asks or pays for a link; others link only to sites that have met certain criteria.

What information about users does the website collect and why?

Websites routinely track the path users take through their sites to determine what pages are being used. However, many health-related websites ask the user to subscribe or become a member. In some cases, this may be done so they can collect a user fee or select relevant information for the user. In all cases, the subscription or membership will allow personal information about the user to be collected by the website owners.

Any website asking users for personal information should explain exactly what the site will and will not do with the information. Many commercial sites sell aggregate data about their users to other companies—information such as what percent of their users are women with breast cancer. In some cases, they may collect and reuse information that is personally identifiable, such as the user's zip code, gender, and birth date. Users should be certain they read and understand any privacy policy or similar language on the site, and not sign up for anything they do not fully understand.

How does the website manage interactions with users?

There should always be a way for users to contact the website owners with problems, feedback, and questions. If the site hosts a chat room or other online discussion areas, it should tell users about the terms of using the service. Is the service moderated, and if so, by whom, and why? It is always a good idea to spend time reading the discussion without joining in, to feel comfortable with the environment before becoming a participant.

How can people verify the accuracy of information they receive via e-mail?

Any e-mail messages should be carefully evaluated. The origin of the message and its purpose should be considered. Some companies or organizations use e-mail to advertise products or attract people to their websites. The accuracy of health information may be influenced by the desire to promote a product or service.

How does the federal government protect consumers from false or misleading health claims posted on the internet?

The Federal Trade Commission (FTC) enforces consumer protection laws. As part of its mission, the FTC investigates complaints about false or misleading health claims posted on the internet. The Food and Drug Administration (FDA) regulates drugs and medical devices to ensure that they are safe and effective.

Finding Reliable Health Information Online

As internet users quickly discover, an enormous amount of health information is available online. Finding accurate and reliable information among the millions of online sources is a difficult task for almost everyone. These tips may help you perform searches more easily.

Reviewing Scientific and Medical Literature

Information on just about any disease can be obtained from the published scientific literature. Medical and scientific journals publish articles written for scientists and health professionals. In a process called peer-review, other professionals review these articles before they are published.

Several types of articles can be found in scientific literature:

- **Review articles:** These articles present what is known to date about a disease. Such articles may focus on the cause, diagnosis, treatment or other aspects of a disease.

- **Basic science or laboratory research:** These articles present original basic science or laboratory research.

- **Case reports:** These articles describe and discuss the clinical aspects of an individual with a disease. Such articles may also present unusual or unexpected cases.

- **Articles discussing treatment:** These articles discuss the effects in humans of various treatments that have been tested or used in a specific disease. Articles that discuss treatment may be about many different types of studies that are conducted in humans. Some of the more common studies include clinical trials, case-control studies, cohort studies and case reports.

Treatment articles in published scientific literature report human studies with negative outcomes as well as those with positive outcomes. In other words, some articles report studies where a treatment was deemed to have beneficial effects, while others report studies where a treatment was not deemed to have beneficial effects and/or may have been associated with side effects, some of which could be severe.

Some studies report on the safety of a particular treatment, and do not directly address whether the treatment was actually deemed to have had a beneficial effect. The treatment discussed may be already in use, or it may be experimental and not widely available (or not available at all).

Interpreting the results of studies and weighing the evidence can be a very complex task. Because of this complexity, and because of the technical nature of these articles, we strongly recommend that you discuss with your physician any articles that interest you.

Internet Resources

- Genetics information from Gene Tests/Gene Clinics is available at http://www.geneclinics.org. It has comprehensive information on genetic testing and genetic counseling.

- MEDLINEplus at http://www.nlm.nih.gov/medlineplus is a service of the National Library of Medicine (NLM) and the National Institutes of Health (NIH). It offers high-quality information on more than 600 diseases and conditions; a series of documents and links on evaluating health information; and information about the source and currency of online resources.

Online Medical Dictionaries and Encyclopedias

Complex medical terminology can be difficult to understand. The internet provides some excellent resources to aid in our understanding of these terms and medical jargon.

- University of Newcastle-Upon-Tyne's (U.K.) Online Medical Dictionary of the CancerWEB project at http://cancerweb.ncl.ac.uk/omd contains more than 46,000 definitions.

- MEDLINEplus Medical Encyclopedia at http://www.nlm.nih.gov/medlineplus/encyclopedia.html offers the A.D.A.M. (Animated Dissection of Anatomy for Medicine) illustrated health encyclopedia which contains more than 4,000 articles on conditions, treatments, and much more.

National Institutes of Health (NIH) Resources

- PubMed available at http://www.ncbi.nlm.nih.gov/sites/entrez?db=PubMed is NIH's searchable database of published scientific and medical literature. PubMed contains citations from 4,600 journals from the United States and 70 other countries. More than 12 million citations are available in MEDLINE, one component of PubMed. Information for locating an article, its title, authors and when it was published is listed in PubMed search results. Using the condition name as your search term should locate articles that may be of interest to you. PubMed searches provide citations on journal articles. Citations may include links to article summaries, or links to full articles. For copies of full articles, you can contact a medical or university library, your local library for interlibrary loan, or order them online.

- National Network of Libraries of Medicine (NNLM) at http://nnlm.gov/members is designed to help you find health information from libraries in your area.

- LinkOut at http://www.ncbi.nlm.nih.gov/projects/linkout provides access to full-text articles at journal websites and other related internet resources.

- ClinicalTrials.gov at http://www.clinicaltrials.gov was developed by NIH and the Food and Drug Administration (FDA) to provide patients, family members, and members of the public with current information about clinical research studies and clinical trials that are enrolling individuals. From the home page, you can enter terms such as condition names, study locations (cities or states), and descriptive terms for patients (such as adult or adolescent). After performing a search, there is a list of search results. Click on a study to review the study's eligibility criteria to determine if you or someone else would qualify. To learn more about the study, refer to the study's contact information. Be sure to check ClinicalTrials.gov often for updates to study information.

- Computer Retrieval of Information on Scientific Projects (CRISP) at http://crisp.cit.nih.gov is NIH's searchable database of federally funded biomedical research projects conducted at universities, hospitals, and other research institutions. CRISP includes projects funded by NIH, the Substance Abuse and Mental Health Services Administration (SAMHSA), the Health Resources and Services Administration (HRSA), the Food and Drug Administration (FDA), the Centers for Disease Control and Prevention (CDC), the Agency for Healthcare Research and Quality (AHRQ), and the Office of the Assistant Secretary of Health (OASH), all government agencies. To search CRISP for studies on a specific disease or condition, enter the condition name in the "Enter Search Terms" box and click the "and" button below the box. Then click "Submit Query." Using other search field boxes, you can narrow your search by looking for information from specific years and states.

- Online Mendelian Inheritance in Man (OMIM) at http://www.ncbi.nlm.nih.gov/sites/entrez?db=OMIM is an electronic catalog of human genes and genetic disorders. The website was developed by the National Center for Biotechnology Information (NCBI), and contains text and reference information. Although the language is technical, OMIM is considered to be a very comprehensive source of information. Based on the complex information found in OMIM, you may benefit from discussing its contents with a medical professional. As with PubMed, you can search OMIM using terms and setting search limits.

- The National Human Genome Research Institute (NHGRI) at http://www.genome.gov, and the Office of Rare Diseases (ORD) at http://rarediseases.info.nih.gov are websites that provide helpful information on genetic and rare diseases research and conditions, patient support groups, and much more. Both websites provide general information about clinical trials.

- Genetics Home Reference at http://ghr.nlm.nih.gov is the National Library of Medicine's website for consumer information about genetic conditions and the genes responsible for those conditions. It offers summaries on more than 70 diseases and more than 50 genes.

Other Sources of Information

Other organizations are dedicated to helping individuals with genetic and rare diseases and provide an array of information.

- The Genetic Alliance at http://www.geneticalliance.org is a broad-based coalition that partners to promote healthy lives for all those living with genetic conditions. It offers information on genetic conditions and issues related to genetic conditions.

- The National Organization for Rare Disorders (NORD) at http://www.rarediseases.org is a federation of not-for-profit voluntary health organizations serving people with rare disorders. You can search their site or obtain a printed report for a specific disorder.

Additional Information

Federal Trade Commission (FTC)
Consumer Response Center
600 Pennsylvania Ave., N.W.
Washington, DC 20580
Toll-Free: 877-382-4357, Toll-Free TTY: 866-653-4261
Website: http://www.ftc.gov

National Institutes of Health (NIH)
9000 Rockville Pike
Bethesda, MD 20892
Phone: 301-496-4000, TTY: 301-402-9612
Website: http://www.nih.gov
E-mail: NIHinfo@od.nih.gov

U.S. Food and Drug Administration (FDA)
Office of Consumer Affairs
5600 Fishers Lane, HFE-50
Rockville, MD 20857
Toll-Free: 888-463-6332, Phone: 301-827-4420, Fax: 301-443-9767
Website: http://www.fda.gov

Chapter 23

Understanding Medical Research Studies: What Do Those Headlines Really Mean?

Lately it seems to happen almost every day—you hear about a new result of medical research on television or read about it in the paper. Often it's about your risk or chance of having a disease or health problem. After reading the story did you worry because the numbers made your chance of getting sick seem high? Or, did the story confuse you because you remember a news item not too long ago about the same health problem, but with a very different finding? What does it all mean?

Which stories can you trust?

The first step in understanding medical research reports is to know the difference between types of research studies. Some projects involve laboratory studies using microscopic cells or creatures such as yeasts, viruses, or bacteria. Some of these studies may not immediately seem relevant to humans, but very often studying other organisms helps us to understand our own bodies and what can go wrong with them to cause diseases and disorders. Some studies involve animals like mice which can serve as a model system for how the human body works. Investigators looking at human diseases, though, eventually need to turn to studies in people.

When studying people, scientists often use observational studies. In these, researchers keep track of a group of people for several years

Excerpted from "Understanding Risk: What Do Those Headlines Really Mean?" by Karin Kolsky, *Word on Health,* National Institutes of Health (NIH), April 2004.

without trying to change their lives or provide special treatment. This can help scientists find out who develops a disease, what those people have in common, and how they differ from the group that did not get sick. What they learn can suggest a path for more research. However, observational studies have certain weaknesses. Sometimes differences between groups are caused by something the investigators are not aware of. Only further research can prove for sure whether their finding is the actual cause of illness or not.

A randomized controlled clinical trial (RCT) is considered the best way to learn whether a certain treatment works or not. A clinical trial can involve thousands of human volunteers. They are assigned to two or more study groups by chance (randomly). One of the groups, the control group, receives a preparation such as a pill that looks just like the treatment or drug being tested, but actually does nothing (a placebo). This is the only way to really compare and see if the treatment is effective.

Clinical trials are usually conducted in phases. The trials at each phase have a different purpose and help scientists answer different questions: In Phase I trials, researchers test a new drug or treatment in a small group of people (usually 20–80) for the first time to evaluate its safety, determine a safe dosage range, and identify possible side effects. In Phase II trials, the study drug or treatment is given to a larger group of people (often 100–300) to see if it is effective and to further evaluate its safety. In Phase III trials, the study drug or treatment is given to even larger groups of people to confirm its effectiveness, monitor side effects, compare it to commonly used treatments, and collect information that will allow the drug or treatment to be used safely. In Phase IV trials, post-marketing studies gather additional information about the drug's risks, benefits, and optimal use.

A clinical trial, especially a larger one, sometimes yields different results than earlier studies in laboratories, in animals, or even in people. But, the clinical trial results will be more meaningful to you because the research involved people and because of the way these studies are designed.

Understanding Scientific Results

How do you understand the results you read in a news story? Different types of numbers can be used to explain the same facts, and the way these numbers are presented can change how you feel about the results. For example, let's say you heard that only one percent of people in the U.S. had a disease. You might not think that was very much until you realize that that's almost three million people. When you hear numbers like these, it's important to try to put them in context to understand how important they really are.

When investigators report their findings, especially from large clinical trials, they often talk about risk. They might mention relative risk, absolute risk, or both. These are different ways to explain how likely someone is to have a certain health problem. Relative risk is usually shown as a ratio or a percent. An absolute risk is nothing more than a number found by subtraction. How these numbers are presented to you can sway how you feel about the finding and affect whether you change your behavior.

Consider an imaginary new drug. After testing this fictitious drug in a large clinical trial, the investigators learn that the relative risk of getting a certain side effect from the medicine is 2.0, which means the risk is increased by 100%. It does sound serious. But that doesn't mean that all of the people using the drug will have that side effect. It means that twice as many people on the drug get the symptom as those not taking the drug (news reports often phrase it this way, too). So, if six people out of every 10,000 normally have a symptom in one year, then twelve people out of 10,000 using the medicine might have it. The absolute risk of this side effect is twelve minus six, or six more people out of every 10,000 using the medicine. Many people who really need a new medicine might not consider six in 10,000 a large enough risk to prevent them from taking it, even if the side effect is quite serious.

It is important to be critical when reading or listening to reports of new medical findings. The next time you read or hear about a medical study in the news, ask yourself questions to see how important the finding may be to you. If you're not sure, turn to your health care provider for help.

A Word to the Wise—Ask Yourself

When you learn about a new medical finding, ask yourself:

- Was it a study in the laboratory, in animals, or in people? The results of research in people are more likely to be meaningful for you.

- Does the study include enough people like you? You should check to see if the people in the study were the same age, sex, education level, income group, and ethnic background as yourself and had the same health concerns.

- Was it a randomized controlled clinical trial involving thousands of people? They are the most expensive to do, but they also give scientists the most reliable results.

- Where was the research done? Scientists at a medical school or large hospital, for example, might be better equipped to conduct complex experiments or have more experience with the topic. Many large clinical trials involve several institutions, but the results may be reported by one coordinating group.

- Are the results presented in an easy-to-understand way? They should use absolute risk, relative risk, or some other easy-to-understand number.

- If a new treatment was being tested, were there side effects? Sometimes the side effects are almost as serious as the disease. Or, they could mean that the drug could worsen a different health problem.

- Who paid for the research? Do those providing support stand to gain financially from positive or negative results? Sometimes the federal government or a large foundation contributes funding towards research costs. This means they looked at the plans for the project and decided it was worthy of funding, but they will not make money as a result. If a drug is being tested, the study might be partly or fully paid for by the company that will make and sell the drug.

- Who is reporting the results? Is the newspaper, magazine, or radio or television station a reliable source of medical news? Some large publications and broadcast stations have special science reporters on staff who are trained to interpret medical findings. You might want to talk to your health care provider to help you judge how correct the reports are.

The bottom line is: Talk to your doctor. He or she can help you understand the results and what they could mean for your health. Remember that progress in medical research takes many years. The results of one study often need to be duplicated by other scientists at different locations before they are accepted as general medical practice. Every step along the research path provides a clue to the final answer-and probably sparks some new questions also.

Chapter 24

Creating a Personal Health Record

Why Should You Have a Personal Health Record (PHR)?

All individuals should be able to readily access, understand, and use their personal health information. Your health information is scattered across many different providers and facilities. Keeping your own complete, updated, and easily accessible health record means you can play a more active role in your health care. You wouldn't write checks without keeping a check register. The same level of responsibility makes sense for your health care.

Your own personal health record (PHR) offers a different perspective, showing all your health-related information. It can include any information that you think affects your health, including information that your doctor may not have, such as your exercise routines, dietary habits, or glucose levels if you are diabetic.

In a medical emergency, quick access to your health information is vital so that you can receive the best possible care. If you are in an accident, the emergency responder needs three things: quick access to your medical information, the delivery of that information by trained professionals, and accurate, up-to-date information. Most people think that an emergency room can obtain their medical information, but almost none can.

Also, the PHR is a critical tool that enables you to partner with your providers. It can reduce or eliminate duplicate procedures or processes, which saves health care dollars, your time, and the provider's time.

And the PHR empowers you, the patient. The information you gather gives you knowledge that assists your preparation for appointments. Overall, it gives you more intimate knowledge of your health information, including an active role in preventive care and care management. This way, you are more involved in your own care.

The American Health Information Management Association demonstrated its advocacy for the empowerment of individuals to manage their healthcare by issuing a joint Position Statement for Consumers of Health Care on the Value of Personal Health Records with the American Medical Informatics Association in February 2007.

Step-by-Step Guide to Creating a PHR

To start your personal health record, you will need to request a copy of your health records from all your health care providers, including your general practitioner, plus your eye doctor, dentist, and any other specialist you have seen.

Don't feel that you must gather all your health information at once. If you like, the next time you visit the doctor, simply ask for recent records, and do so each time you visit a health care provider.

Following are steps for creating a complete personal health record (PHR), but feel free to create your PHR at your own pace.

Step 1: Contact your doctors' offices or the health information management (HIM) or medical records staff at each facility where you received treatment. Find out if your provider has his or her own plan for helping patients to create PHR. Ask if your records are in an electronic format that you can access yourself, or if you need to request copies. Also, ask your physician or the HIM professional to help you determine which parts of your record you need. If you want medical records kept by your health plan, contact the plan's customer service department.

Step 2: Ask for an "authorization for the release of information" form. Complete the form and return it to the facility as directed. Most facilities do charge for copies. The fee can only include the cost of copying (including supplies and labor), as well as postage if you request the copy to be mailed. It can take up to 60 days to receive your medical records, so ask when you can expect to receive the information you requested.

Step 3: Once you've gathered the information you are seeking, there are a few different ways you can maintain your PHR. To get started, you can simply gather your information in a file folder. Since not all information may be available to you in an electronic format, an old-fashioned file folder or three-ring binder may be the easiest and most inclusive format for now. You can divide the binder into sections by family members. Then within each family member's section, divide information by year or illness.

Step 4: There are many great PHR tools and services to help you get organized. You can transfer electronic information to a computer disk and carry that with you. Also, portable devices are available that allow you to carry information on a memory chip inside something called a key chain universal serial bus (USB) drive, which plugs into most computers. Then there are internet-based services you can access from your home computer where you can store and retrieve your health information. Some services can even help you collect the information you need from your doctors and other health care providers.

Some PHR tools are available free of charge and others are products you purchase or pay a subscription fee to use. You need to research PHR options and decide which method is best for you.

Step 5: Bring your PHR to all visits so you have the information with you and to remember to keep adding and updating it with entries from providers, yourself, or your family members.

Step 6: Create and carry a card that has vital information on it—such as medication needs or allergies—with you at all times. You won't always have your PHR with you.

Step 7: Remember, this is your private information, so protect it and maintain confidentiality. Let trusted family members know that you are compiling it, and where you keep it, but beyond that, keep it safe and protected.

Information for Caregivers

If you are a caregiver for someone else, don't assume you automatically have rights to that person's information, even if you are an immediate family member. Parents take note: Even dependent children under the age of 18 have special rights in certain circumstances.

To access another adult's information:

- Have the person you are caring for submit written authorization to his or her doctors and health care facilities.

- In that authorization, the patient should include language that gives permission to release all information regarding treatment and care to you, and anyone else the patient wants to have access.

- This document might also include the names of people the information should not be shared with. An example might be a domestic abuse case where the wife would request that a husband not have access to any information.

- Then you'll need to give this authorization to the health care facility's Health Information Management Department.

In cases of lengthy or permanent incapacity, a legal guardian for the patient may be appointed through court proceedings. In that case, the legal guardian can access the patient's health records and decide who else can see them.

When incapacity is anticipated, a person may grant power of attorney to another person. Power of attorney is the legally recognized authority to act and make decisions on behalf of another party. This authorizes the designee to act on behalf of the person who is now incapacitated. The person with power of attorney is often responsible for making decisions regarding the disclosure of health information to others.

But, there are different types of power of attorney. Some grant very broad powers to the holder; others are limited to specific issues, such as consenting to health care. Be sure you and your loved one understand what sort of power of attorney will serve you both best.

Different Ways to Keep Your PHR

Individuals are encouraged to begin tracking their health information in whatever format works best for them, even if the choice is paper. We recommend that individuals use an electronic media to facilitate a timely, accurate, and secure exchange of information across health care institutions and providers. PHR information should always be stored in a secure manner just as you would store other confidential personal information such as financial information.

Once you've gathered the information you're seeking, there are a few different ways you can maintain your PHR:

- You can simply gather your information in a file folder.

- You can transfer the information to a computer disk and carry that with you.

- Portable devices are available that allow you to carry the information on a chip inside something called a USB drive that plugs into most computers.

- Internet-based services offer secure servers that you access from a computer and on which you enter your information. Some of these are free, and for others you may have to pay a fee or subscription.

Your doctor may use electronic health records, and have what's called a web portal or patient gateway that allows you to view and track some of your health information on the internet. You may also be able to e-mail your doctor, schedule appointments, or get a prescription refilled. This is a great start to giving you access to your information, but it is not your complete personal health record. You'll still need to be proactive to collect all the information you need.

Evolving Conceptions of Personal Health Records

This is a time of lively experimentation in which there are many models of personal health records (PHR). Two broad types of PHR are evolving in the private and public sectors, distinguished primarily by their relationship to electronic health records (EHR). One is a patient-facing extension of clinician-controlled EHR; the other is not routinely linked to the patient's EHR.

Large health care organizations such as Kaiser-Permanente, Intermountain Health Care and Geisinger are driving much of the momentum in PHR development by developing models in the first category. These PHR give enrollees a view of their EHR along with other functions that facilitate administrative tasks (for example, appointments and medication refills), health and disease self-management (exercise or blood pressure records), communication with physicians, and access to health information resources. Among a sampling of larger early rollouts of PHR of this kind, it is roughly estimated that some 15 percent of the target population in these organizations typically register to use PHR.

Free-standing PHR products are offered by several dozen companies (for example, Cap-Med, WebMD). In general, there is greater variety among these products, which typically are made available to consumers through a third-party sponsor such as a health plan, employer, or disease management program. By definition, the PHR in this group do not derive from EHR, although some are designed to link to users' EHR through voluntary participation by their health care providers.

It is possible that these two types of PHR will converge over time, if producers of free-standing PHR products find a sustainable path toward greater connectivity with providers. One approach would be to make PHR that are used primarily in a free-standing mode capable of interfacing to provider EHR that use common data standards.

No uniform understanding yet exists about what threshold a personal e-health tool must cross to be called a PHR, or about the boundary between the PHR and the many functions it enables. Another source of confusion is the lack of a clear dividing line between the EHR and the PHR. Opinions also vary as to whether the PHR consists only of the health record—an index or document—or encompasses a set of interactive functions and activities that might be called a personal health system (a term some in the field prefer). These functions can help consumers and family caregivers manage health across a continuum that includes staying healthy, managing illness, and handling transitions such as the end of life. This discussion uses the term "personal health record" to connote both the record and health management functions.

Opinions and practice also vary with respect to interoperability. While there is no question that many forms of interoperability are critical in the long run, people hold differing views about whether interoperability is a necessary precondition for moving ahead meaningfully with PHR, and also about what in particular needs to be interoperable. Data in the PHR come primarily from consumers themselves and (at least for professionally-sourced PHR) from their clinicians or industry sources such as payers and pharmacies. Although the ideal PHR would encompass clinical data from all providers across a person's lifetime, today's reality falls considerably short of this ideal. To make matters more complicated, many data sources besides EHR are being considered, including claims data from payers and prescription data from pharmacies or pharmacy benefit managers. In the absence of a common framework for exchange of patient data into PHR, each data source represents interoperability challenges as well as significant issues about privacy and business models.

Additional Information

American Health Information Management Association (AHIMA)
233 N. Michigan Ave., 21st Floor
Chicago, IL 60601-5800
Phone: 312-233-1100
Fax: 312-233-1090
Website: http://www.myphr.com
E-mail: info@ahima.org

AHIMA does not make, sell, or endorse any PHR products, but has compiled a list of PHR tools and services. You need to research your PHR options and decide which method is best for you. Access this information at: http://www.myphr.com/resources/phr_search.asp.

Chapter 25

Patient Rights and Responsibilities

What to Expect during Your Hospital Stay

Understanding Expectations, Rights, and Responsibilities

When you need hospital care, your doctor and the nurses and other professionals at the hospital are committed to working with you and your family to meet your health care needs. The dedicated doctors and staff serve the community in all its ethnic, religious, and economic diversity. The goal is for you and your family to have the same care and attention they would want for their families and themselves.

The sections explain some of the basics about how you can expect to be treated during your hospital stay. They also cover what will be needed from you to care for you better. If you have questions at any time, please ask them. Unasked or unanswered questions can add to the stress of being in the hospital. Your comfort and confidence in your care are very important.

High Quality Hospital Care

The hospital staff's first priority is to provide you the care you need, when you need it, with skill, compassion, and respect. Tell your caregivers if you have concerns about your care or if you have pain. You

---

"The Patient Care Partnership," reprinted with permission of the American Hospital Association, copyright © 2003.

have the right to know the identity of doctors, nurses, and others involved in your care, and you have the right to know when they are students, residents, or other trainees.

A Clean and Safe Environment.

The hospital works hard to keep you safe. They use special policies and procedures to avoid mistakes in your care and keep you free from abuse or neglect. If anything unexpected and significant happens during your hospital stay, you will be told what happened, and any resulting changes in your care will be discussed with you.

Involvement in Your Care

You and your doctor often make decisions about your care before you go to the hospital. Other times, especially in emergencies, those decisions are made during your hospital stay. When decision-making takes place, it should include:

Discussing your medical condition and information about medically appropriate treatment choices: To make informed decisions with your doctor, you need to understand:

- the benefits and risks of each treatment;
- whether your treatment is experimental or part of a research study;
- what you can reasonably expect from your treatment and any long-term effects it might have on your quality of life;
- what you and your family will need to do after you leave the hospital; and
- the financial consequences of using uncovered services or out-of-network providers.

Please tell your caregivers if you need more information about treatment choices.

Discussing your treatment plan: When you enter the hospital, you sign a general consent to treatment. In some cases, such as surgery or experimental treatment, you may be asked to confirm in writing that you understand what is planned and agree to it. This process protects your right to consent to or refuse a treatment. Your doctor will explain the medical consequences of refusing recommended treatment. It also protects your right to decide if you want to participate in a research study.

Getting information from you: Your caregivers need complete and correct information about your health and coverage so that they can make good decisions about your care. That includes:

- past illnesses, surgeries or hospital stays;

- past allergic reactions;

- any medicines or dietary supplements (such as vitamins and herbs) that you are taking; and

- any network or admission requirements under your health plan.

Understanding your health care goals and values: You may have health care goals and values or spiritual beliefs that are important to your well-being. They will be taken into account as much as possible throughout your hospital stay. Make sure your doctor, your family, and your care team know your wishes.

Understanding who should make decisions when you cannot: If you have signed a health care power of attorney stating who should speak for you if you become unable to make health care decisions for yourself, or a living will or advance directive that states your wishes about end-of-life care, give copies to your doctor, your family and your care team. If you or your family need help making difficult decisions, counselors, chaplains, and others are available to help.

Protection of Your Privacy

The staff respect the confidentiality of your relationship with your doctor and other caregivers, and the sensitive information about your health and health care that are part of that relationship. State and federal laws and hospital operating policies protect the privacy of your medical information. You will receive a Notice of Privacy Practices that describes the ways that they use, disclose, and safeguard patient information and that explains how you can obtain a copy of information from hospital records about your care.

Preparing You and Your Family for when You Leave the Hospital

Your doctor works with hospital staff and professionals in your community. You and your family also play an important role in your care. The success of your treatment often depends on your efforts to follow medication, diet, and therapy plans. Your family may need to help care for you at home. You can expect staff to help you identify sources of follow-up care and to let you know if the hospital has a financial interest in any referrals. As long as you agree that they can share information about your care with them, staff will coordinate their activities with your caregivers outside the hospital. You can also expect to receive information and, where possible, training about the self-care you will need when you go home.

Help with Your Bill and Filing Insurance Claims

The staff will file claims for you with health care insurers or other programs such as Medicare and Medicaid. They also will help your doctor with needed documentation. Hospital bills and insurance coverage are often confusing. If you have questions about your bill, contact the business office. If you need help understanding your insurance coverage or health plan, start with your insurance company or health benefits manager. If you do not have health coverage, staff will try to help you and your family find financial help or make other arrangements. They need your help with collecting needed information and other requirements to obtain coverage or assistance.

While you are at the hospital, you will receive more detailed notices about some of the rights you have as a hospital patient and how to exercise them. Hospitals are always interested in improving.

Chapter 26

Patient Rights to Health Information Privacy

Common Privacy Myths

With the new federal laws protecting the privacy of your health information, there has been much confusion and misinformation. Here are the truths to some of these common myths:

- **Health information cannot be faxed—False.** Your information may be shared between health care providers by faxing the information. But, the organizations that send and receive your information by fax must have security policies regarding faxing.

- **E-mail cannot be used to transmit health information— False.** E-mail can be used to transmit information, as long as organizations have a means of protecting the electronic health information, such as encryption and decryption which protect the information from unwanted access or tampering.

- **Health care providers cannot leave messages for patients on answering machines or with someone who answers the telephone—False.** As long as the patient has given the okay for someone else to receive a message, and as long as the answering machine has an outgoing message that gives the person's name or number for verification, a message may be left. Your provider will determine what the message may include, but a message can be left.

- **Your name and location while in the hospital may not be given out without your consent—False.** You must specifically ask not to be listed in a hospital's directory if you do not want it known that you are a patient there.

- **Your health care provider must have your approval to disclose your personal health information to another health care provider—False.** Your provider can share your health information with another provider if there is a reason to believe you will receive care there.

- **Your doctor cannot discuss your care with your family members—False.** The Privacy Rule permits health care providers to share information that is directly relevant to the involvement of a spouse, family members, friends, or other persons identified by you regarding your care or payment for health care. Your provider may also share relevant information with your family or other persons if it can reasonably infer, based on professional judgment that you do not object.

Your Health Information Privacy Rights

Privacy Is Important to All of Us

You have privacy rights under a federal law that protects your health information. These rights are important for you to know. You can exercise these rights, ask questions about them, and file a complaint if you think your rights are being denied or your health information isn't being protected.

This law must be followed by:

- most doctors, nurses, pharmacies, hospitals, clinics, nursing homes, and many other health care providers;

- health insurance companies, health maintenance organizations (HMO), most employer group health plans; and

- certain government programs that pay for health care, such as Medicare and Medicaid.

The notice you receive should also make clear other health information rights you may have under your state's laws when these laws affect how your health information can be used or shared.

Your Privacy Rights

Providers and health insurers who are required to follow this law must comply with your right to:

Ask to see and get a copy of your health records. You can ask to see and get a copy of your medical record and other health information. You may not be able to get all of your information in a few special cases. For example, if your doctor decides something in your file might endanger you or someone else, the doctor may not have to give this information to you.

- In most cases, your copies must be given to you within 30 days, but this can be extended for another 30 days if you are given a reason.

- You may have to pay for the cost of copying and mailing if you request copies and mailing.

Have corrections added to your health information. You can ask to change any wrong information in your file or add information to your file if it is incomplete. For example, if you and your hospital agree that your file has the wrong result for a test, the hospital must change it. Even if the hospital believes the test result is correct, you still have the right to have your disagreement noted in your file.

- In most cases the file should be changed within 60 days, but the hospital can take an extra 30 days if you are given a reason.

Receive a notice that tells you how your health information is used and shared. You can learn how your health information is used and shared by your provider or health insurer. They must give you a notice that tells you how they may use and share your health information and how you can exercise your rights. In most cases, you should get this notice on your first visit to a provider or in the mail from your health insurer, and you can ask for a copy at any time.

Decide whether to give your permission before your information can be used or shared for certain purposes. In general, your health information cannot be given to your employer, used or shared for things like sales calls or advertising, or used or shared for many other purposes unless you give your permission by signing an authorization form. This authorization form must tell you who will get your information and for what your information will be used.

Get a report on when and why your health information was shared. Under the law, your health information may be used and shared for particular reasons, like making sure doctors give good care, making sure nursing homes are clean and safe, reporting when the flu is in your area, or making required reports to the police, such as reporting gunshot wounds. In many cases, you can ask for and get a list of who your health information has been shared with for these reasons.

- You can get this report for free once a year.

- In most cases you should get the report within 60 days, but it can take an extra 30 days if you are given a reason.

Ask to be reached somewhere other than home. You can make reasonable requests to be contacted at different places or in a different way. For example, you can have the nurse call you at your office instead of your home, or send mail to you in an envelope instead of on a postcard. If sending information to you at home might put you in danger, your health insurer must talk, call, or write to you where you ask and in the way you ask, if the request is reasonable.

Ask that your information not be shared. You can ask your provider or health insurer not to share your health information with certain people, groups, or companies. For example, if you go to a clinic, you could ask the doctor not to share your medical record with other doctors or nurses in the clinic. However, they do not have to agree to do what you ask.

File complaints. If you believe your information was used or shared in a way that is not allowed under the privacy law, or if you were not able to exercise your rights, you can file a complaint with your provider or health insurer. The privacy notice you receive from them will tell you who to talk to and how to file a complaint. You can also file a complaint with the U.S. government.

How to File a Health Information Privacy Complaint with the Office for Civil Rights

If you believe that a person, agency, or organization covered under the Health Insurance Portability and Accountability Act (HIPAA) Privacy Rule (a covered entity) violated your own or someone else's health information privacy rights or committed another violation of the Privacy Rule, you may file a complaint with the Office for Civil Rights (OCR). OCR has authority to receive and investigate complaints against covered entities related to the Privacy Rule. A covered entity is a health plan, health care clearinghouse, and any health care provider who conducts certain health care transactions electronically.

Complaints to the Office for Civil Rights must: (1) Be filed in writing, either on paper or electronically; (2) name the entity that is the subject of the complaint and describe the acts or omissions believed to be in violation of the applicable requirements of the Privacy Rule; and (3) be filed within 180 days of when you knew that the act or omission complained of occurred. OCR may extend the 180-day period if you can show good cause. Any alleged violation must have occurred on or after April 14, 2003 (on or after April 14, 2004 for small health plans) for OCR to have authority to investigate.

Anyone can file written complaints with OCR by mail, fax, or e-mail. If you need help filing a complaint or have a question about the complaint form, please call this OCR toll-free number: 800-368-1019. OCR has ten regional offices, and each regional office covers certain states. You should send your complaint to the appropriate OCR regional office, based on the region where the alleged violation took place. Use the OCR regions list at the end of this chapter. Complaints should be sent to the attention off the appropriate OCR regional manager.

You can submit your complaint in any written format. The OCR Health Information Privacy Complaint Form is available on the OCR website or at an OCR regional office. If you prefer, you may submit a written complaint in your own format. Be sure to include the following information in your written complaint:

- Begin with your name, full address, home and work telephone numbers, and e-mail address.

- If you are filing a complaint on someone's behalf, also provide the name of the person on whose behalf you are filing.

- Include the name, full address, and phone of the person, agency, or organization you believe violated your (or someone else's) health information privacy rights or committed another violation of the Privacy Rule.

- Briefly describe what happened. How, why, and when you believe your (or someone else's) health information privacy rights were violated, or the Privacy Rule otherwise was violated?

- Add any other relevant information.

- Remember to sign your name and date your letter.

The following information is optional:

- Do you need special accommodations for OCR to communicate with you about this complaint?

- If OCR cannot reach you directly, is there someone else they can contact to help them reach you?

- Have you filed your complaint somewhere else?

The Privacy Rule, developed under authority of the Health Insurance Portability and Accountability Act of 1996 (HIPAA), prohibits the alleged violating party from taking retaliatory action against anyone for filing a complaint with the Office for Civil Rights. You should notify OCR immediately in the event of any retaliatory action.

To File a Privacy Rule Complaint

Office for Civil Rights (OCR)
Toll-Free: 866-627-7748
Website: http://www.hhs.gov/ocr/hipaa
E-mail: OCRComplaint@hhs.gov

This toll-free number (866-627-7748) will connect you to the OCR regional office of the area code from which you are calling.

Region I—CT, ME, MA, NH, RI, VT
Office for Civil Rights
U.S. Department of Health and Human Services
JFK Federal Bldg., Rm. 1875
Boston, MA 02203
Phone: 617-565-1340
TDD: 617-565-1343
Fax: 617-565-3809

Region II—NJ, NY, PR, VI
Office for Civil Rights
U.S. Department of Health and Human Services
26 Federal Plaza, Suite 3312
New York, NY 10278
Phone: 212-264-3313
TDD: 212-264-2355
Fax: 212-264-3039

Region III—DE, DC, MD, PA, VA, WV
Office for Civil Rights
U.S. Department of Health and Human Services
150 S. Independence Mall W., Suite 372
Philadelphia, PA 19106-3499
Phone: 215-861-4441
TDD: 215-861-4440
Fax: 215-861-4431

Region IV—AL, FL, GA, KY, MS, NC, SC, TN
Office for Civil Rights
U.S. Department of Health and Human Services
61 Forsyth St., S.W., Suite 3B70
Atlanta, GA 30323
Phone: 404-562-7886
TDD: 404-331-2867
Fax: 404-562-7881

Region V—IL, IN, MI, MN, OH, WI
Office for Civil Rights
U.S. Department of Health and Human Services
233 N. Michigan Ave., Suite 240
Chicago, IL 60601
Phone: 312-886-2359
TDD: 312-353-5693
Fax: 312-886-1807

Region VI—AR, LA, NM, OK, TX
Office for Civil Rights
U.S. Department of Health and Human Services
1301 Young St., Suite 1169
Dallas, TX 75202
Phone: 214-767-4056

TDD: 214-767-8940
Fax: 214-767-0432

Region VII—IA, KS, MO, NE
Office for Civil Rights
U.S. Department of Health and Human Services
601 East 12th St., Rm. 248
Kansas City, MO 64106
Phone: 816-426-7277
TDD: 816-426-7065
Fax: 816-426-3686

Region VIII—CO, MT, ND, SD, UT, WY
Office for Civil Rights
U.S. Department of Health and Human Services
1961 Stout St., Rm. 1426
Denver, CO 80294
Phone: 303-844-2024
TDD: 303-844-3439
Fax: 303-844-2025

Region IX—AZ, CA, HI, NV, AS, GU, The U.S. Affiliated Pacific Island Jurisdictions
Office for Civil Rights
U.S. Department of Health and Human Services
90 7th St., Suite 4-100
San Francisco, CA 94103
Phone: 415-437-8310
TDD: 415-437-8311
Fax: 415-437-8329

Region X—AK, ID, OR, WA
Office for Civil Rights
U.S. Department of Health and Human Services
2201 6th Ave., Mail Stop RX-11
Seattle, WA 98121
Phone: 206-615-2290
TDD: 206-615-2296
Fax: 206-615-2297

Chapter 27

Informed Consent

Many people think informed consent is just the formality of signing a written consent form before a medical procedure, but it is much more than that. Informed consent involves ongoing communication with your doctor so that you can make a fully informed decision on your treatment. This process is meant to protect you as the patient, and to make sure that you have been given adequate information and understand your options. For your doctor, informed consent is both an ethical obligation and legal requirement.

You may be given material to read or videos to watch about a procedure, but talking with your doctor is the most important component of informed consent. You should not hesitate to bring up any questions or concerns you have.

Before Giving Consent

For all non-emergency medical procedures, whether a preventive health screening in your doctor's office or a major surgery in the hospital, you should not give consent until you have a full understanding of what procedure is being done and why.

Before signing a consent form, you should have answers to the following questions:

"Giving Informed Consent," *Journal of Patient Safety*, Volume 1, Issue 3, p. 177, September 2005. © Lippincott Williams and Wilkins, Inc. Reprinted with permission.

- How is the procedure done?

- What are the reasons for having this treatment?

- What are the benefits of having this treatment?

- What complications may occur (and the likelihood of these happening)?

- What might happen if I do not have this treatment?

- Are there alternative options?

- Is this treatment part of a study or is it considered experimental?

- What kind of care will be necessary after the procedure?

Communicating with Your Doctor about Consent

Good communication between you and your doctor takes a team effort. You should tell your doctor and other members of your health care team (nurses, technicians, physical therapists) if they use words that you do not know. Your doctor should spend whatever time is necessary to answer your questions.

If you have discussed a treatment in the doctor's office, but have additional questions once you are home, you should follow up with a phone call or appointment.

If you do not feel comfortable with your doctor, you can seek another opinion from someone who may be better able to explain the risks and benefits of the procedure you are agreeing to undertake.

If your questions have not been answered when you sign the form, it may be consent, but it is not informed consent.

Remember that informed consent is an ongoing process. At any point before, during, or after your treatment, you shouldn't hesitate to ask questions. After all, you are asking questions about a procedure that is being done to you. A good way to ensure that you understand the information you have been given is to repeat it back to your doctor in your own words.

While no one can ensure the outcome of a treatment before it is performed, your doctor should be able to provide you with good information on what to expect. In partnership with your doctor, you can be an active participant of your care, making informed decisions about your treatments.

Make sure your health team knows about your health, including:

- any allergies you have to medications or materials (such as latex);

- all illnesses and conditions you have, including asthma;

- any herbal preparations or over-the-counter or prescription medications you are taking (this is especially important before surgery); and

- if your condition changes or you experience side effects.

Chapter 28

What Consumers Can Do to Make Health Care Safer

If a medical error occurs, it is often a result of a series of small failures that are individually not big enough to cause an accident, but combined can result in an error. Patients can ensure a safer experience with the health care system by being involved and informed about their treatment. Improving patient safety requires continuous learning and constant communication between caregivers, organizations, and patients. Everyone has a role in patient safety, and everyone will benefit from its successes.

What can consumers do to make sure they have a safer experience with the health care system?

National Patient Safety Foundation (NPSF) suggests these steps to help make your health care experience safer:

Become a more informed health care consumer.

- Seek information about illnesses or conditions that affect you.

- Research options and possible treatment plans.

- Choose a doctor, clinic, pharmacy, and hospital experienced in the type of care you require.

- Ask questions of your doctor, nurse, pharmacist, or benefits plan coordinator.

- Seek more than one opinion.

Keep track of your history.

- Write down your medical history including any medical conditions you have, illnesses, immunizations, allergies, hospitalizations, all medications and dietary supplements you're taking, and any reactions or sensitivities you've experienced.

- Write down the names and phone numbers of your doctors, clinics, and pharmacies, for quick and easy reference.

Work with your doctor and other health care professionals as a team.

- Share your health history with your care team.

- Share up-to-date information about your care with everyone who's treating you.

- Make sure you understand the care and treatment you'll be receiving. Ask questions if you're not clear on your care.

- Pay attention. If something doesn't seem right, call it to the attention of your doctor or health care professional.

- Discuss any concerns about your safety with your health care team.

Involve a family member or friend in your care.

- If you're not able to observe or participate fully in your care, ask a family member or friend to assist. They can accompany you on appointments or stay with you, help you ask questions, understand care instructions, and suggest your preferences.

Follow the treatment plan agreed upon by you and your doctor.

- Be sure you receive all instructions verbally and in writing that you can read and understand. Ask questions about any instructions that are confusing or unclear.

- Take medications exactly as prescribed.

- Use home medical equipment and supplies only as instructed.

- Report anything unusual to your doctor.

For More Information

National Patient Safety Foundation
132 MASS MoCA Way
North Adams, MA 01247
Phone: 413-663-8900
Fax: 413-663-8905
Website: http://www.npsf.org
E-mail: info@npsf.org

Chapter 29

Preventing Medical Errors

A Patient's Role in Reducing Test Errors: A Guide for Patients

Medical tests are a modern wonder. They can identify diseases in their earliest stages when treatment is most effective, allow us to see inside a mother's womb, and tell us where a bone is broken. They can help us determine how our bodies are working and whether or not medical treatment is needed. Simply put, medical tests can help save lives.

Most medical tests involve several steps, including scheduling, collecting a specimen (a blood sample, for example), sending it to the laboratory, interpreting and reporting results, and identifying any additional steps necessary. A breakdown in one of these steps can lead to a testing error. For example: Your doctor orders a stress test for your heart; it's a hectic month and you forget to schedule it. You have a blood test at your doctor's office, but the results are filed in the wrong chart and you never hear back. You go for allergy testing but are unaware that you need to stop taking your allergy medicine prior to the test, so the results are inaccurate.

This chapter includes: "A Patient's Role in Reducing Test Errors: A Guide for Patients," *Journal of Patient Safety*, Volume 1, Issue 1, p. 72, March 2005. © 2005 Lippincott Williams and Wilkins, Inc. Reprinted with permission. And, "20 Tips to Help Prevent Medical Errors," Agency for Healthcare Research and Quality (AHRQ), Publication No. 00-PO38, February 2000. Reviewed in November 2007 by Dr. David A. Cooke, M.D., Diplomate, American Board of Internal Medicine.

Most testing errors are the result of a complex health care system. Communication with your health care team can be a powerful tool. The better the communication, the less chance for errors to occur. Below are quick tips allowing you to take an active role when having medical tests.

When Your Physician Orders a Test

- If you do not understand why a test is being ordered, ask. Don't be afraid to bring up concerns and questions.

- Schedule the test as soon as you can so you don't forget.

- Ask if there are any special preparations you need to make for the test, such as fasting or discontinuing certain medications.

- If your physician has given you written orders for a test, make sure you can read them.

- If you have a choice on the facility at which a test will be done, ask your physician for a recommendation. Choose a facility that has experience in the particular test you are having done.

When You Go In for the Test

- If the test is being done somewhere other than the doctor's office where the test was originally ordered, check with the facility to make sure the ordering physician will receive a copy of the results.

- Make sure that both your physician's office and the facility running the test know of any allergies, and all prescription and over-the-counter medications you are taking, including herbal and vitamin supplements.

- Make sure the testing facility has your name and other identifying information correctly recorded.

- Make sure that the test being performed is the one your physician ordered. If you have any doubts, speak up.

- If the test is one that will be repeated at specific intervals, ask the facility to send you a reminder when you are due for your next test.

After the Test

- Ask how you will receive the test results and when to expect them. If you do not receive the results by the expected date, be proactive and follow up. Do not accept a policy of "no news is good news"—where your doctor only calls if test results are abnormal.

- If you receive test results but do not understand what they mean, call the physician who ordered the test for an explanation. If your physician uses terms you do not understand, ask him or her to explain again using plain language.

- Consider asking for and keeping your own file of test results. It may prevent having duplicate tests done and will give you a personal record.

20 Tips to Help Prevent Medical Errors

Medical errors are one of the nation's leading causes of death and injury. A report by the Institute of Medicine estimates that as many as 44,000 to 98,000 people die in U.S. hospitals each year as the result of medical errors. This means that more people die from medical errors than from motor vehicle accidents, breast cancer, or acquired immune deficiency virus (AIDS).

What Are Medical Errors?

Medical errors happen when something that was planned as a part of medical care doesn't work out, or when the wrong plan was used in the first place. Medical errors can occur anywhere in the health care system, including:

- hospitals,
- clinics,
- outpatient surgery centers,
- doctors' offices,
- nursing homes,
- pharmacies, or at
- patients' homes.

Errors can involve:

- medicines,
- surgery,

- diagnosis,

- equipment, or

- lab reports.

They can happen during even the most routine tasks, such as when a hospital patient on a salt-free diet is given a high-salt meal.

Most errors result from problems created by today's complex health care system. But errors also happen when doctors and their patients have problems communicating. For example, a study supported by the Agency for Healthcare Research and Quality (AHRQ) found that doctors often do not do enough to help their patients make informed decisions. Uninvolved and uninformed patients are less likely to accept the doctor's choice of treatment and less likely to do what they need to do to make the treatment work.

What Can You Do? Be Involved in Your Health Care

1. The single most important way you can help to prevent errors is to be an active member of your health care team. That means taking part in every decision about your health care. Research shows that patients who are more involved with their care tend to get better results. Some specific tips, based on the latest scientific evidence about what works best, follow.

Medicines

2. Make sure that all of your doctors know about everything you are taking. This includes prescription and over-the-counter medicines, and dietary supplements such as vitamins and herbs. At least once a year, bring all of your medicines and supplements with you to your doctor. "Brown bagging" your medicines can help you and your doctor talk about them and find out if there are any problems. It can also help your doctor keep your records up to date, which can help you get better quality care.

3. Make sure your doctor knows about any allergies and adverse reactions you have had to medicines. This can help you avoid getting a medicine that can harm you.

4. When your doctor writes you a prescription, make sure you can read it. If you can't read your doctor's handwriting, your pharmacist might not be able to either.

5. Ask for information about your medicines in terms you can understand—both when your medicines are prescribed and when you receive them.

    - What is the medicine for?

    - How am I supposed to take it, and for how long?

    - What side effects are likely? What do I do if they occur?

    - Is this medicine safe to take with other medicines or dietary supplements I am taking?

    - What food, drink, or activities should I avoid while taking this medicine?

6. When you pick up your medicine from the pharmacy, ask: Is this the medicine that my doctor prescribed? A study by the Massachusetts College of Pharmacy and Allied Health Sciences found that 88 percent of medicine errors involved the wrong drug or the wrong dose.

7. If you have any questions about the directions on your medicine labels, ask. Medicine labels can be hard to understand. For example, ask if "four doses daily" means taking a dose every six hours around the clock or just during regular waking hours.

8. Ask your pharmacist for the best device to measure your liquid medicine. Also, ask questions if you're not sure how to use it. Research shows that many people do not understand the right way to measure liquid medicines. For example, many use household teaspoons which often do not hold a true teaspoon of liquid. Special devices, like marked syringes, help people to measure the right dose. Being told how to use the devices helps even more.

9. Ask for written information about the side effects your medicine could cause. If you know what might happen, you will be better prepared if it does—or, if something unexpected happens instead. That way, you can report the problem right away and get help before it gets worse. A study found that written information about medicines can help patients recognize problem side effects and then give that information to their doctor or pharmacist.

Hospital Stays

10. If you have a choice, choose a hospital at which many patients have the procedure or surgery you need. Research shows that

patients tend to have better results when they are treated in hospitals that have a great deal of experience with their condition.

11. If you are in a hospital, consider asking all health care workers who have direct contact with you whether they have washed their hands. Handwashing is an important way to prevent the spread of infections in hospitals. Yet, it is not done regularly or thoroughly enough. A recent study found that when patients checked whether health care workers washed their hands, the workers washed their hands more often and used more soap.

12. When you are being discharged from the hospital, ask your doctor to explain the treatment plan you will use at home. This includes learning about your medicines and finding out when you can get back to your regular activities. Research shows that at discharge time, doctors think their patients understand more than they really do about what they should or should not do when they return home.

Surgery

13. If you are having surgery, make sure that you, your doctor, and your surgeon all agree and are clear on exactly what will be done. Doing surgery at the wrong site (for example, operating on the left knee instead of the right) is rare. But even once is too often. The good news is that wrong-site surgery is 100 percent preventable. The American Academy of Orthopaedic Surgeons urges its members to sign their initials directly on the site to be operated on before the surgery.

Other Steps You Can Take

14. Speak up if you have questions or concerns. You have a right to question anyone who is involved with your care.

15. Make sure that someone, such as your personal doctor, is in charge of your care. This is especially important if you have many health problems or are in a hospital.

16. Make sure that all health professionals involved in your care have important health information about you. Do not assume that everyone knows everything they need to.

17. Ask a family member or friend to be there with you and to be your advocate (someone who can help get things done and speak up for you if you can't). Even if you think you don't need help now, you might need it later.

18. Know that more is not always better. It is a good idea to find out why a test or treatment is needed and how it can help you. You could be better off without it.

19. If you have a test, don't assume that no news is good news. Ask about the results.

20. Learn about your condition and treatments by asking your doctor and nurse and by using other reliable sources. For example, treatment recommendations based on the latest scientific evidence are available from the National Guidelines Clearinghouse™ at http://www.guideline.gov. Ask your doctor if your treatment is based on the latest evidence.

For More Information

Agency for Healthcare Research and Quality (AHRQ) Publications Clearinghouse
P.O. Box 8547
Silver Spring, MD 20907-8547
Toll-Free: 800-358-9295
Website: http://www.ahrq.gov
E-mail: AHRQPubs@ahrq.hhs.gov

Chapter 30

Health Care Fraud

The Problem of Health Care Fraud: A Serious and Costly Reality for All Americans

Since the early 1990s, health care fraud—for example, the deliberate submittal of false claims to private health insurance plans or tax-funded public health insurance programs such as Medicare and Medicaid—has been viewed as a serious and still-growing nationwide crime phenomenon, linked directly to the nation's ever-growing annual health care outlay, which in calendar-year 2003 alone amounted to $1.7 trillion (Office of the Actuary, Centers for Medicare and Medicaid Services). This represents a growth of 7.7 percent over the prior year.

That Some Health Insurance Claims Are Fraudulent Is beyond Dispute

It is an undisputed reality that some of the more than four billion health insurance benefit transactions processed in the United States every year are fraudulent. Although they constitute only a small fraction, those fraudulent claims carry a very high price tag.

Each year, for example, the Office of Inspector General (OIG) of the U.S. Department of Health and Human Services (HHS) conducts a formal audit of the Medicare program's fee-for-service claim payment system. On February 21, 2002, the HHS-OIG reported its finding that of the $191.8 billion such claims paid in 2001, 6.3 percent—amounting to $12.1 billion—should not have been paid due to erroneous billing or payment, inadequate provider documentation of services to back up the claims, or outright fraud.

In May, 2004, the National Health Care Anti-Fraud Association (NHCAA) reported in its *Anti-Fraud Management Survey* that 52 of its member insurers collectively recovered or prevented payment of $503 million in 2003 as a direct result of their anti-fraud activities— a great deal of money, but barely a measurable fraction of the total estimated loss.

The bottom line: The NHCAA estimates that of the nation's annual health care outlay, at least three percent—or $51 billion in calendar-year 2003—is lost to outright fraud. Other estimates by government and law enforcement agencies place the loss as high as ten percent of our annual expenditure—or $170 billion—each year.

Although the immediate targets and victims of that fraud are private health payers and government-funded health plans, all of us ultimately pay for the crime—through higher health insurance premiums (or fewer benefits) for employers and individuals, higher taxes, and higher insurance co-payments for privately and publicly insured patients.

The Involvement of Organized Criminal Groups

So strong an invitation to some is the country's ever larger pool of health care money that in certain areas—Florida, for example—law enforcement agencies and health insurers have witnessed in recent years the migration of some criminals from illegal drug trafficking into the safer and far more lucrative business of perpetrating fraud schemes against Medicare, Medicaid, and private health insurance companies.

In South Florida alone, government programs and private insurers have lost hundreds of millions of dollars in recent years to criminal rings—some of them based in Central and South America—that fabricate claims from non-existent clinics, using genuine patient-insurance and provider-billing information that the perpetrators have bought or stolen for that purpose. When the bogus claims are paid, the mailing address in most instances belongs to a freight forwarder that bundles up the mail and ships it offshore.

A Federal Crime with Stiff Penalties

In response to these realities, Congress—through the Health Insurance Portability and Accountability Act of 1996 (HIPAA)—specifically established health care fraud as a federal criminal offense, with the basic crime carrying a federal prison term of up to ten years in addition to significant financial penalties. (United States Code, Title 18, Section 1347.)

The federal law also provides that should a perpetrator's fraud result in the injury of a patient, the prison term can double, to twenty years; and, should it result in a patient's death, a perpetrator can be sentenced to life in federal prison.

Congress also mandated the establishment of a nationwide "Coordinated Fraud and Abuse Control Program," to coordinate federal, state, and local law enforcement efforts against health care fraud and to include "the coordination and sharing of data" with private health insurers.

In their capacities as health insurance regulators, many states also have responded vigorously since the early 1990s, not only by strengthening their insurance fraud laws and penalties, but also by requiring health insurers to meet certain standards of fraud detection, investigation and referral as a condition of maintaining their insurance or health maintenance organization (HMO) licenses.

Dishonest Health Care Providers Take the Greatest Toll

Individual patients can, and in some cases do, commit health care fraud—either on their own or in collusion with dishonest health care providers. By far the greatest damage, though, is attributable to fraud committed by dishonest health care providers. This is not because large numbers of physicians and other health care professionals are dishonest. On the contrary, the vast majority are honest and ethical, and they too are victimized both by the dishonest few within their professions and by the increasing number of professional criminal operations that pose as health care providers for purposes of committing fraud.

The few who make up that dishonest minority, however, have all the necessary tools with which to commit ongoing fraud on a very broad scale including:

- the entire population of insured patients to attract and exploit;

- the entire range of potential medical conditions and treatments on which to base false claims; and

- the ability to spread false billings among many insurers simultaneously, increasing their fraud proceeds while lessening their chances of being detected by any one insurer.

The most common types of fraud committed by dishonest providers are:

- billing for services that were never rendered—either by using genuine patient information to fabricate entire claims or by padding claims with charges for procedures or services that did not take place;

- billing for more expensive services or procedures than were actually provided or performed, commonly known as up-coding—for example, falsely billing for a higher-priced treatment than was actually provided (which often requires the accompanying inflation of the patient's diagnosis code to a more serious condition consistent with the false procedure code);

- performing medically unnecessary services solely for the purpose of generating insurance payments—seen very often in nerve-conduction and other diagnostic-testing schemes (recently, the Rent-a-Patient schemes in Southern California have resulted in clinics performing unnecessary, and sometime harmful, surgeries on patients who have been recruited, and paid, to have these unnecessary surgeries performed); and

- misrepresenting non-covered treatments as medically necessary covered treatments for purposes of obtaining insurance payments—widely seen in cosmetic surgery schemes, in which non-covered cosmetic procedures such as nose jobs, tummy tucks, liposuction, or breast augmentations, for example, are billed to patients' insurers as deviated-septum repairs, hernia repairs, or lumpectomies.

The illicit proceeds of such schemes typically amount to very significant sums of money. In cases involving individual dishonest providers, it is not uncommon to see schemes in which the thefts have ranged from a few hundred thousand dollars to several million dollars in a relatively short period—that is two, three, or four years—prior to their detection.

In November, 2001, for example, an Arlington, Texas chiropractor was sentenced to five years in prison after pleading guilty to masterminding a broad-based scheme responsible for submitting $5.7 million in false claims—of which $3.2 million were paid—to a variety of health insurers over a five-year period. (In the same scheme, one physician was convicted, two more submitted guilty pleas, and two former physicians were indicted.)

In institutional cases, involving such perpetrators as hospital chains, national laboratory companies, transportation, pharmaceutical and medical equipment companies, the totals in various federal criminal and civil fraud cases of recent years have ranged from tens of millions to hundreds of millions of dollars. Several recent high-profile fraud cases involving hospital chains and pharmaceutical companies, for example, have resulted in criminal or civil settlements ranging from $600 million to $850 million.

Fraud's Impact Goes Far beyond Financial Loss

Health care fraud features the theft of very large amounts of money. However, the damage it does goes well beyond financial losses. More important is its inherent exploitation of individuals and their insurance information as the basis for falsified claims.

Falsification of Patients' Diagnoses or Treatment Histories

By its nature, one cannot commit health care fraud without falsifying something about a patient's medical condition or treatment history. Thus, fraud perpetrators routinely assign to the patients, whom they exploit, false diagnoses of medical conditions they do not have, or of more severe conditions than they actually have.

Unless and until discovered (perhaps under adverse circumstances) those phony or inflated diagnoses become part of the patient's medical history, at least in the health insurer's records.

A Boston-area psychiatrist, for example, forfeited $1.3 million and was sentenced to several years in federal prison following his late-1990s conviction on 136 counts of mail fraud, money laundering, and witness intimidation related to his fraudulent billing of several health insurers for psychiatric therapy sessions that never took place—using the names and insurance information of many people whom he actually had never met, let alone treated. (He also went so far as to write fictitious longhand session notes to ensure phony backup for his phony claims.)

In fabricating the claims, the psychiatrist also fabricated diagnoses for those "patients"—many of them adolescents. The phony conditions he assigned to them included depressive psychosis, suicidal ideation, sexual identity problems, and behavioral problems in school.

Theft of Patients' Finite Health Insurance Benefits

Privately insured patients typically have lifetime caps or other limits on benefits under their policies. Every time a false claim is paid in a given patient's name, the dollar amount counts toward that patient's lifetime or other limits.

Part of the aforementioned psychiatrist's fraud involved routinely billing for the maximum number of therapy sessions covered by patients' health insurance, even if he had seen them only a handful of times—a fact that some patients discovered only when their claims for treatment by different psychiatrists were denied on the basis that they had already used all of their available benefits.

Physical Risk to Patients

Finally, the perpetrators of some types of fraud schemes (for example, involving medical transportation, surgeries, invasive testing, certain drug therapies) deliberately and callously place their trusting patients at significant physical risk—illustrating vividly why federal law provides for longer potential prison terms in health care fraud cases that result in a patient's injury or death.

In June, 2002, for example, a Chicago cardiologist was sentenced to 12½ years in federal prison and was ordered to pay $16.5 million in fines and restitution after pleading guilty to performing 750 medically unnecessary heart catheterizations, along with unnecessary angioplasties and other tests as part of a ten-year fraud scheme.

Three other physicians and a hospital administrator also pleaded guilty and received prison sentences for their part in the scheme, which resulted in the deaths of at least two patients.

The physicians and hospital induced hundreds of homeless persons, substance abusers, and elderly men and women to feign symptoms and be admitted to the hospital for the unnecessary procedures. How? They did it by offering them such incentives as food, cash, and cigarettes.

"There were 750 people who had needles stuck into their hearts purely for profit, not because they needed it," said one of the federal prosecutors.

At the bottom line, health care fraud is a serious crime that legitimately concerns all parties to our health care system—insurers and premium-payers, government and taxpayers, and patients and health care providers—and it is a costly reality that government and society cannot afford to overlook.

Private-Public Cooperation against Fraud Is Essential

Founded in 1985 by a handful of private insurers and law enforcement personnel, the National Health Care Anti-Fraud Association is a private-public non-profit organization focused solely on improving the private and public sectors' ability to detect, investigate, prosecute, and ultimately, prevent fraud against our private and public health insurance systems.

Today it represents the combined efforts of the anti-fraud units of over 90 private health payers and the entire spectrum of federal and some state law enforcement agencies that have jurisdiction over the crime, along with hundreds of individual members from the private health insurance sector and from federal, state and local law enforcement.

The NHCAA pursues its mission by fostering private-public cooperation against health care fraud at both the case and policy making levels, by facilitating the sharing of investigative information among health insurers and law enforcement agencies and by providing information on health care fraud to all interested parties.

The NHCAA Institute for Health Care Fraud Prevention, a non-profit educational foundation, provides professional education and training to industry and government anti-fraud investigators and other personnel.

What can the public do? How can you help to detect and prevent health care fraud?

Read your benefit and billing statements. If you receive an "Explanation of Benefits" after your health insurance plan has paid a claim on your behalf, or if you receive a bill directly, read it carefully to ensure that you actually received the treatments that were paid for, and report apparent discrepancies to the special investigations unit of your insurance company or its hotline. Many such statements list toll-free numbers that you may call to report suspicious charges.

Beware of free medical treatments. Various community-based service organizations periodically offer perfectly legitimate free screenings of vision, cholesterol, blood pressure, or other basic health indicators. However, other, sometimes heavily advertised offers of free medical treatments (for example, free footcare, dental treatments, chiropractic visits) often are the lure with which fraud perpetrators seek to obtain patient names and insurance information for use in fraudulent billings. Question any free treatment that features no out-of-pocket expense or no deductibles, or for which you are required to provide your health insurance coverage information.

Protect your health insurance information. It pays to treat your health insurance card as you do your credit cards, and never give your health insurance number to telephone or door-to-door solicitors.

Additional Information

National Health Care Anti-Fraud Association
1201 New York Ave., N.W., Suite 1120
Washington, DC 20005
Phone: 202-659-5955
Fax: 202-785-6764
Website: http://www.nhcaa.org
E-mail: nhcaa@nhcaa.org

Part Four

Prescription (Rx) and Over-the-Counter (OTC) Medications

Chapter 31

Understanding Medications and What They Do

Sometimes it seems like there are more medicines than there are diseases. Some medications can be bought over the counter at pharmacies or other stores. Others require a doctor's prescription. A few medicines are available only in hospitals. Medicines can cure, stop, or prevent disease; ease symptoms; or help in the diagnosis of certain illnesses.

What Are Medicines?

Medicines are chemicals or compounds used to prevent or treat diseases and the symptoms you might have as a result of those diseases. During the past century, advances in medications have enabled doctors to cure many diseases and save lives.

These days, medicines come from a variety of sources. Many have been developed from substances found in nature, and even today many are extracted from plants. For example, one medicine that is used to treat cancer comes from the Pacific yew tree.

Some medicines are produced in a laboratory by mixing together a number of chemicals; others, like penicillin, are a byproduct of organisms such as fungus. And a few medicines are even biologically engineered by inserting genes into bacteria that make them produce the desired substance.

This information was provided by TeensHealth, one of the largest resources online for medically reviewed health information written for teens, kids, and parents. For more articles like this one, visit www.TeensHealth.org, or www.KidsHealth .org. © 2006 The Nemours Foundation.

When we think about taking medications, we often think of pills. The truth is there are many ways in which medications can be delivered, such as:

- liquids that are swallowed (like cough syrup);
- drops that are put into ears or eyes;
- creams, gels, or ointments that are rubbed onto the skin;
- inhalers (like nasal sprays or asthma inhalers);
- patches that are stuck to skin (called transdermal patches);
- tablets that are placed under the tongue (called sublingual medicines; the medication is absorbed into blood vessels and enters the bloodstream);
- shots.

No medicine can be sold for use unless it has first been approved by the U.S. Food and Drug Administration (FDA). The manufacturers of the medication perform tests on all new medicines and send the results to the FDA.

The FDA allows new medicines to be used only if they work and if they are safe enough. When a medicine's benefits outweigh its known risks, the FDA usually approves the sale of the drug. The FDA can withdraw a medication from the market at any time if it later is found to cause harmful side effects.

Different Types of Medicines

Medicines act in a variety of ways. Some can cure an illness by killing or halting the spread of invading germs, such as bacteria and viruses. Others are used to treat cancer by killing cells as they divide or preventing them from multiplying. Some drugs simply replace missing substances or correct abnormally low levels of natural body chemicals such as certain hormones or vitamins. Medicines can even affect parts of the nervous system that control a particular body process.

Nearly everyone has taken an antibiotic. This type of medicine fights bacterial infections. Your doctor may prescribe an antibiotic for things like strep throat or an ear infection. These medicines work either by killing bacteria or halting their multiplication so that the body's immune system can fight off the infection.

Sometimes a part of the body can't produce enough of a certain chemical. That can also make you sick. Someone with insulin-dependent diabetes, for instance, has a pancreas that can't produce enough insulin. Some people have a low production of thyroid hormone, which helps control how the body uses energy. In each case, doctors can prescribe medicines to replace the missing chemical.

Some medicines treat symptoms but can't cure the illness that causes the symptoms. (A symptom is anything you feel while you're sick, such as a cough or nausea.) So taking a lozenge may soothe a sore throat, but it won't kill that nasty strep bacteria.

Certain medicines are designed to relieve pain. If you pull a muscle, your doctor might tell you to take ibuprofen or acetaminophen. These analgesics don't get rid of the source of the pain—your muscle will still be pulled. What they do is block the pathways that transmit pain signals from the injured or irritated body part to the brain (in other words, they affect the way the brain reads the pain signal) so that you don't hurt as much.

As people get older, they sometimes develop chronic or long-term conditions. Medicines can help control certain conditions like high blood pressure or high cholesterol. These drugs don't fix the basic problem, but they can help prevent some of the body-damaging effects of the disease or condition over time.

Among the most important medicines are immunizations. These keep people from getting sick in the first place by immunizing, or protecting, the body against certain infectious diseases. Vaccines contain parts or products of infectious organisms or whole germs that have been modified or killed. When a vaccine is given, it primes the body's immune system to fight off infection by that germ.

Most immunizations that prevent you from catching diseases like measles, whooping cough, and chickenpox are given by injection. No one thinks shots are fun. But when your friends get the flu and you don't, thanks to your flu shot, that injection isn't so bad.

Although some medications require a prescription, some are available in stores. For example, many medications for pain, fever, cough, or allergies can be purchased without a prescription. But just because a medicine is available over-the-counter (OTC), that doesn't mean it's free of side effects. Take over-the-counter medicines with the same caution as those that are prescribed by your doctor.

Taking Medicines

No matter what type of medicine your doctor prescribes, it's always important to be safe and follow some basic rules:

- If you feel worse after taking a medicine, tell your doctor right away.

- Double-check that you have the right medicine. If you get the same prescription filled more than once, check that it's the same shape, size, and color as the last time. If not, be sure to ask the pharmacist about it.

- Read the label and follow directions. Ask if you have questions.

- Take medicines as prescribed. If the instructions say take one tablet four times a day, don't take two tablets twice a day. It's not the same.

- Ask if the medicine is likely to affect everyday tasks such as driving or concentrating in school.

- Don't take more medication than is recommended. It won't make you heal faster or feel better quicker. In fact, an overdose of medication can make you sick.

- Always follow your doctor's or pharmacist's instructions. For instance, he or she may tell you to take a medicine with food to help lessen the stomach upset it may cause or take the medicine on an empty stomach so as not to interfere with the medicine's absorption into your body.

- Never share prescription medicine with anyone else, even if that person has the same thing as you do. Today's medications are very complex, and the dosages tend to be precisely prescribed for each person's needs. Either under-dosing or overdosing can be harmful. Additionally, someone else's body may react differently to the same medication—for example, if they have an allergy to one of the components of the medication.

- If you're already taking a medication but also want to take something you can buy over-the-counter, ask the pharmacist. There could be a bad interaction between the medications.

- Remember that drinking alcohol can dramatically worsen the side effects of many medications.

- Always tell your doctor and pharmacist if you're taking any other medicines or any herbal supplements so that he or she can check for any interactions between the medications.

- Even if you get sick with what you think is the same old thing, don't decide on your own that you know what's wrong and take some leftover medicine. Taking that medicine for a different disease may not work—and it can even be harmful. Talk to your doctor first.

- Take antibiotics for the full time prescribed, even if you start to be feel better, so that all the germs are killed and the infection doesn't bounce back.

- Keep medicines in their original labeled containers, if possible.

- Don't use medicine that has expired, especially prescription medicine.

- Medicines should not be stored in your bathroom because heat and humidity can affect the potency of the drug. Most medicines should be kept at room temperature and away from sunlight. Some must be refrigerated. Check with your pharmacist or doctor if you aren't sure.

- Make sure all medicines are stored safely and out of the reach of younger brothers or sisters and pets.

- If you have any allergies, tell your doctor and pharmacist before they start you on a new medicine.

- If you get a rash, start itching, or have trouble breathing after starting a medication, tell your parents or doctor immediately. Breathing difficulty, breaking out in hives, or suddenly developing swelling of the tongue, lips, face, or other body parts may be signs of a severe allergic reaction—get emergency medical care right away.

Taking medicines may feel like a hassle sometimes. But medicines are the most effective treatments available for many illnesses. If you ever have any questions about what a medicine does or how you should take it, talk with your doctor or the pharmacist.

Chapter 32

Medicines and Your Body

Taking Medicines

Medicines can enter the body in many different ways. As drugs make their way through the body, many steps happen along the way. Understanding how medicines work in your body can help you learn why it is important to use medicines safely and effectively.

Drugs in the Body

Drugs are absorbed into the body when they travel from their point of entry into the blood. When you take medicines by mouth, they move through the digestive tract to the liver, the place where the body processes chemicals. When you take medicines in other ways—getting a shot, using an inhaler, or applying a skin patch, for instance—the medicine bypasses the liver and enters the bloodstream directly or through the skin or lungs. The bloodstream carries medicines throughout the body in a process called distribution. Drugs often interact with many body organs. Side effects can occur if a drug has an effect in an organ other than its target organ.

After a medicine has done its job in the body, the drug is broken down through a process called metabolism. Drug metabolism is the

This chapter includes text from "Taking Medicines: Medicines and Your Body," National Institute of General Medical Sciences (NIGMS), reviewed March 2007; and "Understanding a Drug's Journey Through the Body Fact Sheet," NIGMS, updated July 14, 2007.

chemical alteration of a medicine by the body. Often, when a drug is broken down (or chemically altered by the body), it produces products called metabolites. These metabolites are not usually as strong as the original drug, but sometimes they can have effects that are stronger than the original drug. Because most metabolites are broken down in the liver, scientists refer to the liver as a detoxifying organ. As such, the liver can be prone to damage caused by too much medicine in the body. Once the liver is finished working on a medicine, the now-inactive drug enters the excretion stage and exits the body in the urine or feces. Age-related changes in kidney function can have significant effects on how fast a drug is eliminated from the body.

Side Effects

While everyone needs to be careful when taking a medicine, older adults frequently take more than one medication at a time, and anyone taking several medications at the same time should be extra careful. Also, as the body ages its ability to absorb foods and drugs changes. As people age, the body's ability to break down substances can decrease, so that older people may not be able to metabolize drugs as well as they once did. Thus, older people sometimes need smaller doses of medicine per pound of body weight than young or middle-aged adults do.

All medicines have risks as well as benefits. The benefits of medicines are the helpful effects you get when you take them, such as curing infection or relieving pain. The risks are the chances that something unwanted or unexpected will happen when you use medicines. Unwanted or unexpected symptoms or feelings that occur when you take medicine are called side effects.

Side effects can be relatively minor, such as a headache or a dry mouth. They can also be life-threatening, such as severe bleeding or irreversible damage to the liver or kidneys. Stomach upset, including diarrhea or constipation, is a side effect common to many medications. Often, this side effect can be lessened by taking the drug with meals. Always check with your doctor, nurse, or pharmacist to see if you should take a particular medication with food.

Here are some more tips to help you avoid side effects:

- Always inform your doctor or pharmacist about all medicines you are already taking, including herbal products and over-the-counter medications.

- Tell your doctor, nurse, or pharmacist about past problems you have had with medicines, such as rashes, indigestion, dizziness, or not feeling hungry.

Avoid Side Effects

- Ask whether the drug may interact with any foods or other over-the-counter drugs or supplements you are taking.

- Read the prescription label on the container carefully and follow directions. Make sure you understand when to take the medicine and how much to take each time.

- If you experience side effects, write them down so you can report them to your doctor accurately.

- Call your doctor right away if you have any problems with your medicines or if you are worried that the medicine might be doing more harm than good. He or she may be able to change your medicine to another one that will work just as well.

- Don't mix alcohol and medicine unless your doctor or pharmacist says it's okay. Some medicines may not work well or may make you sick if taken with alcohol.

You should always be sure to tell your doctor and pharmacist about any and all medications that you take every day or even once in a while. Unwanted effects can occur when a drug interacts, or interferes with, another drug or with certain foods. These chemical interactions change the way your body handles one or both medicines. In some cases, the overall effect of an interaction is greater than desired. Combining aspirin with blood-thinning drugs such as Coumadin® (also called warfarin) can cause serious bleeding. Mixing Viagra® (also called sildenafil) and the heart drug nitroglycerin can cause blood pressure to plunge to dangerously low levels.

A single glass of grapefruit juice can raise the level of some medications in the blood. This can occur with several types of drugs commonly used to treat heart conditions. Years ago, scientists discovered this grapefruit juice effect by luck, after giving volunteers grapefruit juice to mask the taste of a medicine. Nearly a decade later, researchers figured out that grapefruit juice blunts the effects of an enzyme that breaks down drugs. This leads to higher levels of medicine remaining in the blood, which can cause health problems. Be sure to ask your doctor or pharmacist if it is safe to consume foods or beverages that contain grapefruit with the medication you are taking.

Mixing drugs also can cause effects that are less than what is desired. For example, calcium-rich dairy products or certain antacids can prevent antibiotics from being properly absorbed into the bloodstream. Ginkgo biloba can reduce the effectiveness of blood-thinning medications and raise the risk for serious complications such as stroke.

Learn what active ingredients are in the prescription and over-the-counter medicines you are taking. An active ingredient is the chemical compound in the medicine that works with your body to bring relief to your symptoms. For example, over-the-counter pain relievers usually contain one or more of four different active pain relief ingredients—acetaminophen, ibuprofen, naproxen sodium, or aspirin. Many prescription or over-the-counter medicines intended for relief of multiple symptoms, such as cold and flu medications, also include these pain relievers as active ingredients.

Don't combine pain relievers, prescription drugs, or multi-symptom medicines that have the same active pain relief ingredient—this could result in taking too much of that ingredient, and too much of any one ingredient might damage your liver or lead to other serious health problems. Also, it is a good idea to check what other active ingredients may be present in the over-the-counter medications you are taking. Some may also contain antihistamines, which can cause drowsiness. Caffeine, which is present in some over-the-counter medicines, can interact with certain drugs or with underlying conditions such as high blood pressure.

Understanding a Drug's Journey through the Body

As recently as 10–15 years ago, up to 40 percent of drugs failed to work properly because they were poorly absorbed, were destroyed by the body, failed to get to the right place, or were excreted from the body too quickly. Today, fewer than ten percent of medicines fail for these reasons. In part, that is because scientists are able to identify which enzymes metabolize a candidate drug and what the end products will be. The Food and Drug Administration now requires this information before it considers approving a new drug.

Researchers have characterized dozens of human drug-metabolizing enzymes and transport proteins that regulate the activity and levels of drugs in the body. Scientists also have identified certain medicines, vitamins, herbal remedies, nutritional supplements, and other compounds that interact with these enzymes and transporters, possibly causing adverse cross-reactions. To minimize dangerous interactions, doctors and pharmacists maintain lists of such substances. Pharmaceutical scientists are able to detect potentially troublesome compounds early in drug discovery so they can prevent these compounds from moving forward in development.

By analyzing the genetic sequences of drug-metabolizing enzymes from many people, researchers have identified more than 100 slightly different versions of the enzymes. Although most of these genetic variations are rare, some of them can markedly alter the activity and side effects of drugs.

As scientists learn more about drug-metabolizing enzymes, particularly those called P450s, they are able to design and develop drugs that influence the activity of the enzymes. Advances in technology allow researchers to determine the detailed, three-dimensional structures of some human P450 enzymes. By examining the shapes and biochemical properties of these molecules, researchers learn how medicines and other compounds interact with them.

Scientists are now able to use human, rather than animal, enzymes to predict whether a drug candidate or any of its byproducts will be toxic to humans. However, rare, serious drug reactions remain difficult to predict before testing experimental medicines in humans.

The formulation, packaging, and delivery of drugs are tailored to ensure optimal effectiveness, safety, and convenience. Therapeutics ranging from cold remedies to anti-cancer treatments are dispensed in time-release capsules that provide a constant level of a drug over several hours. Acid-sensitive drugs like some antibiotics and antihistamines are packaged so they can pass unscathed through the stomach into the small intestine, where they are absorbed. Other delivery systems include pumps (insulin), inhalers (asthma medications), implants (anticancer and pain medications), patches (estrogen replacement and smoking cessation treatments), and the covering of stents (the blood thinner heparin). The patient instructions routinely indicate whether a drug should be taken at a particular time of day and whether oral medications should be consumed with a meal or on an empty stomach.

Future Research

Researchers are working towards these goals:

- Scientists will understand drug transporters and drug-metabolizing enzymes well enough that they will be able to predict accurately the effect these proteins will have on the action and distribution of drug candidates in the body.

- Better animal models and sensitive protein markers that detect cellular damage in specific organs will allow scientists to predict toxicity early in drug development.

- Researchers will better understand how a person's genetic makeup influences whether specific medicines are effective, ineffective, or even dangerous.

- Doctors will be able to calculate the amount of drug at its site of action, not just the concentration in a patient's blood.

- Technical advances will allow doctors to deliver pharmaceuticals to specific organs or disease sites. This will increase the therapeutic benefit and reduce the bad side effects of drugs.

- Scientists and engineers will develop new, automated devices for drugs.

Chapter 33

Pharmacogenomics: Genes Affect Individual Responses to Medicines

What are pharmacogenomics and pharmacogenetics?

Your genes determine a lot about how you look. They also play a key role in how your body responds to medicines. The terms pharmacogenomics and pharmacogenetics are often used interchangeably to describe a field of research focused on how genes affect individual responses to medicines. Whether a medicine works well for you—or whether it causes serious side effects—depends, to a certain extent, on your genes.

Just as genes contribute to whether you will be tall or short, black-haired or blond, your genes also determine how you will respond to medicines. Genes are like recipes—they carry instructions for making protein molecules. As medicines travel through your body, they interact with thousands of proteins. Small differences in the composition or quantities of these molecules can affect how medicines do their jobs. These differences can be due to diet, level of activity, or the medicines a person takes, but they can also be due to differences in genes. By understanding the genetic basis of drug responses, scientists hope to enable doctors to prescribe the drugs and doses best suited for each individual.

Aren't prescribed medicines already safe and effective?

While standard doses of most medicines work well for most people, some medicines do not work at all in certain people or cause annoying

"Frequently Asked Questions about Pharmacogenetics." National Institute of General Medical Sciences, updated July 26, 2007.

and sometimes dangerous side effects. For example, codeine is useless as a painkiller in nearly ten percent of people, and an anticancer drug, 6-mercaptopurine, is extremely toxic in a small fraction of the population.

How do scientists gather pharmacogenetic information?

Many pharmacogenetic findings are based on knowledge of biochemical pathways within cells. For example, scientists already knew a lot about the enzymes that break down the anticancer drug irinotecan when its toxic effects in certain patients came to light. This knowledge allowed researchers to rapidly pinpoint a genetic variant of one of these enzymes as the cause of the dangerous reaction. Scientists have developed a genetic test for this variant so that doctors can adjust the dosage for those at risk for serious side effects.

Pharmacogenetic advances can also come from studies that accompany clinical drug trials. After obtaining permission from participants, some pharmaceutical companies collect deoxyribonucleic acid (DNA) samples from people in clinical trials. Scientists then analyze the samples together with results of the clinical trial to identify genetic variations that correlate with a drug's effectiveness or toxicity.

Pharmacogenetic researchers have already identified many genes whose variations affect drug responses. They also know where to look for the numerous others they are bound to discover in the future. The availability of the human genome sequence, which was completed in 2003, led to the HapMap project, an international effort to catalog common genetic differences among human beings. These resources are providing a treasure trove of genetic information that is expected to speed advances in pharmacogenetics.

In what ways can doctors use pharmacogenetics to help them treat their patients?

For many diseases, there are a variety of treatment options. Pharmacogenetics can help doctors pick the right one for each patient. Pharmacogenetics can be used by doctors to identify the optimal dose and medicine for each patient.

The right dose: Dosage is usually based on factors such as age, weight, and liver and kidney function. But for someone who breaks down a drug quickly, a typical dose may be ineffective. In contrast, someone who breaks down a drug more slowly may need a lower dose to avoid accumulating toxic levels of the drug in the bloodstream. A pharmacogenetic test can help reveal the right dose for individual patients.

The right drug—for cancer: Pharmacogenetics is used in targeted therapy for cancer to identify the best drug regimen for a particular tumor. Even tumors of the same type (such as lung, breast, or liver) vary at the genetic level. Cancer is fundamentally a genetic disease, but most of the genetic differences between cancer cells and normal cells are not inherited—they accumulate as the cancer develops. Analyzing specific genes in a patient's tumor helps doctors identify the drug combination to which the tumor will most likely respond. For example, the breast cancer drug Herceptin® is only effective when the tumor cells have accumulated extra copies of the human epidermal growth factor receptor-2 (HER2) gene and have high levels of the protein this gene encodes on their surfaces.

The right drug—for human immunodeficiency virus (HIV): For patients with a bacterial or viral infection, analyzing the genes of the infectious agent can reveal the most suitable drug treatment. For example, the Food and Drug Administration (FDA) has approved a genotyping kit that detects genetic variations in HIV that make the virus resistant to some antiretroviral drugs. If drug resistance is discovered, doctors can prescribe other medications.

The right drug—for depression: Depression can be treated with a variety of different medicines, and it is often time-consuming and difficult to find the drug(s) that works best for each person. In the future, genetic testing may take some of the guesswork out of choosing a drug regimen. These tests are likely to involve analyzing a person's liver enzymes, especially those in the cytochrome P450 family, which are largely responsible for processing antidepressants.

Other tests that may prove useful to psychiatrists will detect differences in the molecules targeted by antidepressants, such as the serotonin transporters targeted by a large class of antidepressants called selective serotonin reuptake inhibitors (SSRIs). Scientists have uncovered evidence for a link between a person's response to SSRIs and variations in serotonin transporters and other biological molecules that act on serotonin.

The right drug—for cardiovascular disease: Statins, the most widely prescribed drugs worldwide, help prevent cardiovascular disease by reducing the level of bad cholesterol in the bloodstream. While statins work well for many patients, responses are highly variable and doctors must adjust the dosage for each person.

Researchers have discovered that variants in a number of molecules—including those that break down or transport statins, as well as the statins' molecular target in the cholesterol production pathway—contribute to the variable response among individuals. Using results of genetic tests, doctors may one day be able to prescribe the right dose from the start and more quickly reduce their patients' risk of dangerous cardiovascular events such as heart attack and stroke.

Does the FDA require that doctors test patients for genetic differences before prescribing any drugs currently on the market?

The labels of more than 20 medications now mention the availability of tests for genetic variations that impact the drug's action. However, in many cases, such as the anticancer drugs azathioprine and irinotecan, which can build up to toxic levels in a small fraction of people, testing is optional.

How do I get a pharmacogenetic test?

Ask your doctor, who can order a test from a medical laboratory. Some major institutions, such as the Mayo Clinic, the Indiana University School of Medicine, and St. Jude Children's Hospital, also offer pharmacogenetic testing. If you take a test, a technician will draw a sample of your blood or rub a cotton swab along the inside of your cheek to collect cells. The lab will extract genetic material from the sample and carry out the test. These tests typically cost a few hundred dollars and may be covered by your health insurance company.

Cancer biopsy samples are also often subjected to genetic tests. The results can help guide therapy and predict the likelihood of recurrence. Several such tests have been approved by the FDA.

Are the results of pharmacogenetic tests confidential?

While pharmacogenetic tests are designed to help people, some fear that the results could be used against them, such as to discriminate against them in a job setting or to deny them health insurance coverage. A person's genetic information is protected through the Health Insurance Portability and Accountability Act (HIPAA), which was passed by Congress in 1996. Many states also have laws in place that protect the privacy of health information, including genetic data.

How will pharmacogenetics affect the design, development, and availability of new medicines?

Pharmacogenetic knowledge will enable pharmaceutical companies to design, develop, and market drugs for people with specific genetic profiles. Testing a drug only in those likely to benefit from it could streamline its development and maximize its therapeutic benefit.

The FDA, which monitors the safety of all drugs in the United States, considers pharmacogenetics to be a valuable tool in the development of new medical products. To date, the FDA has approved a number of genotyping kits relevant to pharmacogenetics, including one that screens for variants in the cytochrome P450 enzymes, which process many kinds of drugs. In most cases the FDA encourages, but does not require, companies to submit pharmacogenetic data with new drug applications. This data is only required for medicines that were developed based on pharmacogenetics.

How will pharmacogenetics affect the quality of health care?

In the future, pharmacogenetics will increasingly enable doctors to prescribe the right dose of the right medicine the first time for everyone. This would mean that patients will receive medicines that are safer and more effective, leading to better health care overall. Also, if scientists could identify the genetic basis for certain toxic side effects, drugs could be prescribed only to those who are not genetically at risk for these effects. This could maintain the availability of potentially lifesaving medications that might otherwise be taken off the market.

What are some of the challenges that face pharmacogenetics?

While pharmacogenetics is expected to be a useful tool to find the best dose of the right medicine for each patient, doctors are unlikely to be able to rely on it alone. Other factors will remain important, and may sometimes overshadow pharmacogenetics. These other factors include characteristics of the disease itself as well as the patient's diet, weight, lifestyle, and other medicines he or she is taking.

As with many new medical advances, it will take time before pharmacogenetics enters the mainstream and becomes a standard tool for making treatment decisions. Overcoming this barrier may be particularly tricky for pharmacogenetics because most medicines work well for most people and adverse reactions are rare.

Another challenge facing pharmacogenetics is the number and complexity of interactions a drug has with biological molecules in the body. Variations in many different molecules may influence how someone responds to a medicine. Teasing out the genetic patterns associated with particular drug responses could involve some intricate and time-consuming scientific detective work.

While routine pharmacogenetic testing could ultimately save our health care system billions of dollars by improving drug effectiveness and safety, the savings could be offset by the additional cost of genetic tests.

What is the role of the National Institutes of Health (NIH)?

In April 2000, NIH launched the Pharmacogenetics Research Network (PGRN), a nationwide collaboration of hundreds of scientists focused on understanding how genes affect the way a person responds to medicines. Since its inception, PGRN scientists have studied genes and medications relevant to a wide range of diseases, including asthma, depression, cancer, and heart disease. A key component of the PGRN is the Pharmacogenetics Knowledge Base, an online resource that contains pharmacogenetic data from the PGRN and others, and is freely available to the research community.

NIH takes seriously the ethical and legal implications of pharmacogenetics research and is working closely with several task forces and associations to maximize the benefits of this research and to prevent any potential harm to individuals or society.

National Institute of General Medical Sciences
45 Center Dr., MSC 6200
Bethesda, MD 20892-6200
Phone: 301-496-7301
Website: http://www.nigms.nih.gov
E-mail: info@nigms.nih.gov

The NIH Pharmacogenetics Research Network has made many advances in understanding the way genes affect individual responses to medicines, including those for heart disease, asthma, depression, cancer, and many other diseases. For more information about this nationwide research team visit, http://www.nigms.nih.gov/Initiatives/PGRN.

Chapter 34

Using Medicines Safely

Managing the Benefits and Risks of Medicines

Although medicines can make you feel better and help you get well, it is important to know that all medicines, both prescription and over-the-counter, have risks as well as benefits.

The benefits of medicines are the helpful effects you get when you use them, such as lowering blood pressure, curing infection, or relieving pain. The risks of medicines are the chances that something unwanted or unexpected could happen to you when you use them. Risks could be less serious things, such as an upset stomach, or more serious things, such as liver damage.

When a medicine's benefits outweigh its known risks, the U.S. Food and Drug Administration (FDA) considers it safe enough to approve. But before using any medicine—as with many things that you do every day—you should think through the benefits and the risks in order to make the best choice for you.

There are several types of risks from medicine use:

This chapter includes text from "Think It Through: A Guide to Managing the Benefits and Risks of Medicines," and "Using Medicines Wisely," U.S. Food and Drug Administration (FDA), August 2005; and text from the Agency for Healthcare Research and Quality (AHRQ) documents "Check Your Medicines: Tips for Taking Medicines Safely," AHRQ Pub. No. 07-M0008-1, December 2006, and "Women and Medicines: What You Need to Know," AHRQ Publication No. 03(05)-0019-A, April 2005.

- The possibility of a harmful interaction between the medicine and a food, beverage, dietary supplement (including vitamins and herbals), or another medicine. Combinations of any of these products could increase the chance that there may be interactions.

- The chance that the medicine may not work as expected.

- The possibility that the medicine may cause additional problems.

For example, every time you get into a car, there are risks—the possibility that unwanted or unexpected things could happen. You could have an accident, causing costly damage to your car, or injury to yourself or a loved one. But there are also benefits to riding in a car: you can travel farther and faster than walking, bring home more groceries from the store, and travel in cold or wet weather in greater comfort.

To obtain the benefits of riding in a car, you think through the risks. You consider the condition of your car and the road, for instance, before deciding to make that trip to the store.

The same is true before using any medicine. Every choice to take a medicine involves thinking through the helpful effects as well as the possible unwanted effects.

Weighing the Risks, Making the Choice

The benefit to risk decision is sometimes difficult to make. The best choice depends on your particular situation. You must decide what risks you can and will accept in order to get the benefits you want. For example, if facing a life-threatening illness, you might choose to accept more risk in the hope of getting the benefits of a cure or living a longer life. On the other hand, if you are facing a minor illness, you might decide that you want to take very little risk. In many situations, the expert advice of your doctor, pharmacist, or other health care professionals can help you make the decision.

Talk with Your Doctor, Pharmacist, or Other Health Care Professionals

- Keep an up-to-date, written list of all of the medicines (prescription and over-the-counter) and dietary supplements, including vitamins and herbals, that you use—even those you only use occasionally.

- Share this list with all of your health care professionals.

- Tell about any allergies or sensitivities that you may have.

- Tell about anything that could affect your ability to take medicines, such as difficulty swallowing or remembering to take them.

- Tell if you are or might become pregnant, or if you are nursing a baby.

- Always ask questions about any concerns or thoughts that you may have.

Using Medicines Wisely

Today we have many medicines to choose from. Medicine can help you, but no drug is totally safe. There are things you can do to lower your chances of having problems, and make sure your medicine works the best it can.

Ask Questions

- Why am I using this medicine?

- How long should I use it?

- When should I start to feel better?

- What problems should I watch for?

- What should I do if I have problems or side effects?

- When should I use this medicine?

- Should I take it on an empty stomach or with food?

- Is it safe to drink alcohol with it?

- What should I do if I forget to use it?

Know the Medicine

- What is the brand name? Does the drug have any other names?

- What does the drug look like? Look at the color, shape, and package. If it looks different next time, ask why. It could be the wrong medicine.

Read the Label

- Find out what is in the drug. Do not use the medicine if you are allergic to anything in it. Ask your doctor, nurse or pharmacist about changing your medicine.

- Don't use two drugs with the same or similar ingredients.
- Don't use two drugs for the same problem unless your doctor, nurse or pharmacist suggests it.
- Read the warnings carefully.

Follow Directions

- Do not skip taking your medicines.
- Don't take more than the suggested dose.
- Do not share medicines.
- Do not take medicine in the dark. It's too easy to make a mistake.

Keep a List of All the Medicines You Use

- List all of your prescription medicines.
- List any over-the-counter medicines you use.
- List any vitamins, minerals, herbs, amino acids, and other products you use.
- Carry the list with you to show your doctor, pharmacist, or nurse.

How do you feel?

- If you are not feeling better, or start to feel worse, call your doctor or clinic. You might need a different medicine or a different dose.

Check Your Medicines: Tips for Taking Medicines Safely

Use these tips to help avoid medication errors. Simple checks could save your life.

Bring a list or a bag with all your medicines when you go to your doctor's office, the pharmacy, or the hospital. Include all prescription and over-the-counter medicines, vitamins, and herbal supplements that you use. If your doctor prescribes a new medicine, ask if it is safe to use with your other medicines. Remind your doctor and pharmacist if you are allergic to any medicines.

Ask questions about your medicines. Make sure you understand the answers. Choose a pharmacist and doctor you feel comfortable talking with about your health and medicines. Take a relative or friend with you to ask questions and remind you about the answers later. Write down the answers.

Make sure your medicine is what the doctor ordered. Does the medicine seem different than what your doctor wrote on the prescription, or look different than what you expected? Does a refill look like it is a different shape, color, or size than what you were given before? If something seems wrong, ask the pharmacist to double check it. Most errors are first found by patients.

Ask how to use the medicine correctly. Read the directions on the label and other information you get with your medicine. Have the pharmacist or doctor explain anything you do not understand. Are there other medicines, foods, or activities (such as driving, drinking alcohol, or using tobacco) that you should avoid while using the medicine? Ask if you need lab tests to check how the medicine is working or to make sure it doesn't cause harmful side effects.

Ask about possible side effects. Side effects can occur with many medicines. Ask your doctor or pharmacist what side effects to expect and which ones are serious. Some side effects may bother you but will get better after you have been using the medicine for a while. Call your doctor right away if you have a serious side effect or if a side effect does not get better. A change in the medicine or the dose may be needed.

Women and Medicines: What You Need to Know

Be aware of how your medicines—both prescription and non-prescription medicines—affect your body. Discuss any questions or symptoms you may have with your pharmacist or provider. Work together to keep your medicine safe and effective. Remember:

- Women's bodies are different from men's. This affects the way chemicals are processed in the body.

- Hormones can affect how medicines work in women's bodies. For example, medication levels vary at different times of the menstrual cycle.

- Pregnant women need to consult their health care provider before taking any medicine to avoid risks to the fetus.

- As women age, their bodies process medicines differently, including the same medicines they used at younger ages.

Tips for Safe Medicine Use

Tell your health care provider:

- about allergies or bad reactions to medicines, and
- if you are pregnant or plan to get pregnant soon.

Ask about your medicines.

- What are they used for?
- Are there any side effects you should watch for?
- Are they safe to take with your other medicines and supplements?
- What is the correct way to take them—whole, crushed, with food, with water, at the same time every day?
- Should you drive while taking this medicine?
- Are there certain foods or drinks you should avoid while using this medicine?

Make a list of your medicines, including nonprescription medicines and supplements.

- Keep the list current.
- Show it to your doctor and pharmacist at every visit.

Try to get all your medicines at the same pharmacy and ask your pharmacist to be sure they are safe if you take them together. Tell your provider or pharmacist if:

- there's a change in how your medicines are working; or
- your medicines seem to work differently during different parts of your menstrual cycle.

Be informed. Learn about the medicines you are taking.

- Carefully read the printed information that comes with your medicine.
- Use reliable book and internet sources such as MEDLINEplus®.

If you need surgery or a procedure, ask if you should stop taking medicines beforehand.

Chapter 35

Over-the-Counter (OTC) Medicines

Advice for Americans about Self-Care

American medicine cabinets contain a growing choice of nonprescription, over-the-counter (OTC) medicines to treat an expanding range of ailments. OTC medicines often do more than relieve aches, pains, and itches. Some can prevent diseases like tooth decay, cure diseases like athlete's foot, and with a doctor's guidance, help manage recurring conditions like vaginal yeast infection, migraine, and minor pain in arthritis.

The U.S. Food and Drug Administration (FDA) determines whether medicines are prescription or nonprescription. The term prescription (Rx) refers to medicines that are safe and effective when used under a doctor's care. Nonprescription or OTC drugs are medicines FDA decides are safe and effective for use without a doctor's prescription.

FDA also has the authority to decide when a prescription drug is safe enough to be sold directly to consumers over the counter. This regulatory process allowing Americans to take a more active role in their health care is known as Rx-to-OTC switch. As a result of this process, more than 700 products sold over the counter today use ingredients or dosage strengths available only by prescription 30 years ago.

This chapter includes "Over-the-Counter Medicine: What's Right for You?" Center for Drug Evaluation and Research (CDER), U.S. Food and Drug Administration (FDA), March 7, 2006; excerpts from "The New Over-the-Counter Medicine Label: Take a Look," FDA-CDER, March 7, 2006; and "What's on the Label," FDA-CDER, 2006.

Increased access to OTC medicines is especially important for our maturing population. Two out of three older Americans rate their health as excellent to good, but four out of five report at least one chronic condition.

The fact is, today's OTC medicines offer greater opportunity to treat more of the aches and illnesses most likely to appear in our later years. As we live longer, work longer, and take a more active role in our own health care, the need grows to become better informed about self-care.

The best way to become better informed—for young and old alike—is to read and understand the information on OTC labels. Next to the medicine itself, label comprehension is the most important part of self-care with OTC medicines.

With new opportunities in self-medication come new responsibilities and an increased need for knowledge. FDA and the Consumer Healthcare Products Association (CHPA) have prepared the following information to help Americans take advantage of self-care opportunities.

OTC Know-How: It's on the Label

You would not ignore your doctor's instructions for using a prescription drug; so don't ignore the label when taking an OTC medicine. Here's what to look for:

- product name
- active ingredients—therapeutic substances in medicine
- purpose—product category (such as antihistamine, antacid, or cough suppressant)
- uses—symptoms or diseases the product will treat or prevent
- warnings—when not to use the product, when to stop taking it, when to see a doctor, and possible side effects
- directions—how much to take, how to take it, and how long to take it
- other information—such as storage information
- inactive ingredients—substances such as binders, colors, or flavoring

You can help yourself read the label. Always use enough light. It usually takes three times more light to read the same line at age 60 than at age 30. If necessary, use your glasses or contact lenses when reading labels.

Always remember to look for the statement describing the tamper-evident feature(s) before you buy the product and when you use it.

When it comes to medicines, more does not necessarily mean better. You should never misuse OTC medicines by taking them longer or in higher doses than the label recommends. Symptoms that persist are a clear signal it's time to see a doctor.

Be sure to read the label each time you purchase a product. Just because two or more products are from the same brand family does not mean they are meant to treat the same conditions or contain the same ingredients.

Remember, if you read the label and still have questions, talk to a doctor, nurse, or pharmacist.

Drug Interactions: A Word to the Wise

Although mild and relatively uncommon, interactions involving OTC drugs can produce unwanted results or make medicines less effective. It is especially important to know about drug interactions if you are taking Rx and OTC drugs at the same time.

Some drugs can also interact with foods and beverages, as well as with health conditions such as diabetes, kidney disease, and high blood pressure. Here are a few drug interaction cautions for some common OTC ingredients:

- Avoid alcohol if you are taking antihistamines, cough-cold products with the ingredient dextromethorphan, or drugs that treat sleeplessness.

- Do not use drugs that treat sleeplessness if you are taking prescription sedatives or tranquilizers.

- Check with your doctor before taking products containing aspirin if you are taking a prescription blood thinner or if you have diabetes or gout.

- Do not use laxatives when you have stomach pain, nausea, or vomiting.

- Unless directed by a doctor, do not use a nasal decongestant if you are taking a prescription drug for high blood pressure or depression, or if you have heart or thyroid disease, diabetes, or prostate problems.

This is not a complete list. Read the label. Drug labels change as new information becomes available. That's why it is important to read the label each time you take medicine.

Time for a Medicine Cabinet Checkup

- Be sure to look through your medicine supply at least once a year.

- Always store medicines in a cool, dry place or as stated on the label.

- Throw away any medicines that are past the expiration date.

- To make sure no one takes the wrong medicine, keep all medicines in their original containers.

Pregnancy and Breast Feeding

Drugs can pass from a pregnant woman to her unborn baby. A safe amount of medicine for the mother may be too much for the unborn baby. If you are pregnant, always talk with your doctor before taking any drugs, Rx or OTC.

Although most drugs pass into breast milk in concentrations too low to have any unwanted effects on the baby, breast feeding mothers still need to be careful. Always ask your doctor or pharmacist before taking any medicine while breast feeding. A doctor or pharmacist can tell you how to adjust the timing and dosing of most medicines so the baby is exposed to the lowest amount possible, or whether the drugs should be avoided altogether.

Kids Are Not Just Small Adults

OTC drugs rarely come in one-size-fits-all. Here are some tips about giving OTC medicines to children:

- Children are not just small adults, so do not estimate the dose based on their size.

- Read the label. Follow all directions.

- Follow any age limits on the label.

- Some OTC products come in different strengths. Be aware.

- Know the difference between abbreviations for tablespoon (Tbsp) and teaspoon (tsp). They are very different doses.

- Be careful about converting dose instructions. If the label says two teaspoons, it is best to use a measuring spoon or a dosing cup marked in teaspoons, not a common kitchen spoon.

- Do not play doctor. Do not double the dose just because your child seems sicker than last time.

- Before you give your child two medicines at the same time, talk to your doctor or pharmacist.

- Never let children take medicine by themselves.

- Never call medicine candy to get your kids to take it. If they come across the medicine on their own, they are likely to remember that you called it candy.

Child-Resistant Packaging

Child-resistant closures are designed for repeated use to make it difficult for children to open. Remember, if you do not re-lock the closure after each use, the child-resistant device cannot do its job—keeping children out.

It is best to store all medicines and dietary supplements where children can neither see nor reach them. Containers of pills should not be left on the kitchen counter as a reminder. Purses and briefcases are among the worst places to hide medicines from curious kids. And since children are natural mimics, it is a good idea not to take medicine in front of them. They may be tempted to play house with your medicine later on.

If you find some packages too difficult to open—and do not have young children living with you or visiting—you should know the law allows one package size for each OTC medicine to be sold without child-resistant features. If you do not see it on the store shelf, ask.

Protect Yourself against Tampering

Makers of OTC medicines seal most products in tamper-evident packaging (TEP) to help protect against criminal tampering. TEP works by providing visible evidence if the package has been disturbed. But OTC packaging cannot be 100 percent tamperproof. Here is how to help protect yourself:

- Be alert to the tamper-evident features on the package before you open it. These features are described on the label.

263

- Inspect the outer packaging before you buy it. When you get home, inspect the medicine inside.

- Do not buy an OTC product if the packaging is damaged.

- Do not use any medicine that looks discolored or different in any way.

- If anything looks suspicious, be suspicious. Contact the store where you bought the product. Take it back.

- Never take medicines in the dark.

The New Over-the-Counter Medicine Label: Take a Look

Always Read the Label

Reading the product label is the most important part of taking care of yourself or your family when using over-the-counter (OTC) medicines (available without a prescription). This is especially true because many OTC medicines are taken without seeing a doctor. The OTC medicine label has always contained important usage and safety information for consumers, but now that information will be more consistent and even easier to read and to understand. The U.S. Food and Drug Administration (FDA) has issued a regulation to make sure the labels on all OTC medicines (from a tube of fluoride toothpaste to a bottle of cough syrup) have information listed in the same order; are arranged in a simpler eye-catching, consistent style; and may contain easier to understand words. While the new labels on a majority of OTC drug products are on store shelves now, some products and companies have additional time to comply with the new labeling regulations. If you read the OTC medicine label and still have questions about the product, talk to your doctor, pharmacist, or other health care professional.

What Is on the New Label?

All nonprescription, over-the-counter (OTC) medicine labels have detailed usage and warning information so consumers can properly choose and use the products.

The new Drug Facts labeling requirements do not apply to dietary supplements, which are regulated as food products, and are labeled with a Supplement Facts panel.

Reading the Label: The Key to Proper Medicine Use

The label tells you what a medicine is supposed to do, who should or should not take it, and how to use it. But efforts to provide good labeling cannot help unless you read and use the information. It is up to you to be informed and to use OTC drug products wisely and responsibly.

The manufacturers of OTC medicines sometimes make changes to their products or labeling (new ingredients, dosages, or warnings). Make

WHAT'S ON THE **LABEL**

All nonprescription, over-the-counter (OTC) medicine labels have detailed usage and warning information so consumers can properly choose and use the products.

Below is an example of what the new OTC medicine label looks like.

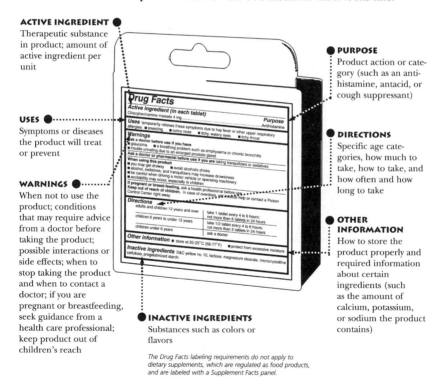

ACTIVE INGREDIENT
Therapeutic substance in product; amount of active ingredient per unit

USES
Symptoms or diseases the product will treat or prevent

WARNINGS
When not to use the product; conditions that may require advice from a doctor before taking the product; possible interactions or side effects; when to stop taking the product and when to contact a doctor; if you are pregnant or breastfeeding, seek guidance from a health care professional; keep product out of children's reach

INACTIVE INGREDIENTS
Substances such as colors or flavors

PURPOSE
Product action or category (such as an antihistamine, antacid, or cough suppressant)

DIRECTIONS
Specific age categories, how much to take, how to take, and how often and how long to take

OTHER INFORMATION
How to store the product properly and required information about certain ingredients (such as the amount of calcium, potassium, or sodium the product contains)

The Drug Facts labeling requirements do not apply to dietary supplements, which are regulated as food products, and are labeled with a Supplement Facts panel.

Figure 35.1. *New Over-the-Counter Medicine Label. For more information visit: www.fda.gov/cder or call 1-888-INFO-FDA.*

sure to read the label each time you use the product. Always look for special flags or banners on the front product label alerting you to such changes. If you read the label and still have questions, ask your doctor, pharmacist, or other health care professional for advice.

The label also tells you:

- the expiration date, when applicable (date after which you should not use the product);

- lot or batch code (manufacturer information to help identify the product);

- name and address of manufacturer, packer, or distributor;

- net quantity of contents (how much of the product is in each package); and

- what to do if an overdose occurs.

Many OTC medicines are sold in containers with child safety closures. Use them properly. Remember—keep all medicines out of the sight and reach of children.

Additional Information

Consumer Healthcare Products Association
Publications Department
900 19th St., N.W., Suite 700
Washington, DC 20006
Phone: 202-429-9260
Fax: 202-223-6835
Website: http://www.chpa-info.org

U.S. Food and Drug Administration
Office of Consumer Affairs
5600 Fishers Lane
HFE-50
Rockville, MD 20857
Toll-Free: 888-463-6332
Phone: 301-827-4420
Fax: 301-443-9767
Website: http://www.fda.gov

Chapter 36

What Value Do Prescription Drugs Provide to Patients?

How do you put a value on good health? What is the value of the smile of a child no longer feeling the pain of cancer? What is the value of giving a grandfather with congestive heart failure the energy to go camping with his grandson?

Quantifying the value of good health is difficult. But, we can often quantify the value of medicines to patients, to society, and to the health care system. Here are a few examples.

Stroke: A study sponsored by the Agency for Health Care Policy and Research found that increased use of a blood-thinning drug would prevent 40,000 strokes a year, saving $600 million annually.

Human immunodeficiency virus (HIV)/acquired immunodeficiency syndrome (AIDS): New medicines have made a major contribution to the decline in the death rate from HIV/AIDS in the U.S. over the last ten years. Since the mid-1990s, when researchers developed a new wave of medicines to treat HIV/AIDS, the U.S. death rate from AIDS has dropped about 70 percent.

High cholesterol: Changes in the recommended use of statins reflects the increasingly important role that they can play in reducing the incidence of heart disease. Several studies have found that using statin therapy to treat people with high cholesterol reduces hospital admissions and invasive cardiac surgeries. For example, a study of one statin showed that it reduced hospital admissions by a third during five years of treatment. It also reduced the number of days that patients had to spend in the hospital when they were admitted, and it reduced the need for bypass surgery and angioplasty.

Cancer: A February 2004 study by Columbia University professor Frank R. Lichtenberg found that new cancer drugs have accounted for 50 to 60 percent of the gains we have made in cancer survival rates since 1975. Since 1971, when the U.S. declared war on cancer, our arsenal of cancer medicines has tripled. During that time, the survival rate has risen from 50 percent to 62.7 percent. Overall, new cancer drugs have contributed a remarkable 10.7 percent of the increase in life expectancy at birth in the U.S.

Heart failure: A January 2004 study by Duke University researchers found that five years of treatment for heart failure without beta-blockers cost a total of $52,999. With beta-blockers added to treatment, total treatment costs fell by $3,959, patient survival increased by an average of about three-and a-half months, and patients needed fewer overnight hospital stays.

Diabetes: One recent study published in the *Journal of the American Medical Association* found that effective treatment of diabetes with medicines and other therapy yields annual health care savings of $685 to $950 per patient within one to two years.

Alzheimer disease: A study of the effects of a new Alzheimer medicine, donepezil, on costs in a Medicare managed care plan showed that, although the prescription costs for the group receiving the drug were over $1,000 higher per patient, the overall medical costs fell to $8,056 compared with $11,947 for the group not receiving drug treatment.

Depression: A December 2003 study in the *Journal of Clinical Psychiatry* showed that newer, better medicines are reducing the cost of treating people with depression. The study found that per patient spending on depression had fallen by 19 percent over the course of the previous decade.

Aging: A recent study of the National Bureau of Economic Research noted that new medicines account for 40 percent of the increase in longevity. Between 1980 and 2000 alone, life expectancy in women increased from 77 to 79, and in men from 70 to 74.

What Role Do Prescription Drugs Play in Improving Health Care?

Significant under-diagnosis and under-treatment of serious diseases is a growing health care problem in America. Americans would be healthier—and overall health care costs might actually decrease—if more patients were properly diagnosed and treated.

Prescription medicines play an important and growing role in basic health care. They are helping patients remain independent and productive. For example, the need for more expensive health care services such as long hospitalizations and surgeries can be reduced by using prescription medicines.

Currently, prescription drug expenditures account for less than eleven cents of every health care dollar. The good news is that while that percentage has increased in recent years, this increase means that more people are benefiting from more and better medicines. In fact, a study by Columbia University economist Frank Lichtenberg found that while treating conditions with newer medicines instead of older ones increases medicine costs, it significantly lowers non-drug medical spending. The study found that each additional dollar spent on using a newer prescription medicine (instead of an older one) saves roughly $7.20 in other health care costs.

Utilization Versus Price Increases

There are several factors behind increasing medicine expenditures:

A steady stream of new medicines: Many new medicines replace higher-cost surgeries and hospital care. In 2004 alone, pharmaceutical companies added 38 new treatments to the nation's medicine chest. Over the last decade, 330 new medicines have become available for treating patients. These include important new medicines for some of the most devastating and costly diseases including: AIDS, cancer, glaucoma, heart disease, schizophrenia, and Alzheimer disease. Additionally, there are over 1,000 new medicines in the research and development pipeline.

Greater treatment of previously undiagnosed and untreated patients: For example, over 19 million American adults are annually affected by depression. Unfortunately, despite therapeutic advances and efforts to increase depression awareness and diagnosis, depression remains widely untreated. However, the federal government's 2003 report *Healthy People 2010 Psychiatry* found that per-patient spending on depression fell by 19 percent during the 1990s, largely as a result of a switch from hospitalization to medication as a first line treatment.

An aging population: The nation's population is aging, and the elderly use more medicines than do younger people. People 65 and older, on average, fill their prescriptions more than 25 times a year compared to those 64 and younger who average around seven refills per year.

New guidelines on the use of medicines: For example, the National Institutes of Health (NIH) has recommended that more Americans take cholesterol-lowering drugs. According to an NIH official, if these recommendations were followed, heart disease would cease to be the leading cause of death in the U.S. Despite the fact that more people are benefiting from medicines, under-treatment continues to be a major health care concern. For example:

- More than 23 million Americans who should be taking cholesterol-lowering drugs are not taking them, according to the National Institutes of Health.

- Over 19 million Americans suffer from depression and fewer than half seek treatment.

- Almost 6 million Americans have diabetes but do not know it or are not being treated for it.

Chapter 37

Buying Prescription Drugs

Chapter Contents

Section 37.1

Saving Money on Prescription Drugs

Excerpted from "Saving Money on Prescription Drugs," *FDA Consumer magazine*, September-October 2005, U.S. Food and Drug Administration (FDA).

Consumers can save money on prescription drugs by becoming smart shoppers and knowing what to discuss with their doctor or pharmacist. Having discussions on whether a less expensive drug will work, comparing prices among U.S. pharmacies in the area or online, and finding out about assistance programs and how to qualify can help.

"The FDA also encourages consumers to learn about potential savings through Medicare's outpatient prescription drug coverage," U.S. Food and Drug Administration (FDA) Commissioner Lester Crawford says. "This program comes at a time when five out of six people aged 65 and older are taking at least one medication, and almost half of all elderly people take three or more." Medicare is the national health insurance program for people ages 65 and older and for people of all ages who have certain disabilities. In January 2006, the 43 million people in Medicare became eligible for prescription drug coverage as part of the Medicare Prescription Drug, Improvement and Modernization Act of 2003 (MMA).

This coverage gives substantial help to beneficiaries in paying for prescription drugs, regardless of their income or how they pay for health care, according to Mark McClellan, M.D., Ph.D., Administrator of the Centers for Medicare and Medicaid Services (CMS). "The MMA also gives Medicare the ability to provide additional comprehensive help to those in greatest need—beneficiaries with very high prescription drug costs and people with low incomes," he says. On average, people with limited incomes who qualify for extra help will save about 95 percent on prescription drug costs, according to CMS spokesman Gary Karr.

Generic Drugs

In 2004, the average price of a generic prescription drug was $28.74, while the average price of a brand-name prescription drug was

$96.01, according to the National Association of Chain Drug Stores. Patent protection gives brand-name manufacturers the right to be the sole source of a drug for a certain time period so they can recoup the money they invested in trying to develop the product. Once the patent protection expires, a generic version of the drug can be marketed.

"Many see generics as the only way they can afford prescription drugs," says Gary Buehler, R.Ph., Director of the FDA's Office of Generic Drugs. "Still, there are some people who doubt generics because they think that anything that costs more must be better. But the reason generic manufacturers can sell the drugs less expensively is not because the quality is lower. It's because there is competition among these generic manufacturers, who don't have to repeat the expensive safety and effectiveness testing that brand companies have already conducted." For a number of years, the FDA has been increasing public awareness and confidence in generic drugs.

Generic drug companies must perform tests and show the FDA that their drugs are equivalent in terms of therapeutic effect to the brand-name drug. These companies must show that the ingredients of the generic drug enter into the blood stream in the same way and in the same length of time as the brand-name drug. The FDA's Orange Book lists drugs and generic counterparts. It is accessible online at http://www.fda.gov/cder/ob. It lists approved drug products with therapeutic equivalence evaluations.

Physicians and patients should discuss which drug is the best therapy. Even when a particular branded drug has no generic, a very similar member of the same drug class may be available. For this reason, instead of asking doctors whether a particular brand-name drug has a generic version, patients should ask whether there is a generic available to treat their problem, suggests Jack Billi, M.D., associate vice president for medical affairs at the University of Michigan. "Patients should ask if there is a generic in the class of drugs they are taking," he says.

For people who have insurance that pays for drugs, use of generics can make a big difference, Billi says. "Tiered co-payment structures through insurance plans encourage the use of generics," he says. "For example, there might be a co-pay of $7.00 for generics and $14.00 for brand drugs."

"Even if you have a fixed co-pay," Billi says, "choosing generics saves your employer money, and that makes it more likely the employer will continue offering coverage. And if you don't have health insurance and you're paying out-of-pocket, generics will bring you big savings."

Communicating with Your Doctor

It's a good idea to tell your doctors whether paying for medicine is a problem, says Edward Langston, M.D., a family physician in Lafayette, Indiana, and an American Medical Association trustee. That doesn't mean physicians can fix all the problems, Langston says, but not being able to afford medication clearly affects your health.

"I think most physicians would want to help if they knew a patient won't be able to follow the treatment," Langston says. "But many patients find it a hard subject to bring up." When Langston writes a prescription, he asks patients, "Are you going to have any trouble getting this medication?"

So what can patients struggling with drug costs reasonably expect from their doctors? Patients should feel free to ask about whether a generic can be used instead of a brand-name drug or whether there is a similar drug that is less expensive. But some doctors don't know the price of drugs, so patients might have to do their own research, says Paul Hunter, M.D., a physician with Community Care for the Elderly in Milwaukee. In some cases, there may be nonprescription drugs that might work. Loratadine for allergies is a good example of an over-the-counter (OTC) medicine that is less expensive than brand-name prescription alternatives, Hunter says. Loratadine is the active ingredient in Claritin, Alavert, and some generic allergy medicines.

The doctor's office also can serve as a valuable resource for patients for such activities as informing them about the Medicare prescription drug benefit, signing application forms for patient assistance programs, and referring patients to state-sponsored services and community assistance programs.

In a survey of 519 cardiologists and general internists, nearly all reported that doctors should consider these costs when writing prescriptions. The study appeared in the March 28, 2005, issue of the *Archives of Internal Medicine*. One-third reported knowing how much patients are spending out of pocket for prescriptions. Commonly cited barriers to discussing drug costs with patients were insufficient time and concern over possible patient discomfort.

The researchers found that switching patients to a generic or a less expensive brand-name drug, the most frequently used strategy, was likely to be beneficial. But they noted that other approaches, such as tablet splitting, needed caution. Tablet splitting is done because higher-strength tablets are sometimes not much more expensive than lower-dose tablets. For example, tablet splitting involves splitting a 40 milligram (mg) tablet to get a 20 mg dose. The researchers said that while tablet splitting can reduce costs, it can also complicate prescription regimens and can be technically difficult to do.

"We don't advocate splitting pills to save money, and this isn't something patients should do on their own," says Tom McGinnis, R.Ph., the FDA's Director of Pharmacy Affairs. "We leave it up to the doctors. If the prescriber thinks a patient could benefit from a lower dose of medication than is available or if it's the only way a patient can afford the treatment, then the doctor can direct that a patient split the tablet. Pharmacies sell inexpensive devices that help consumers easily split tablets of all shapes." McGinnis says. The major concerns over tablet splitting are that the patient may not split the pills accurately and that some tablets, such as time-release versions, should never be split.

The practice of physicians distributing free samples of brand-name drugs—another area that isn't clear-cut—was the second most likely strategy used by doctors in the study to help ease cost concerns. Hunter says he thinks free samples influence doctors to prescribe expensive, new medications, but he has also worked in clinics where patients rely on free samples to reduce their drug costs.

"The intended use of a free sample is to allow a patient to evaluate side effects and effectiveness for a couple of weeks before actually buying the drug," Hunter says. "So patients can ask for free samples, but know that they are a temporary fix." Patients can't usually expect samples to provide long-term treatment. Patients who receive free samples should still ask their physicians whether a generic drug could be satisfactory.

Nicole Petersen, Pharm.D., a community clinical pharmacist at Schnuck's Pharmacy in St. Louis, says that samples aren't always the ideal solution, but sometimes they are all a patient has. When an 86-year-old woman walked out of the pharmacy without her medicine because she couldn't afford a $70 brand-name osteoporosis drug, Petersen called the patient's doctor to see what could be done. "There was no generic alternative, so the doctor gave her some free samples," Petersen says. "But patients have to consider how long the physician can provide the free samples and what to do when they run out."

It might make sense for patients to take free samples while they are waiting to receive drugs through a prescription assistance program (PAP), she says. "If you do take free samples, you should still let your pharmacist know so that we can stay on top of drug interactions." Also, consumers should ask their doctors for information about the sample drug's directions, side effects, and warnings.

Some doctors don't stock free samples, which are normally distributed to doctors' offices by pharmaceutical sales representatives. Billi

275

says drug samples have been eliminated at University of Michigan clinics. "The samples are a marketing tool," he says. "They aren't intended for maintenance. Giving them out puts doctors in the position of having to act like a pharmacist because you're supposed to keep up with lot numbers and expiration dates in case there are recalls. You're also getting patients started on a more expensive drug."

Medicare Prescription Drug Coverage

Medicare part D, the new outpatient drug coverage which began on Jan. 1, 2006, works like other health insurance plans. Medicare beneficiaries are able to choose from at least two prescription drug coverage plans. Those plans will cover drugs for all medically necessary treatments, will pay for brand-name and generic drugs, and will enable beneficiaries to get prescriptions at a pharmacy or through mail order.

Assistance from Pharmaceutical Companies

Two main types of assistance are available from pharmaceutical companies. Several companies offer programs that allow consumers to take a discount drug card to the pharmacy to get a discount off of the price of prescription drugs. And most major pharmaceutical companies offer prescription assistance programs (PAP), which give free or low-cost medicines to people in need. These programs typically target people without health insurance and people who don't qualify for government-funded programs.

Maggie Kohn, a spokeswoman for the drug manufacturer Merck, says that unlike many other programs, Merck's discount program offers discounts of 15 percent to 40 percent on many of the company's medicines to uninsured patients, regardless of age or income. About 15,000 people signed up for the program within the first few weeks that it began in April 2005, Kohn says.

Merck's PAP supplied 700,000 patients with 6.7 million prescriptions valued at $490 million in 2004, Kohn says. Patients may qualify if they have a household income below $19,140 for individuals, $25,660 for couples, and $38,700 for a family of four. "We do sometimes make exceptions for patients whose incomes exceed these amounts in special circumstances like if they are taking a number of medicines," Kohn says.

The Partnership for Prescription Assistance (PPA), which was launched in April 2005, is an industry initiative that is helping patients find assistance programs faster. "With one call," GlaxoSmithKline spokeswoman Patty Seif says, "patients are directed to programs that could be most helpful." The PPA provides a single point of access to more than 275 public and private PAP, including more than 150 programs offered by drug companies. The PPA also will show people how to contact Medicare and other government programs.

"We know that medicines, when taken as prescribed, improve lives and decrease overall health care spending," Seif says. "But for people who can't pay for them, any price is too high. That's why GlaxoSmithKline (GSK) and the pharmaceutical industry support programs that make our programs accessible." In 2004, GSK provided 372.5 million dollars' worth of free medicine.

Every company has its own eligibility criteria for PAP, and, in most cases, U.S. citizenship and some proof of income, such as tax records or a record of social security benefits, are required. Patients can initiate the PAP process on their own by printing forms off the internet or by calling pharmaceutical companies directly to request forms. Patients should fill out as much as possible, and then take the form to their doctor's office. PAP forms require a doctor's signature.

Quick Tips

- Tell your doctor whether paying for prescription drugs is a problem.

- Ask your doctor about generics, another brand of the drug that may cost less, and nonprescription options.

- Find out whether Medicare prescription drug coverage can benefit you and your family members.

- Check to see whether you are eligible for drug assistance programs in your state.

- Check with the pharmaceutical companies that manufacture your medicines to find out whether you qualify for assistance programs.

- Shop around your neighborhood or legitimate online pharmacies for the best prices on prescription drugs.

- The FDA recommends making sure that pharmacists are aware of all products being taken to help avoid drug interactions. These products include prescription and nonprescription drugs, drug samples, herbals, vitamins, and other dietary supplements. Whether you shop at local pharmacies or online, the FDA recommends purchasing only from state-licensed pharmacies that are located in the United States.

Section 37.2

Cost May Result in Underuse of Medications

Excerpted from "Underusing Medications Because of Cost May Lead to Adverse Health Outcomes," National Institute on Aging (NIA), June 25, 2004.

Middle-aged and older Americans with heart disease who cut back on their prescribed medications because of cost were 50% more likely to suffer heart attacks, strokes, or angina than those who did not report cost-related medication underuse, according to a study funded in part by the National Institute on Aging, part of the National Institutes of Health. Michele Heisler, M.D., M.P.A., at the Veterans Affairs Ann Arbor Healthcare System, Ann Arbor, Michigan, and colleagues* conducted the study, which appeared in the July 2004 issue of *Medical Care*, a journal of the American Public Health Association.

This is the first nationally representative longitudinal study to demonstrate that patients with serious chronic illnesses experience adverse health events when they restrict their use of prescription drugs due to cost. The downturns in patients' health were observed over a relatively brief (2–3 year) period, suggesting that cost barriers to prescription drug use may have important short-term effects on older patients' health and well-being, Heisler said.

"This study underlines how important medications can be and how important it is for people who need the medications to be able to get them," said U.S. Health and Human Services (HHS) Secretary Tommy G. Thompson. "This is why a new drug benefit for Medicare was so crucial, including the interim drug card with its special benefit for low-income Americans. It's also why FDA is working to make generic products available quickly, as well as rapid review for significant new medications. We need to keep working toward better access to drugs and keep supporting the science that underlies ever-improving products."

After controlling for risk factors for poor health outcomes, 32% of adults in the study who had restricted medications because of cost pressures reported a significant decline in their self-reported health status during their follow-up interviews compared to 21% of adults with no cost-related underuse. Self-reports of health have been found to strongly predict other serious life events, including mortality, according to the study.

"There is a growing array of effective but often expensive prescription medications that clearly improve health outcomes, especially in the field of cardiovascular disease. As medications become even more effective, differences in access to prescriptions drugs because of cost may further worsen disparities in health outcomes between rich and poor Americans," Heisler said.

"This study suggests what can happen when older people cannot get the medications they need and will help inform policy regarding prescription drug insurance coverage," said Richard M. Suzman, Ph.D., NIA Associate Director for the Behavioral and Social Research Program. "The longitudinal design employed in this study suggests that the cost of drugs can lead to drug underuse and that this underuse could in turn contribute to adverse health outcomes. Additional research will be needed to further examine the causal relationship between drug costs and health outcomes."

In addition to cardiovascular declines, older individuals who restricted medication use because of cost had increased rates of depression, according to the study. Researchers found no health differences among people with arthritis and diabetes who said they had restricted drug use due to cost.

*The study was conducted by Michele Heisler, M.D., M.P.A., Kenneth M. Langa, M.D., Ph.D, Elizabeth L. Eby, M.P.H., A. Mark Fendrick, M.D., Mohammed U. Kabeto, M.S., John D. Piette, Ph.D.

Section 37.3

Purchase Prescription Medicine Online Safely

This section includes text from the following U.S. Food and Drug Administration (FDA) documents: "Buying Prescription Medicine Online: A Consumer Safety Guide," October 2006; "FDA Safety Alert: You Should Not Buy the Drugs Listed Below Over the Internet," March 2007; and "FDA Warns Consumers about Counterfeit Drugs from Multiple Internet Sellers," May 2007.

Buying Your Medicine Online Can Be Easy: Just Make Sure You Do It Safely

The internet has changed the way we live, work, and shop. The growth of the internet has made it possible to compare prices and buy products without ever leaving home. But when it comes to buying medicine online, it is important to be very careful. Some websites sell medicine that may not be safe to use and could put your health at risk.

Some websites that sell medicine:

• are not U.S. state-licensed pharmacies or are not pharmacies at all;

• may give a diagnosis that is not correct and sell medicine that is not right for you or your condition; and

• won't protect your personal information.

Some medicines sold online:

• are fake (counterfeit or copycat medicines);

• are too strong or too weak;

• have dangerous ingredients;

• have expired (are out-of-date);

• are not FDA-approved (have not been checked for safety and effectiveness);

• are not made using safe standards;

- are not safe to use with other medicine or products you use; and
- are not labeled, stored, or shipped correctly.

Meet and Talk with Your Doctor

- Talk with your doctor and have a physical exam before you get any new medicine for the first time.
- Use only medicine that has been prescribed by your doctor or another trusted professional who is licensed in the U.S. to write prescriptions for medicine.
- Ask your doctor if there are any special steps you need to take to fill your prescription.

If You Buy Medicine Online: Know Your Source to Make Sure It Is Safe

Make sure a website is a state-licensed pharmacy that is located in the United States. Pharmacies and pharmacists in the United States are licensed by a state's board of pharmacy. Your state board of pharmacy can tell you if a website is a state-licensed pharmacy, is in good standing, and is located in the United States. Find a list of state boards of pharmacy on the National Association of Boards of Pharmacy (NABP) website at http://www.nabp.info.

The NABP is a professional association of the state boards of pharmacy. It has a program to help you find some of the pharmacies that are licensed to sell medicine online. Internet websites that display the seal of this program have been checked to make sure they meet state and federal rules. For more on this program and a list of pharmacies that display the Verified Internet Pharmacy Practice Sites™ Seal, (VIPPS® Seal), go to http://www.vipps.info.

Look for websites with practices that protect you. A safe website should:

- be located in the United States and licensed by the state board of pharmacy where the website is operating (check http://www.nabp.info for a list of state boards of pharmacy);
- have a licensed pharmacist to answer your questions;
- require a prescription from your doctor or other health care professional who is licensed in the United States to write prescriptions for medicine; and
- have a way for you to talk to a person if you have problems.

Be Sure Your Privacy Is Protected

- Look for privacy and security policies that are easy-to-find and easy-to-understand.

- Do not give any personal information (such as social security number, credit card, or medical or health history), unless you are sure the website will keep your information safe and private.

- Make sure that the site will not sell your information, unless you agree.

Protect Yourself and Others

- Report websites you are not sure of, or if you have complaints about a site. Go to http://www.fda.gov/buyonline and click on "Notify FDA about problem websites."

Do Not Buy These Drugs from Internet or Foreign Sources

The drugs on this list have important benefits, but they also have serious known risks. As a result, they are available in the U.S. only under specially created safety controls. If these drugs are bought over the internet or from foreign sources, these safety controls are bypassed, placing patients who use these drugs at higher risk. In addition, drugs bought from foreign sources are generally not FDA approved.

- Accutane (isotretinoin): indicated for the treatment of severe recalcitrant nodular acne.

- Actiq (fentanyl citrate): indicated for the management of severe cancer pain in patients who are tolerant to opioid therapy.

- Clozaril (clozapine): indicated for the management of severe schizophrenia in patients who fail to respond to standard drug treatments for schizophrenia.

- Humatrope (somatropin for injection): indicated for the treatment of non-growth hormone-deficient short stature.

- Lotronex (alosetron hydrochloride): indicated for the treatment of severe irritable bowel syndrome in women.

- Mifeprex (mifepristone or RU-486): indicated for the medical termination of early intrauterine pregnancy.

- Plenaxis (abarelix for injectable suspension): indicated for the treatment of advanced symptomatic prostate cancer in men who are not able to receive other types of treatment.

- Thalomid (thalidomide): indicated for the acute treatment of the cutaneous manifestations of moderate to severe erythema nodosum leprosum.

- Tikosyn (dofetilide): indicated for the maintenance of normal sinus rhythm in patients with certain cardiac arrhythmia.

- Tracleer (bosentan): indicated for the treatment of severe pulmonary arterial hypertension.

- Trovan (trovafloxacin mesylate or alatrofloxacin mesylate injection): an antibiotic administered in in-patient health care settings for the treatment of severe, life-threatening infections.

- Xyrem (sodium oxybate): indicated for the treatment of cataplexy in patients with narcolepsy.

FDA Warns Consumers about Counterfeit Drugs from Multiple Internet Sellers

The Food and Drug Administration (FDA) is cautioning U.S. consumers about dangers associated with buying prescription drugs over the internet. This alert is being issued based on information the agency received showing that 24 apparently related websites may be involved in the distribution of counterfeit prescription drugs.

On three occasions during recent months, FDA received information that counterfeit versions of Xenical 120 milligrams (mg) capsules, a drug manufactured by Hoffmann-La Roche Inc. (Roche), were obtained by three consumers from two different websites. Xenical is an FDA-approved drug used to help obese individuals who meet certain weight and height requirements lose weight and maintain weight loss.

None of the capsules ordered off the websites contained orlistat, the active ingredient in authentic Xenical. In fact, laboratory analysis conducted by Roche and submitted to the FDA confirmed that one capsule contained sibutramine, which is the active ingredient in Meridia, an FDA-approved prescription drug manufactured by Abbott Laboratories.

While this product is also used to help people lose weight and maintain that loss, it should not be used in certain patient populations and therefore is not a substitute for other weight loss products. In addition the drug interactions profile is different between Xenical and sibutramine, as is the dosing frequency; sibutramine is administered once daily while Xenical is dosed three times a day.

Other samples of drug product obtained from two of the internet orders were composed of only talc and starch. According to Roche, these two samples displayed a valid Roche lot number of B2306 and were labeled with an expiration date of April 2007. The correct expiration date for this lot number is actually March 2005.

Roche identified the two websites involved in this incident as brandpills.com and pillspharm.com. Further investigation by FDA disclosed that these websites are two of 24 websites that appear on the pharmacycall365.com home page under the "Our Websites" heading. Four of these websites previously have been identified by FDA's Office of Criminal Investigations as being associated with the distribution of counterfeit Tamiflu and counterfeit Cialis.

At this point, it appears that these websites are operated from outside of the United States. Consumers should be wary, if there is no way to contact the website pharmacy by phone, if prices are dramatically lower than the competition, or if no prescription from your doctor is required. As a result, FDA strongly cautions consumers about purchasing drugs from any of these websites which may be involved in the distribution of counterfeit drugs and reiterates previous public warnings about buying prescription drugs online. Consumers are urged to review the FDA web page at http://www.fda.gov/buyonline for additional information prior to making purchases of prescription drugs over the internet.

The 24 websites that appear on pharmacycall365.com include:

- AllPills.net
- Pharmacy-4U.net
- DirectMedsMall.com
- Brandpills.com
- Emediline.com
- RX-ed.com
- RXePharm.com
- Pharmacea.org
- PillsPharm.com
- MensHealthDrugs.net
- BigXplus.net
- MediClub.md
- InterTab.de
- Pillenpharm.com
- Bigger-X.com
- PillsLand.com
- EZMEDZ.com
- UnitedMedicals.com
- Best-Medz.com
- USAPillsrx.net
- USAMedz.com
- BluePills-Rx.com
- Genericpharmacy.us
- I-Kusuri.jp

Section 37.4

Truth in Advertising: Ads for Prescription Drugs

This section includes excerpts from "Truth in Advertising: Rx Drug Ads Come of Age," by Carol Rados, *FDA Consumer magazine* July-August 2004, U. S. Food and Drug Administration (FDA); and "No Need to Pay for Information on Free (or Low-Cost) Rx Drugs," Federal Trade Commission (FTC), March 2005.

Rx Drug Ads Come of Age

Direct-to-consumer (DTC) advertising of prescription drugs in its varied forms—television, radio, magazines, newspapers—is widely used throughout the United States. DTC advertising is a category of promotional information about specific drug treatments provided directly to consumers by or on behalf of drug companies. According to the U.S. General Accounting Office—the investigational arm of Congress—pharmaceutical manufacturers spent $2.7 billion on DTC advertising in 2001 alone.

The Controversy

Whether it is a 1940s, detective-style film noir of unusual allergy suspects or a middle-aged man throwing a football through a tire swing announcing that he's "back in the game," the DTC approach to advertising prescription drugs has been controversial. Some say that DTC promotion provides useful information to consumers which results in better health outcomes. Others argue that it encourages overuse of prescription drugs and use of the most costly treatments, instead of less expensive treatments that would be just as satisfactory.

There seems to be little doubt that DTC advertising can help advance the public health by encouraging more people to talk with health care professionals about health problems, particularly undertreated conditions such as high blood pressure and high cholesterol. DTC advertising also can help remove the stigma that accompanies diseases that in the past were rarely openly discussed, such as erectile dysfunction or depression. DTC ads also can remind patients to get their prescriptions refilled and help them adhere to their medication regimens.

On the other hand, ads that are false or misleading do not advance—and may even threaten—the public health. While the FDA encourages DTC advertisements that contain accurate information, the agency also has the job of making sure that consumers are not misled or deceived by advertisements that violate the law.

"The goal here is getting truthful, non-misleading information to consumers about safe and effective therapeutic products so they can be partners in their own health care," says Peter Pitts, the FDA's associate commissioner for external relations. "Better-informed consumers are empowered to choose and use the products we regulate to improve their health."

In three FDA surveys conducted in 1999 and 2002, physicians reported that DTC ads had these beneficial effects for patients:

- 53% had better discussions between doctors and patients
- 42% of patients were more aware of treatments
- 10% of patients were better informed
- 10% of patients were more likely to take prescribed medicine
- 9% of patients were more likely to consider a Rx drug
- 6% discovered a new condition
- 2% of patients sought treatment for a serious condition

How Ads Affect Consumers

The FDA surveyed both patients and physicians about their attitudes and experiences with DTC advertising between 1999 and 2002. The agency summarized the findings of these surveys in January 2003 in the report, *Assessment of Physician and Patient Attitudes Toward Direct-to-Consumer Promotion of Prescription Drugs.*

DTC advertising appears to influence certain types of behavior. For example, the FDA surveys found that among patients who visited doctors and asked about a prescription drug by brand name because of an ad they saw, 88 percent actually had the condition the drug treats. This is important, Pitts says, because physician visits that result in earlier detection of a disease, combined with appropriate treatment, could mean that more people will live longer, healthier, more productive lives without the risk of future costly medical interventions.

With the number of ailments Patricia A. Sigler lives with—diabetes, fibromyalgia, high blood pressure, high cholesterol, nerve damage, and a heart defect called mitral valve prolapse—the 64-year-old small business owner in Jefferson, Maryland, says that she's always on the lookout for medicines that might improve her quality of life, and that she pays attention to DTC ads for prescription drugs.

Some Doctors Don't Agree

Michael S. Wilkes, M.D., vice dean of the medical school at the University of California, Davis, says that reasons he doesn't like DTC advertising are that patients may withhold information from their doctors or try to treat themselves. Also, aiming prescription drug ads at consumers can affect the "dynamics of the patient-provider relationship," and ultimately, the patient's quality of care, Wilkes says. DTC advertising can motivate consumers to seek more information about a product or disease, but physicians need to help patients evaluate health-related information they obtain from DTC advertising, he says.

"DTC advertising may cultivate the belief among the public that there is a pill for every ill and contribute to the medicalization of trivial ailments, leading to an even more overmedicated society," Wilkes says. "Patients need to trust that I've got their best interest in mind."

Others who favor DTC ads say that consumer-directed information can be an important educational tool in a time when more patients want to be involved in their own health care. Carol Salzman, M.D., Ph.D., an internist in Chevy Chase, Maryland, emphasizes, however, that physicians still need to remain in control of prescribing medications.

"Doctors shouldn't feel threatened by their patients asking for a medicine by name," she says, "but at the same time, patients shouldn't come in expecting that a drug will be dispensed just because they asked for it." Salzman says she finds it time-consuming "trying to talk people out of something they have their hearts set on." Wilkes agrees. Discussions motivated by ads that focus on specific drugs or trivial complaints, he says, could take time away from subjects such as a patient's symptoms, the range of available treatments, and specific details about a patient's illness.

Education or Promotion

At least one patient advocacy group is concerned about what it says are the downsides of advertising prescription drugs directly to consumers, claiming that DTC ads often masquerade as educational tools, but provide more promotion than education. The ads, they say, provide little access to unbiased information.

"People need to be careful with ads that it isn't just hype that they're going to feel better, with no objectivity of the downsides," says Linda Golodner, president of the National Consumers League in Washington, DC. Although all DTC advertisements must disclose risk information, she says what is typically communicated is a brand name, a reason to use the product, and an impression of the product.

Truth in Advertising

The FDA has regulated the advertising of prescription drugs since 1962, under the Federal Food, Drug, and Cosmetic Act and related regulations. The regulations establish detailed requirements for ad content. Most other advertising, including that of over-the-counter drugs, is regulated by the Federal Trade Commission under a different set of rules.

The FDA's Division of Drug Marketing, Advertising, and Communications (DDMAC) oversees two types of promotion for prescription drugs: promotional labeling and advertising. Advertising includes commercial messages broadcast on television or radio, communicated over the telephone, or printed in magazines and newspapers. Prescription drug ads must contain information in a brief summary relating to both risks and benefits. Recognizing the time constraints of broadcast ads, FDA regulations provide that a broadcast advertisement may include, instead of a brief summary, information relating to the major risks. The ad must also make adequate provision for distributing the FDA-approved labeling in connection with the broadcast ad. This refers to the concept of providing ways for consumers to find more complete information about the drug.

Most ads fulfill this requirement by including a toll-free telephone number, a website address, or a link to a concurrently running print ad. They also encourage consumers to talk to their health care providers. Both print and broadcast ads directed at consumers may only make claims that are supported by scientific evidence.

DDMAC oversight helps ensure that pharmaceutical companies accurately communicate the benefits and risks of an advertised drug. The regulations require that advertising for prescription drugs must disclose certain information about the product's uses and risks.

In addition, advertisements cannot be false or misleading and cannot omit material facts. FDA regulations also call for fair balance in every product-claim ad. This means that the risks and benefits must be presented with comparable scope, depth, and detail; and that information relating to the product's effectiveness must be fairly balanced by risk information.

The FDA does not generally require prior approval of DTC ads, although companies are required to submit their ads to the FDA at the time they begin running. The agency, therefore, routinely examines these commercials and published DTC ads after they become available to the public. FDA, however, also is happy to review proposed ads if a drug company makes a request.

"We look at a lot of DTC ads before they run," says Kathryn J. Aikin, Ph.D., a social scientist in DDMAC. "Manufacturers typically want to be sure they're getting started on the right foot."

The Trouble with Ads

Of the three types of DTC advertisements, the first and most common—product-claim ads—mention a drug's name and the condition it is intended to treat, and describe the risks and benefits associated with taking the drug. Some manufacturers have decided not to present this much information and instead, have made use of two other kinds of ads. Reminder ads give only the name of the product, but not what it is used for, and help-seeking ads contain information about a disease, but do not mention a specific drug. These help-seeking—or disease-awareness—ads can be extremely informative and, because they name no drug, they are not regulated by the FDA. Examples of help-seeking ads are those that mention high cholesterol or diabetes, and then direct you to ask your doctor about treatments. Reminder ads call attention to a drug's name, but say nothing about the condition it is used to treat, its effectiveness, or safety information. A reminder ad is not required to include risk information.

There has been a great deal of discussion about the brief summary that accompanies DTC print ads. The typical brief summary is not brief and uses technical language. This is because it reprints all of the risk information from the physician labeling. People have complained that the brief summary cannot be understood by consumers. Aikin says, "Patients do not typically read the brief summary in DTC print ads unless they're interested in the product." Even then, she says, much information is likely glanced at, rather than fully read.

DTC Ads at a Glance

Product-claim ads:

- mention a drug by name;

- make representations about the drug, such as its safety and effectiveness;

- must have fair balance of information about effectiveness and risks;

- are required to disclose risks in a "brief summary" of benefits and risks (for print ads); and

- are required to give a "major statement" of risks and "adequate provision" for finding out more, such as a toll-free number (for broadcast ads).

Reminder ads:

- provide the name of the medication;

- may provide other minimal information, such as cost and dosage form;

- do not make a representation about the drug, such as the drug's use, effectiveness, or safety; and

- are not required to provide risk information.

Help-seeking ads:

- educate consumers about a disease or medical condition;

- let people know that treatments exist for a medical condition;

- don't name a specific drug; and

- are not required to provide risk information.

No Need to Pay for Information on Free (or Low-Cost) Rx Drugs

Have you gotten spam e-mail claiming that free or low-cost prescription drugs are just a phone call away? Have you visited a website offering to help you get free prescription drugs—for a fee? If so, you may be looking at a scam.

According to the Federal Trade Commission (FTC), America's consumer protection agency, some marketers are using spam e-mail and the web to offer information on free or low-cost prescription drug programs for a fee, sometimes as much as $195. Federal officials encourage you to steer clear of any company that charges for information on free or low-cost prescription drug programs.

While it is true that many prescription drug companies offer free or low-cost drugs for people who do not have prescription drug coverage, cannot afford to pay for medication out of pocket, or have exhausted their insurance's annual allowance, the programs have strict qualification standards. Factors that affect whether you qualify may include your income and the cost of the drugs you need.

If you are trying to get free or low-cost prescription drugs, you do not have to pay for information on how to do it. You just have to know where to look. The information is free—and publicly available—from your physician, pharmacists, and the government.

A drug company trade group sponsors a one stop website at http://www.helpingpatients.org. The site provides information on patient assistance programs for consumers who do not have prescription drug coverage. Industry and government patient assistance programs offer an estimated 1,000 medicines to treat a variety of diseases and conditions, including cancer, high cholesterol, diabetes, high blood pressure, stroke, depression, schizophrenia, and Alzheimer disease.

You can apply for free or low-cost prescription programs or medicines on the website, or you can ask your health care provider to do it for you. A computer program determines whether there might be a match for you among the various programs. Health care providers must approve most applications for these assistance programs.

Additionally, http://www.accesstobenefits.org is a website with information on many programs to help seniors and people with disabilities reduce their prescription drug costs. The site is sponsored by a coalition of organizations serving Medicare beneficiaries. These programs offer the most help if you do not have other prescription drug coverage and if your income is limited.

Finally, you can access the federal government's Medicare information at http://www.medicare.gov or by calling 800-633-2273.

For More Information

Federal Trade Commission (FTC)
Consumer Response Center
600 Pennsylvania Ave., N.W.
Washington, DC 20580
Toll-Free: 877-382-4357, Toll-Free TTY: 866-653-4261
Website: http://www.ftc.gov

The FTC works for the consumer to prevent fraudulent, deceptive, and unfair business practices in the marketplace and to provide information to help consumers spot, stop, and avoid them. The FTC enters internet, telemarketing, identity theft, and other fraud-related complaints into Consumer Sentinel, a secure online database available to hundreds of civil and criminal law enforcement agencies in the U.S. and abroad.

Chapter 38

Facts about Generic Drugs

What are generic drugs?

A generic drug is the same as a brand-name drug in the following:

- dosage
- safety
- strength
- quality
- the way it works
- the way it is taken
- the way it should be used

Are generic drugs as safe as brand-name drugs?

Yes. The FDA says that all drugs must work well and be safe. Generic drugs use the same active ingredients as brand-name drugs and work the same way. So they have the same risks and benefits as the brand-name drugs.

Are generic drugs as strong as brand-name drugs?

Yes. FDA requires that generic drugs be the same as brand-name drugs in the following characteristics:

- high quality
- strong
- pure
- stable

"Facts about Generic Drugs," Center for Drug Evaluation and Research, U.S. Food and Drug Administration (FDA-CDER), updated August 7, 2006.

Are brand-name drugs made in better factories than generic drugs?

No. All factories must meet the same high standards. If the factories do not meet certain standards, the FDA won't allow them to make drugs.

If brand-name drugs and generic drugs have the same active ingredients, why do they look different?

In the United States, trademark laws do not allow generic drugs to look exactly like the brand-name drug. However, the generic drug must have the same active ingredients. Colors, flavors, and certain other parts may be different. But these things do not affect the way the drug works and they are looked at by FDA.

Does every brand-name drug have a generic drug?

No. When new drugs are first made they have drug patents. Most drug patents are protected for 17 years. The patent protects the company that made the drug first. The patent does not allow anyone else to make and sell the drug. When the patent expires, other drug companies can start selling the generic version of the drug. But, first, they must test the drug and the FDA must approve it.

What is the best source of information about generic drugs?

Contact your doctor, pharmacist, or other health care worker for information on your generic drugs. For more information, you can also visit the FDA website at: http://www.fda.gov/cder.

Do generic drugs take longer to work in the body?

No. Generic drugs work in the same way and in the same amount of time as brand-name drugs.

Why are generic drugs less expensive?

Creating a drug costs lots of money. Since generic drug makers do not develop a drug from scratch, the costs to bring the drug to market are less. But they must show that their product performs in the same way as the brand-name drug. All generic drugs are approved by FDA. Your medication guide should be kept with you and up to date. List your prescription and over-the-counter medicines as well as your dietary supplements.

Chapter 39

Taking Medicine

Chapter Contents

Section 39.1

Know when Antibiotics Work

Excerpts from "About Antibiotic Resistance," Centers for Disease
Control and Prevention (CDC), April 2006; and "Frequently Asked
Questions: Know When Antibiotics Work," CDC, February 2007.

What is an antibiotic?

Antibiotics, also known as antimicrobial drugs, are drugs that fight
infections caused by bacteria. Alexander Fleming discovered the first
antibiotic, penicillin, in 1927. After the first use of antibiotics in the
1940s, they transformed medical care and dramatically reduced illness and death from infectious diseases.

The term antibiotic originally referred to a natural compound produced by a fungus or another microorganism that kills bacteria which
cause disease in humans or animals. Some antibiotics may be synthetic compounds (not produced by microorganisms) that can also kill
or inhibit the growth of microbes. Technically, the term antimicrobial
agent refers to both natural and synthetic compounds; however, many
people use the word antibiotic to refer to both. Although antibiotics
have many beneficial effects, their use has created the new problem
of antibiotic resistance.

What is antibiotic resistance?

Antibiotic resistance is the ability of bacteria or other microbes to
resist the effects of an antibiotic. Antibiotic resistance occurs when bacteria change in some way that reduces or eliminates the effectiveness
of drugs, chemicals, or other agents designed to cure or prevent infections. The bacteria survive and continue to multiply causing more harm.

Why should I be concerned about antibiotic resistance?

Antibiotic resistance has been called one of the world's most pressing public health problems. Over the last decade, almost every type of
bacteria has become stronger and less responsive to antibiotic treatment

when it is really needed. These antibiotic-resistant bacteria can quickly spread to family members, schoolmates, and co-workers—threatening the community with a new strain of infectious disease that is more difficult to cure and more expensive to treat. For this reason, antibiotic resistance is among the top concerns of the Centers for Disease Prevention and Control (CDC).

Antibiotic resistance can cause significant danger and suffering for children and adults who have common infections, once easily treatable with antibiotics. Microbes can develop resistance to specific medicines. A common misconception is that a person's body becomes resistant to specific drugs. However, it is the microbes, not people, which become resistant to the drugs.

If a microbe is resistant to many drugs, treating the infections it causes can become difficult or even impossible. Someone with an infection that is resistant to a certain medicine can pass that resistant infection to another person. In this way, a hard-to-treat illness can be spread from person to person. In some cases, the illness can lead to serious disability or even death.

Why are bacteria becoming resistant to antibiotics?

Antibiotic use promotes development of antibiotic-resistant bacteria. Every time a person takes antibiotics, sensitive bacteria are killed, but resistant germs may be left to grow and multiply. Repeated and improper uses of antibiotics are primary causes of the increase in drug-resistant bacteria.

While antibiotics should be used to treat bacterial infections, they are not effective against viral infections like the common cold, most sore throats, and the flu. Widespread use of antibiotics promotes the spread of antibiotic resistance. Smart use of antibiotics is the key to controlling the spread of resistance.

How do bacteria become resistant to antibiotics?

Antibiotic resistance occurs when bacteria change in some way that reduces or eliminates the effectiveness of drugs, chemicals, or other agents designed to cure or prevent infections. The bacteria survive and continue to multiply causing more harm. Bacteria can do this through several mechanisms. Some bacteria develop the ability to neutralize the antibiotic before it can do harm, others can rapidly pump the antibiotic out, and still others can change the antibiotic attack site so it cannot affect the function of the bacteria.

Antibiotics kill or inhibit the growth of susceptible bacteria. Sometimes one of the bacteria survives because it has the ability to neutralize or evade the effect of the antibiotic; that one bacterium can then multiply and replace all the bacteria that were killed off. Exposure to antibiotics therefore provides selective pressure, which makes the surviving bacteria more likely to be resistant. In addition, bacteria that were at one time susceptible to an antibiotic can acquire resistance through mutation of their genetic material or by acquiring pieces of deoxyribonucleic acid (DNA) that code for the resistance properties from other bacteria. The DNA that codes for resistance can be grouped in a single easily transferable package. This means that bacteria can become resistant to many antimicrobial agents because of the transfer of one piece of DNA.

How can I prevent antibiotic-resistant infections?

It is important to understand that, although they are very useful drugs, antibiotics designed for bacterial infections are not useful for viral infections such as a cold, cough, or flu. Some useful tips to remember are:

1. Talk with your health care provider about antibiotic resistance:

   • Ask whether an antibiotic is likely to be beneficial for your illness.

   • Ask what else you can do to feel better sooner.

2. Do not take an antibiotic for a viral infection like a cold or the flu.

3. Do not save some of your antibiotic for the next time you get sick. Discard any leftover medication once you have completed your prescribed course of treatment.

4. Take an antibiotic exactly as the health care provider tells you. Do not skip doses. Complete the prescribed course of treatment even if you are feeling better. If treatment stops too soon, some bacteria may survive and re-infect.

5. Do not take antibiotics prescribed for someone else. The antibiotic may not be appropriate for your illness. Taking the wrong medicine may delay correct treatment and allow bacteria to multiply.

6. If your health care provider determines that you do not have a bacterial infection, ask about ways to help relieve your symptoms. Do not pressure your provider to prescribe an antibiotic.

Frequently Asked Questions about Antibiotic Resistance

What are bacteria and viruses?

Bacteria are single-celled organisms usually found all over the inside and outside of our bodies, except in the blood and spinal fluid. Many bacteria are not harmful. In fact, some are actually beneficial. However, disease-causing bacteria trigger illnesses, such as strep throat and some ear infections. Viruses are even smaller than bacteria. A virus cannot survive outside the body's cells. It causes illnesses by invading healthy cells and reproducing.

What kinds of infections are caused by viruses and should not be treated with antibiotics?

Infections caused by viruses include colds, flu, most coughs, bronchitis, and sore throats (except for those resulting from strep throat). These should not be treated with antibiotics.

How do I know when an illness is caused by a viral or bacterial infection?

Sometimes it is very hard to tell. Consult with your doctor to be sure.

When do I need to take antibiotics?

Antibiotics are very powerful medications. They should only be used when prescribed by a doctor to treat bacterial infections.

Do I need an antibiotic when mucus from the nose changes to yellow or green?

Yellow or green mucus does not indicate a bacterial infection. It is normal for the mucus to get thick and change color during a viral cold.

Should I ask my doctor to prescribe antibiotics?

Talk to your doctor about the best treatment. You should not expect to get a prescription for antibiotics. If you have a viral infection, antibiotics will not cure it, help you feel better, or prevent someone else from getting your virus.

What can I do to avoid antibiotic-resistant infections?

Start by talking with your health care provider about antibiotic resistance.

- Ask whether an antibiotic is likely to be effective in treating your illness.

- Do not demand an antibiotic when your health care provider determines one is not appropriate.

- Ask what else you can do to help relieve your symptoms.

What can I do to protect my child from antibiotic-resistant bacteria?

Use antibiotics only when your doctor has determined that they are likely to be effective. Antibiotics will not cure most colds, coughs, sore throats, or runny noses. Children fight off colds on their own.

Does this mean that I should never give my child antibiotics?

Antibiotics are very powerful medicines and should only be used to treat bacterial infections. If an antibiotic is prescribed, make sure you take the entire course and never save the medication for later use.

How do I know if my child has a viral or bacterial infection?

Ask your doctor. If you think that your child might need treatment, you should contact your doctor. But remember, colds are caused by viruses and should not be treated with antibiotics.

Facts about Antibiotic Resistance

- Antibiotic resistance has been called one of the world's most pressing public health problems.

- The number of bacteria resistant to antibiotics has increased in the last decade. Nearly all significant bacterial infections in the world are becoming resistant to the most commonly prescribed antibiotic treatments.

- Every time a person takes antibiotics, sensitive bacteria are killed, but resistant germs may be left to grow and multiply. Repeated and improper uses of antibiotics are primary causes of the increase in drug-resistant bacteria.

- Misuse of antibiotics jeopardizes the usefulness of essential drugs. Decreasing inappropriate antibiotic use is the best way to control resistance.

- Children are of particular concern because they have the highest rates of antibiotic use. They also have the highest rate of infections caused by antibiotic-resistant pathogens.

- Parent pressure makes a difference. For pediatric care, a recent study showed that doctors prescribe antibiotics 65% of the time if they perceive parents expect them; and 12% of the time if they feel parents do not expect them.

- Antibiotic resistance can cause significant danger and suffering for people who have common infections that once were easily treatable with antibiotics. When antibiotics fail to work, the consequences are longer-lasting illnesses; more doctor visits or extended hospital stays; and the need for more expensive and toxic medications. Some resistant infections can cause death.

Cold and Flu Season: No Reason for Antibiotics

Colds, flu, and most sore throats and bronchitis are caused by viruses. Antibiotics do not help fight viruses. And they may do more harm than good: taking antibiotics when they are not needed—and cannot treat the illness—increases the risk of a resistant infection later.

Section 39.2

Tips for Taking Medications

Excerpted from "Taking Your Medicine," by Harrison Wein, Ph.D., *Word on Health*, April 2001, National Institutes of Health (NIH). Reviewed in November, 2007 by Dr. David A. Cooke, M.D., Diplomate, American Board of Internal Medicine.

Taking Medications

When it comes to following a complicated medication regimen, there are several things you need to be able to do. First, you have to understand the instructions: when to take the medicines and what kinds of restrictions there are on each one, such as taking it with food or avoiding alcohol. You need to be able to plan a schedule, which can be complicated when several medicines are involved, and to understand and remember that schedule. Finally, you need to be able to remember to take each dose.

Medication Aids

There are many things you can do to help you follow a medication regimen. Dr. Denise Park, who has dedicated her career to studying the aging mind, has experimented with bottle tops that beep when you need to take your medicine and found them very effective. But until such things are widely available, a programmable wristwatch can be a good reminder. A phone service or computer scheduling program might be a good substitute if you are usually at home when you need your medications. However, for people taking medicines on different schedules, Dr. Park is reluctant to recommend these simple time reminders without something else to tell them which medicine they are supposed to take each time. Pill organizers with a different compartment for various times of the day can help people stick to a schedule.

But often the most difficult part of taking several medicines is simply figuring out what the regimen is supposed to be in the first place. "I think it would be really useful for a health professional to sit down and ask the person to write out a medication plan," Dr. Park says. It is best for the patient to produce the plan, drawing out a day by day, hour by hour schedule of when they have to take all their medications. It could be a grid with dates and times detailing when to take each medicine, along with any restrictions on them. A plan can be in the form of a poster, a booklet, or just a sheet of paper. Checking off each medicine as it is taken can help you make sure you are following the regimen properly.

"Understand as much about why you're taking these things as you can," Dr. Park advises. "That helps adherence." On drugs that are crucial for a person's health, she says, people are generally very adherent, particularly older people. "One of the reasons is that people's lives depend on this, people's health depends on this, and they know it."

The last advice Dr. Park has is to build a consistent, structured schedule for taking your medications into your daily life. "Behaviors become automatic and almost unconsciously performed over time," she says. "For example, you get to your office and realize you have no memory of how you got there. Taking medications can similarly become just as automatic, having daily routines that are highly structured leads to greater adherence." For example, you might decide to take one medication after you brush your teeth every morning. Dr. Park thinks that people who have a sudden-onset medical condition like a heart attack tend to have a harder time following a complicated regimen than those whose regimens gradually build in complexity. The latter have had time to slowly build these things into their lifestyles and incorporate them into their daily schedules.

A Word to the Wise—Medication Tips

- Keep a daily checklist of all the medicines you take. Include both prescription and over-the-counter (OTC) medicines. Note the name of each medicine, the doctor who prescribed it, the amount you take, and the times of day you take it. Keep a copy in your medicine cabinet and one in your wallet or pocketbook.

- Read and save any written information that comes with the medicine.

- Check the label on your medicine before taking it to make sure that it is for the correct person—you—with the correct directions prescribed for you by your doctor.

- Take your medicine in the exact amount and precise schedule your doctor prescribes.

- Check the expiration dates on your medicine bottles and throw away medicine that has expired.

- Call your doctor right away if you have any problems with your medicines or if you are worried that the medicine might be doing more harm than good. He or she may be able to change your medicine to another one that will work just as well.

Cautions

- Do not take medicines prescribed for another person or give yours to someone else.

- Do not stop taking a prescription drug unless your doctor says it's okay—even if you are feeling better.

- Do not take more or less than the prescribed amount of any medicine.

- Do not use alcohol while taking a medicine unless your doctor says it is okay. Some medicines may not work well or may make you sick if you drink alcohol.

A Complicated Problem

There's no simple solution to helping people follow their medication regimens. People will be healthier if they understand their own health problems and how to manage them. A spoonful of sugar may help the medicine go down, but if you can not remember which of your medicines to take and when to take them, the sugar's not much help.

Helping a Family Member Follow a Medication Regime

Some people are not able to understand why they are taking their medicines and are not capable of making up a daily plan for when to take each one. These people need a health professional or family member to draw up a plan for them and to figure out a system of reminders. If you have a friend or family member in this situation, try to get them as involved in the process as possible.

In designing a schedule and a reminder system, be creative and keep working with your relative to figure out what will work best for them. The more they understand about why they are taking these medicines, the more likely they will be able to follow the regimen.

Remember that it is absolutely crucial for pill organizers to be loaded properly. All the planning in the world won't help your relative take their medicines properly if their organizer is not loaded correctly.

Section 39.3

Kids Aren't Just Small Adults: Advice on Giving Medicine to Your Child

This section includes "Kids Aren't Just Small Adults," U.S. Food and Drug Administration (FDA), March 2006; and an excerpt titled "A Prescription for Parents: Understanding Antibiotic Usage," from "Frequently Asked Questions: Know When Antibiotics Work," Centers for Disease Control and Prevention (CDC), February 2007.

Kids Aren't Just Small Adults

Use care when giving any medicine to an infant or a child. Even over-the-counter (OTC) medicines that you buy are serious medicines. The following is advice for giving OTC medicine to your child, from the U.S. Food and Drug Administration (FDA) and the makers of OTC medicines.

1. **Always read and follow the Drug Facts label on your OTC medicine.** This is important for choosing and safely using all OTC medicines. Read the label every time, before you give the medicine. Be sure you clearly understand how much medicine to give and when the medicine can be taken again.

2. **Know the active ingredient in your child's medicine.** This is what makes the medicine work and is always listed at the top of the Drug Facts label. Sometimes an active ingredient can treat more than one medical condition. For that reason, the same active ingredient can be found in many different medicines that are used to treat different symptoms. For example, a medicine for a cold and a medicine for a headache could each contain the same active ingredient. So, if you're treating a cold and a headache with two medicines and both have the same active ingredient, you could be giving two-times the normal dose. If you are confused about your child's medicines, check with a doctor, nurse, or pharmacist.

3. **Give the right medicine, in the right amount, to your child.** Not all medicines are right for an infant or a child.

305

Medicines with the same brand name can be sold in many different strengths—infant, children, and adult formulas. The amount and directions are also different for children of different ages or weights. Always use the right medicine and follow the directions exactly. Never use more medicine than directed, even if your child seems sicker than the last time.

4. **Talk to your doctor, pharmacist, or nurse to find out what mixes well and what doesn't.** Medicines, vitamins, supplements, foods, and beverages do not always mix well with each other. Your health care professional can help.

5. **Use the dosing tool that comes with the medicine, such as a dropper or a dosing cup.** A different dosing tool, or a kitchen spoon, could hold the wrong amount of medicine.

6. **Know the difference between a tablespoon (Tbs.) and a teaspoon (tsp.).** Do not confuse them. A tablespoon holds three times as much medicine as a teaspoon. On measuring tools, a teaspoon (tsp.) is equal to 5 cubic centimeters (cc) or 5 milliliters (ml).

7. **Know your child's weight.** Directions on some OTC medicines are based on weight. Never guess the amount of medicine to give to your child or try to figure it out from the adult dose instructions. If a dose is not listed for your child's age or weight, call your doctor or other members of your health care team.

8. **Prevent a poison emergency by always using a child-resistant cap.** Re-lock the cap after each use. Be especially careful with any products that contain iron; they are the leading cause of poisoning deaths in young children.

9. **Store all medicines in a safe place.** Today's medicines are tasty, colorful, and many can be chewed. Kids may think that these products are candy. To prevent an overdose or poisoning emergency, store all medicines and vitamins in a safe place out of your child's (and even your pet's) sight and reach. If your child takes too much, call the Poison Center Hotline at 800-222-1222 (open 24 hours every day, 7 days a week) or call 9-1-1.

10. **Check the medicine three times.** First, check the outside packaging for such things as cuts, slices, or tears. Second, once you are at home, check the label on the inside package to be sure you have the right medicine. Make sure the lid and seal

are not broken. Third, check the color, shape, size, and smell of the medicine. If you notice anything different or unusual, talk to a pharmacist or another health care professional.

A Prescription for Parents: Understanding Antibiotic Usage

When are antibiotics necessary? Your doctor can best answer this complicated question and the answer depends on the diagnosis. Here are a few examples:

1. **Ear infections:** There are several types; many need antibiotics, but some do not.

2. **Sinus infections:** Most children with thick or green mucus do not have sinus infections. Antibiotics are needed for some long-lasting or severe cases.

3. **Cough or bronchitis:** Children rarely need antibiotics for bronchitis.

4. **Sore throat:** Viruses cause most cases. Only one major kind, "strep throat," requires antibiotics. This condition must be diagnosed by a laboratory test.

5. **Colds:** Colds are caused by viruses and may last for two weeks or longer. Antibiotics have no effect on colds, but your doctor may have suggestions for obtaining comfort while the illness runs its course.

Cough and Cold Medicines

What can parents do if their children are too young or the health care provider advises against using cough and cold medicines?

Parents might consider clearing nasal congestion in infants with a rubber suction bulb. Also, secretions can be softened with saline nose drops or a cool-mist humidifier.

Are cough and cold medicines safe for children under two years of age?

There are no Food and Drug Administration (FDA)-approved dosing recommendations for children under two years of age. These drugs can, in rare cases, be harmful or even fatal. Parents and health care providers should use caution when giving cough and cold medicines to children under two years of age.

Do cough and cold medicines work in children under two years of age?

There is little evidence that cough and cold medicines work in children under two years of age.

Should parents give cough and cold medicines to children under two years of age?

Parents should consult a health care provider before giving cough and cold medicines to their children and should always tell providers about all prescription and over-the-counter medicines they are giving their child.

Should health care providers prescribe cough and cold medicines to children under two years of age?

Health care providers should exercise caution when recommending or prescribing cough and cold medicines to children under two years of age and should always ask caregivers about any other cough and cold medicines the child might be receiving. No FDA-approved dosing recommendations exist for over-the-counter cough and cold medicines in children under two years of age.

What should parents and doctors be careful of if they want to give cough and cold medicines to children under two years of age?

Be especially careful if giving more than one cough and cold medicine at a time to children under two years of age. Two medicines may have different brand names but may contain the same ingredient. Some cough and cold medicines contain more than one active ingredient.

Remember: It is worth noting that viral infections sometimes lead to bacterial infections. But treating viral infections with antibiotics will not prevent bacterial infections and may trigger infections with resistant bacteria. Keep your doctor informed if the illness gets worse, or lasts a long time, so that the proper treatment can be given as needed.

Section 39.4

Measuring Liquid Medication

Information

- If the product is a suspension, shake well before using.

- Do not use silverware spoons for giving medication. They are not all the same size. A silverware teaspoon could be as small as a half teaspoon or as large as two teaspoons.

- Measuring spoons used for cooking are accurate, but they spill easily.

Oral syringes have some advantages for giving liquid medications:

- They are accurate.

- They are easy to use.

- A child can take a capped syringe containing a dose of medication to daycare or school.

There can be problems with oral syringes, however. The FDA has had reports of young children choking on syringe caps. To be safe, remove the cap before you use an oral syringe. Throw it away if you do not need it for future use. If you need it, keep it out of reach of infants and small children.

Dosing cups are also a handy way to give liquid medications. However, dosing errors have occurred with them. In the past, some product instructions gave the dose in teaspoons, but the measuring cup in the package was marked with tablespoons. Always check to make sure the units (teaspoon, tablespoon, ml, or cc) on the cup or syringe match the units of the dose you want to give.

Liquid medications often don't taste good, but many flavors are now available and can be added to any liquid medication. Ask your pharmacist.

Unit conversions:

- 1 milliliters (ml) = 1 cubic centimeters (cc)
- 2.5 ml = ½ teaspoon
- 5 ml = 1 teaspoon
- 15 ml = 1 tablespoon
- 3 teaspoons = 1 tablespoon

Chapter 40

Adverse Drug Reactions

What is an adverse drug reaction?

Medicines can treat or prevent illness and disease. However, sometimes medicines can cause problems. These problems are called adverse drug reactions. You should know what to do if you think that you or someone you take care of is having an adverse drug reaction.

Can adverse drug reactions happen to everyone?

Yes. Anybody can have an adverse drug reaction. However, people who take more than three or four medicines every day are more likely to have an adverse drug reaction. One medicine might cause an adverse reaction if it is taken with another medicine.

One way to reduce your chances of having adverse drug reactions is to work with your doctor to limit the number of medicines you take. Tell your doctor about all of the medicines you're taking, even if you take something for only a short time. You may also want to use only one drugstore so your pharmacists get to know you and the medicines you take. Pharmacists are trained to look at the medicines you're taking to see whether they might cause an adverse drug reaction.

Reprinted with permission from "Information From Your Family Doctor: Drug Reactions," Reviewed/Updated November 2006, http://familydoctor.org/online/famdocen/home/seniors/seniors-meds/231.html. Copyright © 2006 American Academy of Family Physicians. All Rights Reserved. Additional information at the end of the chapter, "MedWatch Reporting by Consumers," is from the U.S. Food and Drug Administration (FDA), December 2005.

Are prescription medicines the only cause of adverse reactions?

No. Even medicines that don't need a prescription (called over-the-counter medicines) can interact with each other or with prescription drugs and cause problems. Supplements, herbal products in teas or tablets, or vitamins may also cause adverse reactions when taken with certain drugs. Be sure to tell your doctor and pharmacist if you're using any of these products.

Some types of food may also cause adverse drug reactions. For example, grapefruit and grapefruit juice, as well as alcohol and caffeine, may affect how drugs work. Every time your doctor prescribes a new drug, ask about possible interactions with any foods or beverages.

What about medicines I've used in the past?

You might be tempted to save money by taking old medicines that you've used before. However, it's likely that you are taking different medicines now than you were when you were taking the old drug. Even though you didn't have an adverse reaction with the old medicine before, you might have a bad reaction when you take it with the medicines you're taking now.

Is it safe to use a friend or relative's medicine?

No. Using medicines that were prescribed for a friend or relative can cause problems and might lead to adverse drug reactions because:

- Your doctor prescribes medicine according to your size, gender and age. The wrong amount of medicine may cause adverse reactions.

- The medicines you're taking are probably different from the medicines the other person takes. This different combination of drugs may also cause an adverse reaction.

- You might react differently to the medicine than the other person did.

To be safe, never share medicines with anybody.

How will I know I'm having an adverse drug reaction?

When you're taking any medicine, it's important to be aware of any change in your body. Tell your doctor if something unusual happens.

It may be hard to know if an adverse reaction is caused by your illness or by your medicine. Tell your doctor when your symptoms started and whether they are different from other symptoms you have had from an illness. Be sure to remind your doctor of all the medicines you are taking. The following are some adverse drug reactions that you might notice:

- skin rash
- easy bruising
- bleeding
- severe nausea and vomiting
- diarrhea
- constipation
- confusion
- breathing difficulties

The following are some adverse reactions your doctor might notice during a check-up:

- changes in lab test results
- abnormal heartbeat

What will my doctor do if I have an adverse drug reaction?

Your doctor might tell you to stop taking the medicine so the adverse reaction will go away by itself. Or your doctor might have you take another medicine to treat the reaction. If your adverse reaction is serious, you might have to go to a hospital. Never stop taking a medicine on your own; always talk with your doctor first.

MedWatch for Reporting Serious Reactions

MedWatch is the Food and Drug Administration's (FDA) program for reporting serious reactions, product quality problems and product use errors with human medical products, such as drugs and medical devices.

If you think you or someone in your family has experienced a serious reaction to a medical product, you are encouraged to take the reporting form to your doctor. Your health care provider can provide clinical information based on your medical record that can help us evaluate your report.

However, for a variety of reasons, you may not wish to have the form filled out by your health care provider, or your health care provider may choose not to complete the form. Your health care provider is not required to report to the FDA. In these situations, you may complete the Online Reporting Form yourself via the internet.

You will receive an acknowledgement from FDA after they receive your report. You will be personally contacted only if they need additional information.

FDA MedWatch
Toll-Free: 800-332-1088 (to report by phone)
Fax: 800-332-0178 (to fax a report)
Website: http://www.fda.gov/medwatch
To report online: http://www.fda.gov/medwatch/report.htm

Chapter 41

Drug Interactions: What You Should Know

There are more opportunities today than ever before to learn about your health and to take better care of yourself. It is also more important than ever to know about the medicines you take. If you take several different medicines, see more than one doctor, or have certain health conditions, you and your doctors need to be aware of all the medicines you take. Doing so will help you to avoid potential problems such as drug interactions.

Drug interactions may make your drug less effective, cause unexpected side effects, or increase the action of a particular drug. Some drug interactions can even be harmful to you. Reading the label every time you use a nonprescription or prescription drug and taking the time to learn about drug interactions may be critical to your health. You can reduce the risk of potentially harmful drug interactions and side effects with a little bit of knowledge and common sense. Drug interactions fall into three broad categories:

- Drug-drug interactions occur when two or more drugs react with each other. This drug-drug interaction may cause you to experience an unexpected side effect. For example, mixing a drug you take to help you sleep (a sedative) and a drug you take for allergies (an antihistamine) can slow your reactions and make driving a car or operating machinery dangerous.

"Drug Interactions: What You Should Know," U.S. Food and Drug Administration (FDA), updated March 24, 2006.

- Drug-food or beverage interactions result from drugs reacting with foods or beverages. For example, mixing alcohol with some drugs may cause you to feel tired or slow your reactions.

- Drug-condition interactions may occur when an existing medical condition makes certain drugs potentially harmful. For example, if you have high blood pressure you could experience an unwanted reaction if you take a nasal decongestant.

Drug Interactions and Over-the-Counter Medicines

Over-the-counter (OTC) drug labels contain information about ingredients, uses, warnings, and directions that is important to read and understand. The label also includes important information about possible drug interactions. Further, drug labels may change as new information becomes known. That's why it's especially important to read the label every time you use a drug.

The "Active Ingredients" and "Purpose" sections list the name and amount of each active ingredient and the purpose of each active ingredient.

The "Uses" section of the label tells you what the drug is used for and helps you find the best drug for your specific symptoms.

The "Warnings" section of the label provides important drug interaction and precaution information such as:

- when to talk to a doctor or pharmacist before use;
- the medical conditions that may make the drug less effective or not safe;
- under what circumstances the drug should not be used; and
- when to stop taking the drug.

The "Directions" section of the label tells you the length of time and the amount of the product that you may safely use and any special instructions on how to use the product.

The "Other Information" section of the label tells you required information about certain ingredients, such as sodium content, for people with dietary restrictions or allergies.

The **"Inactive Ingredients"** section of the label tells you the name of each inactive ingredient (such as colorings or binders).

The **"Questions?"** or **"Questions or Comments?"** section of the label (if included) provides telephone numbers of a source to answer questions about the product.

Learning More about Drug Interactions

Talk to your doctor or pharmacist about the drugs you take. When your doctor prescribes a new drug, discuss all OTC and prescription drugs, dietary supplements, vitamins, botanicals, minerals and herbals you take, as well as the foods you eat. Ask your pharmacist for the package insert for each prescription drug you take. The package insert provides more information about potential drug interactions.

Before taking a drug, ask your doctor or pharmacist the following questions:

• Can I take it with other drugs?

• Should I avoid certain foods, beverages or other products?

• What are possible drug interaction signs I should know about?

• How will the drug work in my body?

• Is there more information available about the drug or my condition (on the internet or in health and medical literature)?

Know how to take drugs safely and responsibly. Remember, the drug label will tell you:

• what the drug is used for;

• how to take the drug; and

• how to reduce the risk of drug interactions and unwanted side effects.

If you still have questions after reading the drug product label, ask your doctor or pharmacist for more information.

Remember that different OTC drugs may contain the same active ingredient. If you are taking more than one OTC drug, pay attention to the active ingredients used in the products to avoid taking too much of a particular ingredient. Under certain circumstances—such as if you are pregnant or breast feeding—you should talk to your doctor

317

Table 41.1. Examples of Drug Interaction Warnings (continued on the next two pages)

Category	Drug Interaction Information
Acid Reducers: H2 Receptor Antagonists (*drugs that prevent or relieve heartburn associated with acid indigestion and sour stomach*)	**For products containing cimetidine, ask a doctor or pharmacist before use if you are:** • taking theophylline (*oral asthma drug*), warfarin (*blood thinning drug*), or phenytoin (*seizure drug*).
Antacids (*drugs for relief of acid indigestion, heartburn, and/or sour stomach*)	**Ask a doctor or pharmacist before use if you are:** • allergic to milk or milk products if the product contains more than 5 grams lactose in a maximum daily dose; • taking a prescription drug. **Ask a doctor before use if you have:** • kidney disease.
Antiemetics (*drugs for prevention or treatment of nausea, vomiting, or dizziness associated with motion sickness*)	**Ask a doctor or pharmacist before use if you:** • are taking sedatives or tranquilizers. **Ask a doctor before use if you have:** • a breathing problem, such as emphysema or chronic bronchitis; • glaucoma; • difficulty in urination due to an enlarged prostate gland. **When using this product:** • avoid alcoholic beverages.
Antihistamines (*drugs that temporarily relieve runny nose or reduce sneezing, itching of the nose or throat, and itchy watery eyes due to hay fever or other upper respiratory problems*)	**Ask a doctor or pharmacist before use if you are taking:** • sedatives or tranquilizers; • a prescription drug for high blood pressure or depression. **Ask a doctor before use if you have:** • glaucoma or difficulty in urination due to an enlarged prostate gland; • breathing problems, such as emphysema, chronic bronchitis, or asthma. **When using this product:** • alcohol, sedatives, and tranquilizers may increase drowsiness; • avoid alcoholic beverages.

Table 41.1. (continued) Examples of Drug Interaction Warnings (continued on next page)

Category	Drug Interaction Information
Antitussives Cough Medicine (*drugs that temporarily reduce cough due to minor throat and bronchial irritation as may occur with a cold*)	**Ask a doctor or pharmacist before use if you are:** • taking sedatives or tranquilizers. **Ask a doctor before use if you have:** • glaucoma or difficulty in urination due to an enlarged prostate gland.
Bronchodilators (*drugs for the temporary relief of shortness of breath, tightness of chest and wheezing due to bronchial asthma*)	**Ask a doctor before use if you:** • have heart disease, high blood pressure, thyroid disease, diabetes, or difficulty in urination due to an enlarged prostate gland; • have ever been hospitalized for asthma or are taking a prescription drug for asthma.
Laxatives (*drugs for the temporary relief of constipation*)	**Ask a doctor before use if you have:** • kidney disease and the laxative contains phosphates, potassium, or magnesium; • stomach pain, nausea, or vomiting.
Nasal Decongestants (*drugs for the temporary relief of nasal congestion due to a cold, hay fever, or other upper respiratory allergies*)	**Ask a doctor before use if you:** • have heart disease, high blood pressure, thyroid disease, diabetes, or difficulty in urination due to an enlarged prostate gland.
Nicotine Replacement Products (*drugs that reduce withdrawal symptoms associated with quitting smoking, including nicotine craving*)	**Ask a doctor before use if you:** • have high blood pressure not controlled by medication; • have heart disease or have had a recent heart attack or irregular heartbeat, since nicotine can increase your heart rate. **Ask a doctor or pharmacist before use if you are:** • taking a prescription drug for depression or asthma (your dose may need to be adjusted); • using a prescription non-nicotine stop smoking drug. **Do not use:** • if you continue to smoke, chew tobacco, use snuff, or use other nicotine-containing products.

319

Table 41.1. (continued) Examples of Drug Interaction Warnings

Category	Drug Interaction Information
Nighttime Sleep Aids (*drugs for relief of occasional sleeplessness*)	**Ask a doctor or pharmacist before use if you are:** • taking sedatives or tranquilizers. **Ask a doctor before use if you have:** • a breathing problem such as emphysema or chronic bronchitis; • glaucoma; • difficulty in urination due to an enlarged prostate gland. **When using this product:** • avoid alcoholic beverages.
Pain Relievers (*drugs for the temporary relief of minor body aches, pains, and headaches*)	**Ask a doctor before taking if you:** • consume three or more alcohol-containing drinks per day. (*The following ingredients are found in different OTC pain relievers: acetaminophen, aspirin, ibuprofen, ketoprofen, magnesium salicylate, and naproxen. It is important to read the label of pain reliever products to learn about different drug interaction warnings for each ingredient.*)
Stimulants (*drugs that help restore mental alertness or wakefulness during fatigue or drowsiness*)	**When using this product:** • limit the use of foods, beverages, and other drugs that have caffeine. Too much caffeine can cause nervousness, irritability, sleeplessness, and occasional rapid heart beat. • be aware that the recommended dose of this product contains about as much caffeine as a cup of coffee.
Topical Acne (*drugs for the treatment of acne*)	**When using this product:** • increased dryness or irritation of the skin may occur immediately following use of this product or if you are using other topical acne drugs at the same time. If this occurs, only one drug should be used unless directed by your doctor.

before you take any medicine. Also, make sure you know what ingredients are contained in the medicines you take. Doing so will help you to avoid possible allergic reactions.

Drug Interaction Warnings

The following are examples of drug interaction warnings that you may see on certain OTC drug products. These examples do not include all of the warnings for the listed types of products and should not take the place of reading the actual product label.

Additional Information

Express Scripts Drug Digest
Website: http://www.drugdigest.org/DD/Interaction/ChooseDrugs/ 1,4109,,00.html

Online Drug Digest for checking drug interactions.

Chapter 42

Drug Name Confusion: Preventing Medication Errors

An 8-year-old died, it was suspected, after receiving methadone instead of methylphenidate, a drug used to treat attention deficit disorders. A 19-year-old man showed signs of potentially fatal complications after he was given clozapine instead of olanzapine, two drugs used to treat schizophrenia. And a 50-year-old woman was hospitalized after taking Flomax, used to treat the symptoms of an enlarged prostate, instead of Volmax, used to relieve bronchospasm.

In each of these cases reported to the Food and Drug Administration (FDA), the names of the dispensed drugs looked or sounded like those that were prescribed. There have been others: Serzone, an antidepressant, for Seroquel, used to treat schizophrenia, and iodine for Lodine, a non-steroidal anti-inflammatory drug.

Adverse events that can occur when drugs are dispensed as the wrong medications underscore the need for clear interpretation and better communication between the doctors who write prescriptions and the pharmacists who fill them. The FDA says that about ten percent of all medication errors reported result from drug name confusion.

"These errors are not usually due to incompetence," says Carol A. Holquist, R.Ph., director of the Division of Medication Errors and Technical Support in the FDA's Office of Drug Safety. "But they are so underreported because people are afraid of the blame." Errors occur at all levels of the medication-use system, from prescribing to dispensing,

"Drug Name Confusion: Preventing Medication Errors," by Carol Rados, *FDA Consumer magazine*, July–August 2005, U.S. Food and Drug Administration (FDA).

Holquist says, which is why those people who receive the prescriptions must take action, too. "Everybody has a role in minimizing medication errors," she says.

The Problems

Medication errors can occur between brand names, generic names, and brand-to-generic names like Toradol and tramadol. But sometimes, medication errors involve more than just name similarities. Abbreviations, acronyms, dose designations, and other symbols used in medication prescribing also have the potential for causing problems.

For example, the abbreviation "D/C" means both "discharge" and "discontinue." The National Coordinating Council for Medication Error Reporting and Prevention (NCCMERP) notes that patients' medications have been stopped prematurely when D/C—intended to mean discharge—was misinterpreted as discontinue because it was followed by a list of drugs.

Illegible handwriting, unfamiliarity with drug names, newly available products, similar packaging or labeling, and incorrect selection of a similar name from a computerized product list, all compound the problem. And, although some drug names and symbols may not necessarily sound alike or look alike, they could cause confusion in prescribing errors when handwritten or communicated verbally, according to the United States Pharmacopeia (USP).

For example, Holquist says that several errors have occurred involving mix-ups with the oral diabetes drug Avandia and the anticoagulant Coumadin. Although they don't look similar when typed or printed, the names have been confused with each other when poorly written in cursive. The first "A" in Avandia, if not fully formed, can look like a "C," and the final "a" has appeared to be an "n."

The XYZs of Naming Drugs

Names are part of developing a new drug. And coming up with a catchy, snappy moniker that distinguishes one drug from another is not easy. For the most part, drug companies want a name that will boost sales, while consumers long for some indication from the name of what the drug does. The FDA, however, will not allow names that imply medical claims, suggest a use for which a drug is not approved, or promise more than they can deliver.

Naming a drug can be as complicated as creating a rhythmic cacophony of unpronounceable syllables and emphatic-sounding letters, such as C and P. Other naming strategies include letters that when strung together sound like something high-tech—think Zyprexa, Lexapro, and Xanax. But whether it is the sound of certain letters that manufacturers like, or the vision that a name conjures up, the FDA says that selection must take into account concerns for reducing errors and for avoiding trademark infringement.

Because of today's tough trademark requirements, many drug companies are turning to a growing industry of "naming" consultants for the task. These consultants are charged with creating a unique name that will appeal to both doctors and patients, particularly given the recent surge in direct-to-consumer advertising.

"Global companies want a name to be a worldwide mark," says Doug Kapp, vice president of brand strategy at RTi-DFD, a market research company in Stamford, Connecticut. In helping pharmaceutical companies set their products apart from others, Kapp says his company recognizes that the name must resonate with the market target and also must pass worldwide trademark requirements. That recognition, he says, drove his company to develop "relational asemantics," a name-generation process that assists physicians in identifying the nature of a drug. Just as the erectile dysfunction drug Viagra might suggest vitality and vigor, two of RTi-DFD's successes include Advair, linked to "advantage air for asthma," and Amerge, named for "emerging from the pain of a migraine." Kapp says that regardless of how good a name seems, it must be reviewed for potential confusion with other drugs so that "any other associations would not harm the patient in the event of an error."

Satisfying the FDA

Every drug usually has three names: chemical, generic (nonproprietary), and brand (proprietary), and each name is subject to different rules and regulations. The chemical name specifies the chemical structure of the drug. It is not pre-approved by any organization, nor is it recognized in any standard manuals, such as USP publications. Therefore, chemical names are primarily used by researchers, but not in medical practice.

The FDA requires that either the established, or official, name or in the absence of an official name, the common or usual name, appears on labels and labeling of a drug product. The common name, loosely referred to as the generic name, must accompany the brand name, if there is one. The established name for a drug substance is usually found in the originating country's pharmacopeia, an official book or list of drugs and medicines and the standards established for their production, dispensation, and use.

The generic name is usually created for drug substances when a new drug is ready for marketing. It is selected by the United States Adopted Names (USAN) Council, whose expertise is recognized by the FDA, according to principles developed to ensure safety, consistency, and logic. These names are typically used by health care professionals.

Generic names are coined using an established stem, or group of letters, that represents a specific drug class. For example, the USAN stems include suffixes like *-mab* for monoclonal antibodies, such as infliximab, or prefixes like *dopa-* for dopamine receptor agonists. The arthritis medications celecoxib, valdecoxib, and rofecoxib are generic names containing the *-coxib* stem. Each belongs to a class of drugs known as the COX-2 inhibitors.

Names that include such stems, chemistry roots, or any other coded information are easier to remember, and give clues about what a drug is used for. These names, however, typically sound or look so much alike that they contribute to medication errors, especially if the products share common dosage forms and other similarities.

The brand name, also called trademark, can be created as soon as a generic name has been established. Only brand names of products subject to a new drug application or an abbreviated new drug application must be approved by the FDA first. This requirement distinguishes them from generic names. According to a report in the January–February 2004 issue of the *Journal of the American Pharmacists Association*, there are more than 9,000 generic drug names and 33,000 trademarked brand names in use in the United States.

Fixing the Problems

To minimize confusion between drug names that look or sound alike, the FDA reviews about 400 brand names a year before they are marketed. About one-third are rejected. The last time the FDA changed a drug name after it was approved was in 2005, when the diabetes drug Amaryl was being confused with the Alzheimer disease medication Reminyl, and one person died. Now the Alzheimer medicine is called Razadyne.

Generic name confusion also has led to regulatory action, as well as to pharmacy practice recommendations. For example, the USP and the USAN changed the drug name "amrinone" to "inamrinone" after receiving reports of serious outcomes from medication errors involving the similar name pair "amrinone/amiodarone." The generic drug industry also has responded to requests from the FDA to use a mixture of uppercase and lowercase letters to highlight differences in similar generic names, such as vinBLAStine and vinCRIStine. This step also encouraged manufacturers to supplement their new drug applications with revised labels and labeling that visually differentiated their generic names with the so-called "tall man" letters. And the NCCMERP recommendations encourage doctors to write both brand and generic names on prescriptions.

A number of other efforts are underway to reduce the incidence of medical errors stemming from similar-looking or similar-sounding names. The FDA, for example, is encouraging people to talk with their physicians to ensure that they have a complete understanding about their prescription before leaving the doctor's office, and to verify the information with the pharmacist before the medication is dispensed.

FDA health professionals also are requested to interpret both written prescriptions and verbal orders through weekly in-house studies, in an attempt to simulate the prescription ordering process. Holquist says that these studies are a valuable tool used in every review of proposed brand names. It is important, she adds, to be able to detect any potential sound-alike, look-alike confusion with proprietary names before a new drug application is approved. Other efforts strongly encouraged for physicians include writing prescriptions more clearly, printing in block letters rather than writing in cursive, avoiding the use of abbreviations, and indicating the reason for the drug.

According to the FDA, pharmacists can help by keeping look-alike, sound-alike products separated from one another on pharmacy shelves, by avoiding stocking multiple product sizes together, and by verifying with the doctor information that is not clear before filling a prescription.

The FDA encourages pharmacists and other health professionals to report any actual or potential medication errors to the agency's MedWatch Adverse Event Reporting System online at http://www.fda.gov/medwatch, by phone at 800-332-1088, or by fax at 800-332-0178. Caller identification is kept confidential and is protected from disclosure by the Freedom of Information Act.

Reducing Drug-Name Medication Errors

Here's a list of steps you can take:

- Know the name and strength of prescribed drugs before leaving the doctor's office.

- Insist that the doctor include the purpose of the medication on the prescription.

- Ensure that a refill is what it should be.

- Tell your doctor of any medical history changes.

Chapter 43

Unapproved, Counterfeit, and Misused Drugs

Chapter Contents

Section 43.1

Unapproved and Counterfeit Drugs

This section includes text from "The FDA Takes Action Against Unapproved Drugs," by Michelle Meadows, *FDA Consumer magazine*, January–February 2007, U.S. Food and Drug Administration (FDA); and excerpts from "Counterfeit Drugs: Questions and Answers," FDA, July 2003. Reviewed in November, 2007 by Dr. David A. Cooke, M.D., Diplomate, American Board of Internal Medicine.

FDA Action against Unapproved Drugs

Most prescription drugs marketed in the United States have been reviewed and approved by the Food and Drug Administration (FDA) as required by law. Thousands of unapproved prescription drugs, however, are still being prescribed and sold. The FDA, as part of its drug safety efforts, is bolstering its efforts against unapproved drugs in the United States.

"Although we estimate that less than two percent of prescribed drugs are unapproved, we believe that some unapproved products raise safety concerns that warrant regulatory action," says Deborah Autor, director of the Office of Compliance in the FDA's Center for Drug Evaluation and Research (CDER).

There are several reasons why an unapproved drug may be available. One example is when only one company may have approval to market a drug, but other companies are illegally marketing their versions of the drug without having gone through the FDA's approval process. Another scenario is that a combination of ingredients is approved by the FDA, but a company is marketing a single ingredient without approval.

Some older products continue to be marketed illegally for historical reasons. "Many drugs were marketed before Congress made changes to the law requiring drugs to undergo FDA review," Autor says. There are unapproved drugs whose makers claim the drugs are grandfathered under older standards and therefore do not require approval under the current regulatory framework. "But the truly grandfathered drugs represent only a few, at most, of all the unapproved drugs being marketed," Autor says. "Most unapproved drugs do require FDA approval."

Some drugs have been sold for so many years that physicians and pharmacists may not know they are unapproved. They even may be unaware that unapproved drugs are advertised in medical journals and listed in the *Physicians' Desk Reference* (PDR) and other reference books. These practices give the false impression that the drugs were reviewed and approved by the FDA.

"Consumers who discover that they are taking an unapproved drug shouldn't stop treatment without talking to their doctor first," Autor says. The FDA advises consumers and health professionals to carefully consider the medical condition being treated, the patient's previous response to the drug, and the availability of approved alternatives as part of discussing the benefits and risks of any unapproved treatment.

The major categories in which unapproved drugs exist include certain cough and cold preparations with antihistamines, some narcotics, and some types of sedatives. Examples include:

- unapproved prescription cough and cold preparations with antihistamines, such as pheniramine maleate and dexbrompheniramine maleate;

- unapproved prescription single-ingredient narcotics such as codeine phosphate and oxycodone HCL 5 mg; and

- unapproved prescription sedatives such as phenobarbital and chloral hydrate.

Enforcement

In June 2006, the FDA issued a guidance called Marketed Unapproved Drugs—Compliance Policy Guide, which describes plans for enforcement in this area. "The FDA is telling manufacturers to either obtain approval for an unapproved drug or remove it from the market," Autor says. "Even if the drug has been marketed for many years with no known safety problems, companies will still need to comply. The absence of evidence of a safety problem does not mean a product is truly safe."

A patient or physician may believe a drug is safe based on individual experience, but the FDA relies on carefully designed clinical trials that weigh the risks and benefits of taking a drug compared with taking a placebo or another accepted therapy. FDA approval means not only that the product has been reviewed for safety and effectiveness, but that the agency has reviewed manufacturing quality and product labeling to ensure that it adequately conveys the drug's risks and benefits. FDA approval also means that a drug's safety and effectiveness is still monitored after marketing.

Before pursuing regulatory action against unapproved drugs, the FDA plans to consider the effects on the public health, including whether the product is medically necessary. The agency recognizes that some unapproved therapies offer benefits. An example is phenobarbital, a drug used to control seizures. In some cases, FDA action requiring drug approvals will be gradual to avoid shortages of medically necessary products.

The guidance explains that the FDA will continue to focus enforcement actions on unapproved drugs that carry potential safety risks, lack evidence of effectiveness, and constitute health fraud. For example, the FDA has ordered all manufacturers of unapproved carbinoxamine-containing products to stop making them because of safety concerns regarding their use in children younger than two years. Carbinoxamine is a sedating antihistamine. Manufacturers will need to obtain FDA approval to continue marketing these products.

The FDA has received 21 reports of death associated with carbinoxamine-containing drugs in children younger than two years. While it is not clear that the carbinoxamine caused these deaths, the FDA is concerned about the risks. Some of the unapproved products are being promoted for infants and young children, an age group in which carbinoxamine has never been studied. And young children are more susceptible to drug-related adverse events.

Some of these unapproved products are labeled for treatment of cough and cold symptoms, an indication for which carbinoxamine has not been found safe by the FDA. The two carbinoxamine-containing products approved by the FDA are indicated for treating allergic reactions or their symptoms, and are manufactured by Atlanta-based Mikart Inc. The products contain carbinoxamine maleate as the active ingredient without any additional active ingredients.

Visit http://www.accessdata.fda.gov/scripts/cder/drugsatfda to find out whether a drug may be unapproved. If your drug is not listed there, contact your drug's manufacturer and ask whether your drug is approved.

Counterfeit Drugs

What is the definition of a counterfeit medication?

U.S. law defines counterfeit drugs as those sold under a product name without proper authorization. Counterfeiting can apply to both brand name and generic products, where the identity of the source is deliberately and fraudulently mislabeled in a way that suggests that it is the authentic approved product. Counterfeit products may include products without the active ingredient, with an insufficient quantity of the active ingredient, with the wrong active ingredient, or with fake packaging.

What risks are involved with taking counterfeit medications?

An individual who receives a counterfeit medication may be at risk for a number of dangerous health consequences. Patients may experience unexpected side effects, allergic reactions, or a worsening of their medical condition. A number of counterfeits do not contain any active ingredients, and instead contain inert substances, which do not provide the patient any treatment benefit. Counterfeit medications may also contain incorrect ingredients, improper dosages of the correct ingredients, or they may contain hazardous ingredients.

What is the worldwide prevalence of counterfeit medications?

The extent of the problem of counterfeit drugs is unknown. Counterfeiting is difficult to detect, investigate, and quantify. So, it is hard to know or even estimate the true extent of the problem. What is known is that they occur worldwide and are more prevalent in developing countries. It is estimated that upwards of 10% of drugs worldwide are counterfeit, and in some countries more than 50% of the drug supply is made up of counterfeit drugs.

What is the prevalence of counterfeit medications in the U.S.?

Counterfeiting occurs less frequently in the U.S. than in other countries due to the strict guidelines, regulations, and enforcement the FDA provides throughout the production and distribution chain. However, recently FDA has seen two highly publicized examples of counterfeit Lipitor and Procrit within the U.S. distribution system. The FDA continues to believe that the overall quality of drug products that consumers purchase from U.S. pharmacies remains high. The American public can be confident that these medications are safe and effective.

Should consumers who currently purchase medications over the internet or import medications from other countries be concerned about counterfeits?

Consumers can be confident in the quality, safety, and efficacy of medications purchased from a U.S. state licensed pharmacy. For those consumers who purchase medications over the internet, websites that have the Verified Internet Pharmacy Practice Sites (VIPPS) Seal are licensed pharmacies where FDA-approved medications can be purchased. These sites are identified by the VIPPS hyperlink seal displayed on their website. Unless medications have been purchased from a U.S. state licensed pharmacy website, the safety and efficacy of these medications cannot be guaranteed.

What can consumers do to protect themselves from counterfeit drugs?

Consumers can protect themselves from the risks associated with counterfeit drugs by purchasing all prescription and over-the-counter medications from U.S. state licensed pharmacies. Consumers must be vigilant when examining their personal medications, paying attention to the presence of altered or unsealed containers or changes in the packaging of the product. Differences in the physical appearance of the product, taste, and side effects experienced should alert the patient to contact their physician, pharmacist, or other health care professional who is providing treatment.

Are there any promising technologies that have the capability of preventing counterfeiting?

There are several technologies that may prove helpful, including radio frequency chips or tags. For example, radio waves are used to automatically identify items, such as pharmaceutical products, by assigning individual serial numbers to each product. This technology may be capable of ensuring that drugs are not diverted or counterfeited by allowing wholesalers and pharmacists to determine the identity and dosage of individual products.

Will allowing reimports increase the amount of counterfeit drugs in the U.S.? If drugs can be manufactured overseas and sold in the U.S., why can't drugs be reimported?

The number of counterfeits in the U.S. is currently small as a result of the framework of federal-state oversight of the domestic drug distribution system. Currently, drugs entering the U.S. distribution system from other countries are FDA-approved, made in a facility that has been approved by FDA, and imported from the original manufacturer. Therefore, consumers can have high confidence that the medications they receive from their pharmacy are safe and effective. Proposals for reimportation would allow drugs from foreign sources other than the original manufacturer to enter the U.S. market. FDA has no authority to regulate these foreign entities or to determine under what conditions drugs from other countries have been stored and handled. Even FDA-approved drugs sent to another country and then reimported may be contaminated or subpotent due to mishandling. Therefore, wholesalers, pharmacists, consumers, and FDA have no way of knowing if any drug reimported into the U.S. is truly the U.S.-approved product or has been inappropriately stored or handled.

Section 43.2

Misuse of Prescription Pain Relievers

"The Buzz Takes Your Breath Away, Permanently,"
U.S. Food and Drug Administration's (FDA) Center for Drug
Evaluation and Research (CDER), updated August 17, 2005.

The Buzz Takes Your Breath Away, Permanently

How many times has someone told you a party drug could lead to more serious problems—like addiction, brain damage, or even death? You've probably heard it so many times, it's getting hard to believe. Especially when kids around you are smoking, drinking, and rolling. But all drugs have real potential for harm—even prescription pain relievers. When abused alone, or taken with other drugs, prescription pain medications can kill you. And the death toll from misuse and abuse is rising steadily.

Think Twice—Because You Only Die Once

Prescription pain relievers, when used correctly and under a doctor's supervision, are safe and effective. But abuse them, or mix them with illegal drugs or alcohol, and you could wind up in the morgue. Even using prescription pain relievers with other prescription drugs (such as antidepressants) or over-the-counter medications (like cough syrups and antihistamines), can lead to life-threatening respiratory failure. That's why people just like you are dropping pills at parties, and dropping dead. They're not downing handfuls of pills, either. With some prescription pain relievers, all it takes is one pill.

Drugs to Watch Out For

The most dangerous prescription pain relievers are those containing drugs known as opioids, such as morphine and codeine. Some common drugs containing these substances include Darvon, Demerol, Dilaudid, OxyContin, Tylenol with Codeine, and Vicodin. Street names for these drugs include: ac/dc, coties, demmies, dillies, hillbilly heroin, o.c., oxy, oxycotton, percs and vics to name a few. Whatever you call them, remember one thing—they can be killers.

Symptoms of Overdose

If you, or any of your friends, have taken prescription pain relievers, here are the danger signs to watch for:

- slow breathing (less than ten breaths a minute is really serious trouble)
- small, pinpoint pupils
- confusion
- being tired, nodding off, or passing out
- dizziness
- weakness
- apathy (they don't care about anything)
- cold and clammy skin
- nausea
- vomiting
- seizures

A lot of these symptoms can make people think your friend is drunk. And you may be tempted to let them sleep it off, or tell their parents they had too much to drink. But don't. Your friend could go to sleep and never wake up.

If a Friend Is Overdosing

Make an anonymous call to 911 or your friend's parents if you're too scared to identify yourself. Try to get your friend to respond to you by calling out his or her name. Make your friend wake up and talk to you. Shake him or her if you have to. Otherwise, your friend could suffer brain damage, fall into a coma, or die.

Addiction

Addiction can be a living death. If you abuse prescription pain relievers and are lucky enough to cheat death, you are still in big trouble. Prescription pain relievers can be addictive. The longer you take them, the more your body needs. Try to stop, and you could experience withdrawal symptoms. Addiction to prescription pain relievers is like being hooked on heroin and the withdrawal isn't much different: bone and muscle pain, diarrhea, vomiting, cold flashes, and insomnia.

If you, or someone you know, is abusing or is addicted, get professional help. You can ask for help from parents, doctors, relatives, teachers, or school guidance counselors. Substance abuse ruins lives. Don't let it happen to your friends—or you. If you, or someone you know, is hooked on prescription pain relievers, get help.

Remember: Only when used correctly and under a doctor's supervision are prescription pain relievers safe and effective.

Additional Information

National Clearinghouse for Alcohol and Drug Information (NCADI)
Substance Abuse and Mental Health Services Administration (SAMHSA)
P.O. Box 2345
Rockville, MD 20847-2345
Toll-Free: 800-729-6686
Website: http://www.ncadi.samhsa.gov

National Institute on Drug Abuse (NIDA)
National Institutes of Health (NIH)
6001 Executive Blvd., Rm. 5213
Bethesda, MD 20892-9561
Phone: 301-443-1124
Website: http://www.drugabuse.gov

Part Five

Managing Chronic Disease

Chapter 44

Living with a Chronic Illness

Living with a long-lasting health condition (also called a chronic illness) presents a person with new challenges. Learning how to meet those challenges is a process—it doesn't happen right away. But understanding more about your condition, and doing your part to manage it, can help you take health challenges in stride. Many people find that taking an active part in the care of a chronic health condition can help them feel stronger and better equipped to deal with lots of life's trials and tribulations.

What Are Chronic Illnesses?

There are two types of illnesses: acute and chronic. Acute illnesses (like a cold or the flu) are usually over relatively quickly. Chronic illnesses, though, are long-lasting health conditions (the word chronic comes from the Greek word *chronos*, meaning time).

Having a chronic condition doesn't necessarily mean an illness is critical or dangerous—although some chronic illnesses, such as cancer and acquired immunodeficiency syndrome (AIDS), can be life threatening. But chronic illnesses can also include conditions like asthma, arthritis, and diabetes. Although the symptoms of a chronic illness might go away with medical care, usually a person still has

This information was provided by TeensHealth, one of the largest resources online for medically reviewed health information written for teens, kids, and parents. For more articles like this one, visit www.TeensHealth.org, or www.KidsHealth.org. © 2007 The Nemours Foundation.

the underlying condition—even though when properly treated he or she may feel completely healthy and well much of the time.

Each health condition has its own symptoms, treatment, and course. Aside from the fact that they are all relatively long lasting, chronic illnesses aren't necessarily alike in other ways. Most people who have a chronic illness don't think of themselves as "having a chronic illness." They think of themselves as having a specific condition—such as asthma, or arthritis, or diabetes, or lupus, or sickle cell anemia, or hemophilia, or leukemia, or whatever ongoing health condition they have.

If you're living with a chronic illness, you may feel affected not just physically, but also emotionally, socially, and sometimes even financially. The way a person might be affected by a chronic illness depends on the particular illness and how it affects the body, how severe it is, and the kinds of treatments that might be involved. It takes time to adjust to and accept the realities of a long-term illness, but people who are willing to learn, seek support from others, and participate actively in the care of their bodies usually get through the coping process.

The Coping Process

Most people go through stages in learning to cope with a chronic illness. A person who has just been diagnosed with a particular health condition may feel a lot of things. Some people feel vulnerable, confused, and worried about their health and the future. Others feel sad or disappointed in their bodies. For some, the situation seems unfair, causing them to feel angry at themselves and the people they love. These feelings are the start of the coping process. Everyone's reaction is different, but they're all completely normal.

The next stage in the coping process is learning. Most people living with a long-term illness find that knowledge is power: The more they find out about their condition, the more they feel in control and the less frightening it is.

The third stage in coping with a chronic illness is all about taking it in stride. At this stage, people feel comfortable with their treatments and with the tools (like inhalers or shots) they need to use to live a normal life.

So someone with diabetes, for example, may feel a range of emotions when the condition is first diagnosed. The person may believe he or she will never be able to go through the skin prick tests or injections that may be necessary to manage the condition. But after working with doctors and understanding more about the condition, that person will grow to be more practiced at monitoring and managing insulin levels—and it will stop feeling like such a big deal. Over time, managing diabetes will become second nature and the steps involved will seem like just another way to care for one's body, in much the same way that daily teeth brushing or showering help people stay healthy.

There's no definite time limit on the coping process. Everybody's process of coming to terms with and accepting a chronic illness is different. In fact, most people will find that emotions surface at all stages in the process. Even if treatments go well, it's natural to feel sad or worried from time to time. Recognizing and being aware of these emotions as they surface is all part of the coping process.

Tools for Taking Control

People living with chronic illnesses often find that the following actions can help them take control and work through the coping process:

Acknowledge feelings. Emotions may not be easy to identify. For example, sleeping or crying a lot or grouchiness may be signs of sadness or depression. It's also very common for people with chronic illnesses to feel stress as they balance the realities of dealing with a health condition and coping with schoolwork, social events, and other aspects of everyday life.

Many people living with chronic illnesses find that it helps to line up sources of support to deal with the stress and emotions. Some people choose to talk to a therapist or join a support group specifically for people with their condition. It's also important to confide in those you trust, like close friends and family members.

The most important factor when seeking help isn't necessarily finding someone who knows a lot about your illness, but finding someone who is willing to listen when you're depressed, angry, frustrated—or even just plain old happy. Noticing the emotions you have, accepting them as a natural part of what you're going through, and expressing or sharing your emotions in a way that feels comfortable can help you feel better about things.

Play an active role in your health care. The best way to learn about your condition and put yourself in control is to ask questions. There's usually a lot of information to absorb when visiting a doctor. You may need to go over specifics more than once or ask a doctor or nurse to repeat things to be sure you understand everything. This may sound basic, but lots of people hesitate to say, "Hey, can you say that again?" because they don't want to sound stupid. But it takes doctors years of medical school and practice to learn the information they're passing on to you in one office visit.

If you've just been diagnosed with a particular condition, you may want to write down some questions to ask your doctor. For example, some of the things you might want to know are:

- How will this condition affect me?

- What kind of treatment is involved?

- Will it be painful?

- How many treatments will I get?

- Will I miss any school?

- Will I be able to play sports, play a musical instrument, try out for the school play, or participate in other activities I love?

- What can I expect—will my condition be cured? Will my symptoms go away?

- What are the side effects of the treatments and how long will they last?

- Will these treatments make me sleepy, grumpy, or weak?

- What happens if I miss a treatment or forget to take my medicine?

- What if the treatments don't work?

Even though your doctor can't exactly predict how you'll respond to treatment because it varies greatly from one person to the next, knowing how some people react may help you prepare yourself mentally, emotionally, and physically. The more you learn about your illness, the more you'll understand about your treatments, your emotions, and the best ways to create a healthy lifestyle based on your individual needs.

Understand other people's reactions. You may not be the only one who feels emotional about your illness. Parents often struggle with seeing their children sick because they want to prevent anything bad from happening to their kids. Some parents feel guilty or think they've failed their child, others may get mad about how unfair it seems. Everyone else's emotions can seem like an extra burden on people who are sick, when of course it's not their fault. Sometimes it helps to explain to a parent that, when you express anger or fear, you're simply asking for their support—not for them to cure you. Tell your parents you don't expect them to have all the answers, but that it helps if they just listen to how you feel and let you know they understand.

Because the teen years are all about fitting in, it can be hard to feel different around friends and classmates. Many people with chronic illnesses are tempted to try to keep their condition secret. Sometimes, though, trying to hide a condition can cause its own troubles as Melissa, who has Crohn's disease, discovered. Some of Melissa's medications made her look puffy, and her classmates started teasing her about gaining weight. When Melissa explained her condition, she was surprised at how accepting her classmates were.

When talking to friends about your health condition, it can sometimes help to explain that everyone is made differently. For the same reason some people have blue eyes and others brown, some of us are more vulnerable to certain conditions than others.

Depending on the severity of your illness, you may find yourself constantly surrounded by well-meaning adults. Teachers, coaches, and school counselors may all try to help you—perhaps causing you to feel dependent, frustrated, or angry. Talk to these people and explain how you feel. Educating and explaining the facts of your condition can help them understand what you're capable of and allow them to see you as a student or an athlete—not a patient.

Keep things in perspective. It's easy for a health condition to become the main focus of someone's life—especially as that person first learns about and starts dealing with the condition. Many people find that reminding themselves that their condition is only a part of who they are can help put things back in perspective. Keeping up with friends, favorite activities, and everyday things helps a lot.

Living with a Health Condition

There's no doubt the teen years can be a more challenging time to deal with a health condition. In addition to the social pressures to fit in, it's a time of learning about and understanding our bodies. At a time when it's natural to be concerned with body image, it can seem hard to feel different. It's understandable that people can feel just plain sick and tired of dealing with a chronic illness once in a while.

Even people who have lived with an illness since childhood can feel the pull of wanting to lead a "normal" life in which they don't need medicine, have any limitations, or have to care for themselves in any special way. This is a perfectly natural reaction. Sometimes people who have learned to manage their illness feel so healthy and strong that they wonder whether they need to keep following their disease management program. A person with diabetes, for example, may consider skipping a meal when at the mall or checking his or her blood sugar after the game instead of before.

Unfortunately, easing up on taking care of yourself can have disastrous results. The best approach is to tell your doctor how you feel. Talk about what you'd like to be doing and can't. See if there's anything you can work out. This is all part of taking more control and becoming a player in your own medical care.

When you're living with a chronic health condition, it can feel hard at times to love your body. But you don't have to have a perfect body to have a great body image. Body image can improve when you care for your body, appreciate its capabilities, and accept its limitations— a fact that's true for everyone, whether they're living with a chronic condition or not.

Voicing any frustration or sadness to an understanding ear can help when a person feels sick of being sick. At times like this it's important to think of ways others could help and ask for what you'd like. Some people find they can ease their own sense of loss by reaching out and offering to help someone in need. Lending a hand to someone else can help one's own troubles seem easier to manage.

Adjusting to living with a chronic illness takes a little time, patience, support—and willingness to learn and participate. People who deal with unexpected challenges often find an inner resilience they might not have known was there before. Many say that they learn more about themselves through dealing with these challenges and feel they grow to be stronger and more self-aware than they would if they'd never faced their particular challenge. People living with chronic illnesses find that when they take an active role in taking care of their body, they grow to understand and appreciate their strengths—and adapt to their weaknesses—as never before.

Chapter 45

Self-Management of Chronic Illness

Chapter Contents

Section 45.1

Take Charge of Your Health

What is a chronic illness?

There are two main types of illness: acute and chronic. An acute illness doesn't last very long. It goes away either on its own or in response to treatment, such as taking medicine or having surgery. Strep throat is an example of an acute illness.

A chronic illness is ongoing. It affects your health over a long period of time—possibly your entire life. In many cases, there is no way to cure a chronic illness. Diabetes and high blood pressure are examples of chronic illnesses.

What can I do if I have a chronic illness?

It's important to understand that your chronic illness is a serious problem. If you don't believe this, you'll never be motivated to manage your illness effectively. Managing your illness involves making lifestyle choices and using prescribed medical treatments to be as healthy as possible. Unless you take care of your body, your chronic illness can cause more problems in the future.

When you have a chronic health problem, it's easy to feel overwhelmed and helpless, as if the illness has taken over your life. For example, you may need to take daily insulin injections, use an inhaler or monitor your blood pressure. However, you can take steps to control the negative effects of a chronic illness on your health. One method of taking control is called "self-management."

What is self-management of chronic illness?

Self-management of chronic illness means that you take responsibility for doing what it takes to manage your illness effectively. It's important for you to be responsible for your health because the treatment recommendations your doctor makes won't do any good unless you follow them. He or she can't make decisions for you or make you change your behavior. Only you can do these things.

In self-management, you and your doctor are partners in care. Your doctor can provide valuable advice and information to help you deal with your illness. However, the treatment plan that works best for one person with your condition won't necessarily work best for you. Talk to your doctor about the different treatment options available and help him or her create a plan that's right for you. After all, nobody knows more than you do about your feelings, your actions and how your health problems affect you.

As part of self-management, it's also your responsibility to ask for the help you need to deal with your illness. This support can come from friends and family members, as well as from your doctor or a support group for people with your health problem.

How can self-management help a person who has a chronic illness?

Once you've decided to take an active role in managing your illness, you and your doctor can work together to set goals that will lead to better health. These goals will be part of an overall treatment plan.

Pick a problem: Take an honest look at the unhealthy aspects of your lifestyle. Start with a particular behavior that you'd like to change in order to have better control of your illness. For example, you might decide that you don't eat enough vegetables, get enough exercise, or take your medicines as your doctor tells you to.

Get specific: Once you've identified a problem, state a specific goal for dealing with it. The more specific your goal is, the more likely you are to succeed. For example, instead of saying, "I'm going to exercise more," decide what kind of exercise you'll do. Be specific about what days of the week you'll exercise and what times you'll exercise on those days. Your new goal might be: "During my lunch hour on Mondays, Wednesdays, and Fridays, I'm going to walk one mile in the park."

Plan ahead: After you've stated your goal, think of things that could go wrong and plan how you'll deal with them. For example, if it rains and you can't go to the park, where will you go to walk? If you plan how to handle problems in advance, they won't prevent you from meeting your goals.

Check your confidence level: Ask yourself, "How confident am I that I'll be able to meet this goal?" If the answer is "Not very confident," you may need to start with a more realistic goal.

Follow up: As you're working toward your goal, check in regularly with your doctor to let him or her know how you're doing. If you're having trouble following the plan, talk to your doctor to figure out why. Your setbacks can be learning experiences that help you make a new plan for success.

One of the most important things to remember is that you can change your behavior. Even though your illness makes you feel helpless at times, if you work with your doctor to set goals and you take responsibility for following through with them, you can make changes that will lead to better health.

Section 45.2

Exercise Can Improve Some Chronic Disease Conditions

This section includes text from "Components of Physical Fitness," Centers for Disease Control and Prevention (CDC), May 2007; "Is It Safe for Me to Exercise?" National Institute on Aging (NIA), March 2007; and "Tips for Avoiding Activity-Induced Injuries," CDC, May 2007.

What does it mean to be physically fit? Physical fitness is defined as "a set of attributes that people have or achieve that relates to the ability to perform physical activity" (U.S. Department of Health and Human Services [HHS], 1996). In other words, it is more than being able to run a long distance or lift a lot of weight at the gym. Being fit is not defined only by what kind of activity you do, how long you do it, or at what level of intensity. While these are important measures of fitness, they only address single areas. Overall fitness is made up of five main components:

• cardiorespiratory endurance

- muscular strength
- muscular endurance
- body composition
- flexibility

In order to assess your level of fitness, look at all five components together.

What is cardiorespiratory endurance (cardiorespiratory fitness)?

Cardiorespiratory endurance is the ability of the body's circulatory and respiratory systems to supply fuel during sustained physical activity (HHS, 1996 as adapted from Corbin and Lindsey, 1994). To improve your cardiorespiratory endurance, try activities that keep your heart rate elevated at a safe level for a sustained length of time such as walking, swimming, or bicycling. The activity you choose does not have to be strenuous to improve your cardiorespiratory endurance. Start slowly with an activity you enjoy, and gradually work up to a more intense pace.

What is muscular strength?

Muscular strength is the ability of the muscle to exert force during an activity (HHS, 1996 as adapted from Wilmore and Costill, 1994). The key to making your muscles stronger is working them against resistance, whether that be from weights or gravity. If you want to gain muscle strength, try exercises such as lifting weights or rapidly taking the stairs.

What is muscular endurance?

Muscular endurance is the ability of the muscle to continue to perform without fatigue (HHS, 1996 as adapted from Wilmore and Costill, 1994). To improve your muscle endurance, try cardiorespiratory activities such as walking, jogging, bicycling, or dancing.

What is body composition?

Body composition refers to the relative amount of muscle, fat, bone, and other vital parts of the body (HHS, 1996 as adapted from Corbin and Lindsey, 1994). A person's total body weight (what you see on the

351

bathroom scale) may not change over time. But the bathroom scale does not assess how much of that body weight is fat and how much is lean mass (muscle, bone, tendons, and ligaments). Body composition is important to consider for health and managing your weight.

What is flexibility?

Flexibility is the range of motion around a joint (HHS, 1996 as adapted from Wilmore and Costill, 1994). Good flexibility in the joints can help prevent injuries through all stages of life. If you want to improve your flexibility, try activities that lengthen the muscles such as swimming or a basic stretching program.

Is It Safe for Me to Exercise?

Chronic Diseases: Not Necessarily a Barrier

Chronic diseases can't be cured, but usually they can be controlled with medications and other treatments throughout a person's life. They are common among older adults, and include diabetes, cardio-vascular disease (such as high blood pressure), and arthritis, among many others.

Traditionally, exercise has been discouraged in people with certain chronic conditions. But researchers have found that exercise can actually improve some chronic conditions in most older people, as long as it's done when the condition is under control.

Congestive heart failure (CHF) is an example of a serious chronic condition common in older adults. In people with CHF, the heart cannot empty its load of blood with each beat, resulting in a backup of fluid throughout the body, including the lungs. Disturbances in heart rhythm also are common in CHF. Older adults are hospitalized more often for this disease than for any other.

No one is sure why, but muscles tend to waste away badly in people with CHF, leaving them weak, sometimes to the point that they cannot perform everyday tasks. No medicine has a direct muscle-strengthening effect in people with CHF, but muscle-building exercises (lifting weights, for example) can help them improve muscle strength.

Having a chronic disease like CHF probably does not mean you cannot exercise. But it does mean that keeping in touch with your doctor is important if you do exercise. For example, some studies suggest that endurance exercises, like brisk walking, may improve how well the heart and lungs work in people with CHF, but only in people who are in a stable phase of the disease. People with CHF, like those with most chronic diseases, have periods when their disease gets better, then worse, then better again, off and on. The same endurance exercises that might help people in a stable phase of CHF could be very harmful to people who are in an unstable phase; that is, when they have fluid in their lungs or an irregular heart rhythm.

If you have a chronic condition, you need to know how you can tell whether your disease is stable; that is, when exercise would be okay for you and when it would not.

Chances are good that, if you have a chronic disease, you see a doctor regularly (if you don't, you should, for many reasons). Talk with your doctor about symptoms that mean trouble—a flare-up, or what doctors call an acute phase or exacerbation of your disease. If you have CHF, you know by now that the acute phase of this disease should be taken very, very seriously. You should not exercise when warning symptoms of the acute phase of CHF, or any other chronic disease, appear. It could be dangerous. But you and your doctor also should discuss how you feel when you are free of those symptoms—in other words, stable; under control. This is the time to exercise.

Diabetes is another chronic condition common among older people. Too much sugar in the blood is a hallmark of diabetes. It can cause damage throughout the body. Exercise can help your body manage some of the damaging sugar. The most common form of diabetes is linked to physical inactivity. In other words, you are less likely to get it in the first place, if you stay physically active.

If you do have diabetes and it has caused changes in your body—cardiovascular disease, eye disease, or changes in your nervous system, for example—check with your doctor to find out what exercises will help you and whether you should avoid certain activities. If you take insulin or a pill that helps lower your blood sugar, your doctor might need to adjust your dose so that your blood sugar does not get too low. Your doctor might find that you don't have to modify your exercises at all, if you are in the earlier stages of diabetes or if your condition is stable.

If you are a man over 40 or a woman over 50, check with your doctor first if you plan to start doing vigorous, as opposed to moderate, physical activities. Vigorous activity could be a problem for people who have hidden heart disease—that is, people who have heart disease but do not know it because they do not have any symptoms. How can you tell if the activity you plan to do is vigorous? There are a couple of ways. If the activity makes you breathe hard and sweat hard (if you tend to sweat, that is), you can consider it vigorous.

If you have had a heart attack recently, your doctor or cardiac rehabilitation therapist should have given you specific exercises to do.

Research has shown that exercises done as part of a cardiac rehabilitation program can improve fitness and even reduce your risk of dying. If you did not get instructions, call your doctor to discuss exercise before you begin increasing your physical activity.

For some conditions, vigorous exercise is dangerous and should not be done, even in the absence of symptoms. Be sure to check with your physician before beginning any kind of exercise program if you have:

- abdominal aortic aneurysm, a weakness in the wall of the heart's major outgoing artery (unless it has been surgically repaired or is so small that your doctor tells you that you can exercise vigorously); or

- critical aortic stenosis, a narrowing of one of the valves of the heart.

Most adults, regardless of age or condition, will do just fine in increasing their physical activity.

Checkpoints

You have already read about precautions you should take if you have a chronic condition. Other circumstances require caution, too. You should not exercise until checking with a doctor if you have:

- chest pain;
- irregular, rapid, or fluttery heart beat;
- severe shortness of breath;
- significant, ongoing weight loss that hasn't been diagnosed;
- infections, such as pneumonia, accompanied by fever;
- fever, which can cause dehydration and a rapid heart beat;
- acute deep-vein thrombosis (blood clot);
- a hernia that is causing symptoms;
- foot or ankle sores that won't heal;
- joint swelling;
- persistent pain or a problem walking after you have fallen; or
- certain eye conditions, such as bleeding in the retina or detached retina. Before you exercise after a cataract or lens implant, or after laser treatment or other eye surgery, check with your physician.

Tips for Avoiding Activity-Induced Injuries

Keeping the following tips in mind can help prevent common injuries associated with participating in physical activity.

- Listen to your body—monitor your level of fatigue, heart rate, and physical discomfort.

- Be aware of the signs of overexertion. Breathlessness and muscle soreness could be danger signs.

- Be aware of the warning signs and signals of a heart attack, such as sweating, chest and arm pain, dizziness, and lightheadedness.

- Use appropriate equipment and clothing for the activity.

- Take 3–5 minutes at the beginning of any physical activity to properly warm up your muscles through increasingly more intense activity. As you near the end of the activity, cool down by decreasing the level of intensity. (For example, before jogging, walk for 3–5 minutes increasing your pace to a brisk walk. After jogging, walk briskly, decreasing your pace to a slow walk over 3–5 minutes. Finish by stretching the muscles you used—in this case primarily the muscles of the legs.)

- Start at an easy pace—increase time or distance gradually.

- Drink plenty of water throughout the day to replace lost fluids (for example, at least eight to ten 8-oz. cups per day). Drink a glass of water before you get moving, and drink another half cup every 15 minutes that you remain active.

Section 45.3

Adopt a Healthy Eating Plan

Excerpted from, "Better Health and You: Healthy Eating,"
National Institute of Diabetes and Digestive and Kidney Diseases
(NIDDK), NIH Publication No. 04–4992, updated August 2006.

What is a healthy eating plan?

A balanced eating plan and regular physical activity are the building blocks of good health. Poor eating habits and physical inactivity may lead to overweight and related health problems. By eating right and being active, you may reach or maintain a healthy weight. You may also improve your physical health, mental well-being, and set an example for others. Do it for yourself and your family.

A healthy eating plan:

- emphasizes fruits, vegetables, whole grains, and fat-free or low-fat milk and milk products;

- includes lean meats, poultry, fish, beans, eggs, and nuts; and

- is low in saturated fats, trans fats, cholesterol, salt (sodium), and added sugars.

Tips for Healthy Eating

- Eat breakfast every day. People who eat breakfast are less likely to overeat later in the day. Breakfast also gives you energy and helps you get your day off to a healthy start.

- Choose whole grains more often. Try whole-wheat breads and pastas, oatmeal, brown rice, or bulgur.

- Select a mix of colorful vegetables each day. Vegetables of different colors provide different nutrients. Choose dark leafy greens such as spinach, kale, collards, and mustard greens, and reds and oranges such as carrots, sweet potatoes, red peppers, and tomatoes.

- Choose fresh, canned, or frozen fruit more often than fruit juice. Fruit juice has little or no fiber, and the calories may be high. Fresh, canned, or frozen fruit is often better for you. If you eat canned fruit, opt for fruit packed in water rather than syrup.

- Use fats and oils sparingly. Olive, canola, and peanut oils, avocados, nuts and nut butters, olives, and fish provide heart-healthy fat as well as vitamins and minerals.

- Eat sweets sparingly. Limit foods and beverages that are high in added sugars.

- Eat three meals every day. If you skip meals or replace a meal with a snack, you might overeat later on.

- Have low-fat, low-sugar snacks on hand. Whether you are at home, at work, or on the go, healthy snacks may help to combat hunger and prevent overeating.

Quick Breakfast Ideas

- low-fat yogurt sprinkled with low-fat granola
- oatmeal with low-fat or fat-free milk, or soy-based beverage
- a slice of whole-wheat toast with a thin spread of peanut butter
- fruit smoothie made with frozen fruit, low-fat yogurt, and juice
- high-fiber, low-sugar cereal with soy-based beverage or low-fat milk

Easy Snack Ideas

- low-fat or fat-free yogurt
- rice cakes
- fresh or canned fruits
- sliced vegetables or baby carrots
- dried fruit and nut mix (no more than a small handful)
- air-popped popcorn sprinkled with garlic powder or other spices
- high-fiber, low-sugar cereal

Section 45.4

Tips for Dealing with Pain

Pain has been in the news lately, and not always in the ways that we would hope. On the one hand, *Time Magazine* featured the issue of treating chronic pain on its cover in February 2007, and the *Today* show featured a five-part, educational series on chronic pain in March 2007. On the other hand, the Drug Enforcement Administration's (DEA) withdrawal of the "Frequently Asked Questions" document has increased confusion about prescribing proven medications for the treatment of pain, further stigmatizing pain patients. And now, the withdrawal of two COX-2 non-steroidal anti-inflammatory (NSAID) medications and the more stringent, Food and Drug Administration (FDA)-mandated warnings on all NSAIDs have created fear and confusion about what's safe and effective for treating pain.

You may be feeling overwhelmed and confused. You may ask yourself, "What's safe? What medications can I take? Who can I trust to provide accurate and complete information about my condition and my treatment options? What can I do now that I can no longer take this medication? What can I do if my doctor is no longer willing to prescribe to me? What things can I do to improve my quality of life?"

The important thing to remember is that you are not alone. Millions of Americans suffer from chronic pain, and there are many organizations working to address this serious, life-altering and profoundly difficult problem. Overcoming suffering and pain is difficult—sometimes it even seems impossible, but there are things you can do to help yourself. You must be your own best advocate.

Now, more than ever, is the time to educate yourself about your treatment options and empower yourself by doing what you can to care for yourself physically, emotionally, and spiritually.

Unfortunately, there is no magic pill or cure to relieve chronic pain or its underlying conditions. Medication alone often is not enough, especially for people who have chronic pain. As some of your medical options may be disappearing, it may be time to reevaluate what's working for you and what you can do differently to help yourself. Relieving pain requires work both on the part of the physician and on the part of the patient. People with chronic pain must be active participants in their care.

Steps You Can Take to Feel More in Control of Your Pain Condition

Find an Understanding and Knowledgeable Pain Specialist

If you are looking for a pain specialist, you have some different options for your search. First, you can ask for a referral from your primary care physician. This is often the first step that should be taken. You can also ask others to recommend a doctor.

Many professional physician organization websites have listings of their members available to the public. These directories oftentimes can help you locate an appropriate pain medicine physician in your area. You can print the directory and share it with your primary care physician to identify the best physician for your particular needs.

Once you have identified a physician, you should ask specific questions to help you determine whether the physician will best meet your needs. Some of the questions below can help you make an informed decision.

- How many cases of my type of pain condition have you treated?
- What are your special qualifications to treat my pain condition?
- Have you participated in any special training about pain management techniques?
- What is your philosophy of management of my pain condition in terms of medications and alternative therapies?
- What types of medications do you usually prescribe?
- What types of non-medication therapies do you use?
- Where do you refer patients who need additional treatment?
- Is your clinic listed with any professional societies?
- Are you, or is someone in the clinic, available 24 hours a day if I need help?

Finding an understanding and qualified pain specialist is one of the first steps in fighting to regain your life.

Take Care of the Things You Can Control

Part of being an active participant in your care is caring for your body. No one but you can care for your body. Getting adequate rest, eating a healthy diet, and engaging in physical activity are vitally important to maintaining function and health. It may seem like a catch-22—you're in pain, so you don't want to move or you're finally feeling a little better, but you're afraid to move because your pain might come back. Avoiding exercise can be detrimental to your health—you lose muscle tone and strength, your heart and lungs work less efficiently, and your pain can increase.[1] On the other hand, the benefits of incorporating activity into your lifestyle are immeasurable and include increased muscle strength and flexibility, improved sleep, and stress relief.[2]

Following are some suggestions for increasing your activity level:

- Choose exercises that can be incorporated into your daily routine and that you enjoy.

- Set a schedule.

- Ask your doctor about appropriate exercises and activities for your situation.

- Set appropriate goals.[3] No goal is too small—visiting friends or walking around the block may be appropriate goals, depending on your pain and physical condition.

Ask your physician which exercises are safe for you. In addition to a healthy diet and exercise, relaxation techniques such as meditation, visualization, hypnosis, and biofeedback may help you feel better. Your health care provider can help you decide which techniques may be beneficial for you.

Caring for Your Emotional Health

The effect emotions and psychosocial well-being have on pain cannot be ignored as emotions have a direct effect on your health.[4] Pain so often is accompanied by loss—loss of function, loss of employment, loss of money, loss of friends and relationships to name just a few— it's no wonder that people in chronic pain have an increased incidence of depression, anxiety, and sleep disturbances.[5] Research has shown that people in chronic pain suffering from depression have poorer outcomes than those who are not depressed.[6] It is natural for people in pain to grieve for what they've lost, and it is important to remember that your family members and friends grieve too. Your emotions may range from fear, anger, denial, disappointment, guilt, and loneliness to hope and optimism. Every person feels different emotions at different times, which can make relationships and pain control difficult.

Taking care of the emotional aspects of chronic pain is necessary to treat your overall pain condition. Your physician may want to prescribe medication for depression, anxiety, and sleep disturbances and, in addition, may suggest cognitive behavioral therapy (for example, relaxation techniques, coping strategies, psychological therapy).[7] Your doctor does not think you're crazy—he or she is treating you as a whole—not just the part in pain. Following are some suggestions to help you deal with the emotional aspects of pain:

- Keep a journal of your emotions. A journal can help you release some of the emotions you feel.

- Share your thoughts and feelings with loved ones and allow them to share their feelings with you. People cannot read your mind—just as pain is an invisible disease, emotions can be difficult to discern.

- Avoid isolation and loneliness by joining a support group. There are local support groups that you can attend with people who know what you are experiencing and there are online communities that offer support and understanding. The National Pain Foundation's My Community is a good way to share your story and connect with others online. The American Chronic Pain Association has support groups throughout the country. Contact the ACPA at http://www.theacpa.org or 800-533-3231 to find a group near you.

- Be active—exercise can help relieve the stress and emotional pain you feel.

Evaluate Your Treatment Options

Medications such as NSAIDs and selective NSAIDs (COX-2 inhibitors) are important tools in the management of chronic pain, but they are not the only tools available to help you. NSAIDs work by decreasing inflammation and pain. Traditional NSAIDs, such as ibuprofen and naproxen, tend to irritate the stomach and can lead to ulcers and bleeding. The COX-2 NSAIDs have become popular because they are less likely to cause ulcers and bleeding.

News that another NSAID has been withdrawn from the market and the fact that all NSAIDs will now have additional warnings on their labels can be frightening and disheartening for patients dealing with chronic pain. The first step in determining if NSAIDs and COX-2 NSAIDs are still an option for you is to speak with your doctor. All medications have benefits and all medications have side effects and risks. Different people react differently to medications, and choosing to take a medication becomes a very personal decision that must take into account the risks and benefits, your level of functioning without a particular medication, and your overall health. You and your doctor are the only people who can determine whether a specific medication is the right choice for you.

If you are taking any NSAIDs for pain, be sure your doctor knows your medical history, including any history of heart problems, high blood pressure, ulcers, and medication allergies. Be sure your doctor knows about all the medications you currently take, including medications prescribed by other doctors, over-the-counter medications, and supplements. This information will help you and your doctor weigh the overall risk-benefit of a medication.

It is up to you to educate yourself about your health and your treatment options. There are many options for your pain, including:

- prescription and over-the-counter NSAIDs;

- other prescription medications such as opioids, anxiolytics/hypnotics, anticonvulsants, antidepressants, muscle relaxants and more, depending on your pain condition;

- complementary and alternative therapies, such as biofeedback, meditation, relaxation techniques, yoga, acupuncture, and more;

- physical therapy; and

- interventional treatments (for example, for arthritis, injections at the pain site containing a pain reliever and corticosteroid; or for back and neck pain, spinal cord stimulators and intrathecal drug pumps).

Talk with your doctor. Developing an open and trusting relationship with your pain specialist is important to helping you determine which treatment options are best for you.

References

1. "Chronic pain: Exercise can bring relief," Mayo Clinic (April 23, 2001). Available from http://www.mayoclinic.com/invoke .cfm?id=AR00017; M Nicholas et al, *Manage your Pain: Practical and Positive Ways of Adapting to Chronic Pain* (Sydney: ABC Books, 2002) 84–89, 98–127.

2. "Chronic pain," WebMD (March 2001). Available from http:// my.webmd.com/content/article/1832.50232/; "Chronic pain: Exercise can bring relief," Mayo Clinic (April 23, 2001).

3. "Chronic pain: Exercise can bring relief," Mayo Clinic (April 23, 2001); Nicholas et al, *Manage your Pain: Practical and Positive Ways of Adapting to Chronic Pain*, 84–89, 98–127.

4. M McCaffery, C Pasero, *Pain Clinical Manual*, second ed (St. Louis: Mosby, 1999) 499–505.

5. Ibid.

6. Ibid.

7. Ibid.

Section 45.5

Stress and Your Health

Excerpted from "Stress and Your Health,"
National Women's Health Information Center, August 2004.

What are some of the most common causes of stress?

Stress can arise for a variety of reasons. Stress can be brought about by a traumatic accident, death, or emergency situation. Stress can also be a side effect of a serious illness or disease.

There is also stress associated with daily life, the workplace, and family responsibilities. It's hard to stay calm and relaxed in our hectic lives. We have many roles: spouse, parent, caregiver, friend, and worker.

With all we have going on in our lives, it seems almost impossible to find ways to de-stress. But it's important to find those ways. Your health depends on it.

What are some early signs of stress?

Stress can take on many different forms, and can contribute to symptoms of illness. Common symptoms include headache, sleep disorders, difficulty concentrating, short-temper, upset stomach, job dissatisfaction, low morale, depression, and anxiety.

How does stress affect my body and my health?

Everyone has stress. We have short-term stress, like getting lost while driving or missing the bus. Even everyday events, such as planning a meal or making time for errands, can be stressful. This kind of stress can make us feel worried or anxious.

Other times, we face long-term stress, such as racial discrimination, a life-threatening illness, or divorce. These stressful events also affect your health on many levels. Long-term stress is real and can increase your risk for some health problems, like depression.

Both short and long-term stress can have effects on your body. Research is starting to show the serious effects of stress on our bodies. Stress triggers changes in our bodies and makes us more likely to get sick. It can also make problems we already have worse. It can play a part in these problems:

- trouble sleeping
- headaches
- constipation
- diarrhea
- irritability
- lack of energy
- lack of concentration
- eating too much or not at all
- anger
- sadness
- higher risk of asthma and arthritis flare-ups
- tension
- stomach cramping

- stomach bloating
- skin problems, like hives
- depression
- anxiety
- weight gain or loss
- heart problems
- high blood pressure
- irritable bowel syndrome
- diabetes
- neck and/or back pain
- less sexual desire
- fertility difficulties

How can I help handle my stress?

Don't let stress make you sick. We tend to carry a higher burden of stress than we should. Often we aren't even aware of our stress levels. Listen to your body, so that you know when stress is affecting your health. Here are ways to help you handle your stress.

- **Relax:** It's important to unwind. Each person has her own way to relax. Some ways include deep breathing, yoga, meditation, and massage therapy. If you can't do these things, take a few minutes to sit, listen to soothing music, or read a book.

- **Make time for yourself:** It's important to care for yourself. Think of this as an order from your doctor, so you don't feel guilty. No matter how busy you are, you can try to set aside at least 15 minutes each day in your schedule to do something for yourself, like taking a bubble bath, going for a walk, or calling a friend.

- **Sleep:** Sleeping is a great way to help both your body and mind. Your stress could get worse if you don't get enough sleep. You also can't fight off sickness as well when you sleep poorly. With enough sleep, you can tackle your problems better and lower your risk for illness. Try to get seven to nine hours of sleep every night.

- **Eat right:** Try to fuel up with fruits, vegetables, and proteins. Good sources of protein can be peanut butter, chicken, or tuna salad. Eat whole-grains, such as wheat breads and wheat crackers. Don't be fooled by the jolt you get from caffeine or sugar. Your energy will wear off.

- **Get moving:** Believe it or not, getting physical activity not only helps relieve your tense muscles, but helps your mood too. Your body makes certain chemicals, called endorphins, before and after you work out. They relieve stress and improve your mood.

- **Talk to friends:** Talk to your friends to help you work through your stress. Friends are good listeners. Finding someone who will let you talk freely about your problems and feelings without judging you does a world of good. It also helps to hear a different point of view. Friends will remind you that you're not alone.

- **Get help from a professional if you need it:** Talk to a therapist. A therapist can help you work through stress and find better ways to deal with problems. For more serious stress related disorders, like post-traumatic stress disorder (PTSD), therapy can be helpful. There also are medications that can help ease symptoms of depression and anxiety and help promote sleep.

- **Compromise:** Sometimes, it's not always worth the stress to argue. Give in once in awhile.

- **Write down your thoughts:** Have you ever typed an e-mail to a friend about your lousy day and felt better afterward? Why not grab a pen and paper and write down what's going on in your life. Keeping a journal can be a great way to get things off your chest and work through issues. Later, you can go back and read through your journal and see how you've made progress.

- **Help others:** Helping someone else can help you. Help your neighbor, or volunteer in your community.

- **Get a hobby:** Find something you enjoy. Make sure to give yourself time to explore your interests.

- **Set limits:** When it comes to things like work and family, figure out what you can really do. There are only so many hours in the day. Set limits with yourself and others. Don't be afraid to say no to requests for your time and energy.

- **Plan your time:** Think ahead about how you're going to spend your time. Write a to-do list. Figure out what's most important to do.

- **Don't deal with stress in unhealthy ways:** This includes drinking too much alcohol, using drugs, smoking, or overeating.

Chapter 46

Preventing Infection at Home and Work

An Ounce of Prevention Keeps the Germs Away: Seven Keys to a Safer Healthier Home

Staying healthy is important to you and your entire family. Follow these easy, low-cost steps to help stop many infectious diseases before they happen.

Wash Your Hands Often

Keeping your hands clean is one of the best ways to keep from getting sick and spreading illnesses. Cleaning your hands gets rid of germs you pick up from other people, from the surfaces you touch, and from pets or wild animals.

Wash your hands—

- before eating;
- before, during, and after handling or preparing food;
- after contact with blood or body fluids (like vomit, nasal secretions, or saliva);
- after changing a diaper;
- after you use the bathroom;

This chapter includes excerpts from "An Ounce of Prevention Keeps the Germs Away," Centers for Disease Control and Prevention (CDC), 2005; and "Stopping the Spread of Germs at Work," CDC, March 2007.

- after handling animals, their toys, leashes, or waste;
- after touching something that could be contaminated (such as a trash can, cleaning cloth, drain, or soil);
- before dressing a wound, giving medicine, or inserting contact lenses;
- more often when someone in your home is sick; and
- whenever your hands look dirty.

How to Wash?

- Wet your hands and apply liquid, bar, or powder soap.
- Rub hands together vigorously to make a lather and scrub all surfaces.
- Continue rubbing for 20 seconds. It takes that long for the soap and scrubbing action to dislodge and remove stubborn germs. Need a timer? Imagine singing "Happy Birthday" all the way through twice.
- Rinse hands well under running water.
- Dry your hands using a paper towel or air dryer.
- If possible, use your paper towel to turn off the faucet.

Remember: If soap and water are not available, use an alcohol-based wipe or hand gel.

Routinely Clean and Disinfect Surfaces

Cleaning and disinfecting is not the same thing. Cleaning removes germs from surfaces whereas disinfecting actually destroys them. Cleaning with soap and water to remove dirt and most of the germs is usually enough. But sometimes, you may want to disinfect for an extra level of protection from germs.

- While surfaces may look clean, many infectious germs may be lurking around. In some instances, germs can live on surfaces for hours and even days.
- Disinfectants are specifically registered with the U.S. Environmental Protection Agency (EPA) and contain ingredients that actually destroy bacteria and other germs. Check the product label to make sure it says "disinfectant" and has an EPA registration number.

Disinfect those areas where there can be large numbers of dangerous germs and where there is a possibility that these germs could be spread to others.

In the Kitchen

- Clean and disinfect counters and other surfaces before, during, and after preparing food (especially meat and poultry).

- Follow all directions on the product label which usually specifies letting the disinfectant stand for a few minutes.

- When cleaning surfaces, do not let germs hang around on cleaning cloths or towels. Use paper towels that can be thrown away, cloth towels that are later washed in hot water, or disposable sanitizing wipes that both clean and disinfect.

In the Bathroom

- Routinely clean and disinfect all surfaces. This is especially important if someone in the house has a stomach illness, a cold, or the flu.

Handle and Prepare Food Safely

When it comes to preventing food-borne illness, there are four simple steps to food safety that you can practice every day. These steps are easy and they will help protect you and those around you from harmful food-borne bacteria.

Clean Hands and Surfaces Often

Germs that cause food-borne illness can be spread throughout the kitchen and get onto hands from cutting boards, utensils, counter tops, and food. Help stop the spread of these germs.

- Clean your hands with warm water and soap for at least 20 seconds before and after handling food. If soap and water are not available, use an alcohol-based wipe or hand gel.

- Wash your cutting boards, dishes, utensils, and counter tops with hot soapy water after preparing each food item and before you prepare the next food.

- Consider using paper towels to clean up kitchen surfaces. If you use cloth towels, wash them often using the hot cycle of your washing machine. If using a sponge to clean up, microwave it each evening for 30 seconds or place it in the dishwasher.

- Rinse all fresh fruits and vegetables under running tap water. This includes those with skins and rinds that are not eaten. For firm-skin fruits and vegetables, rub with your hands or scrub with a clean vegetable brush while rinsing.

Separate Food

Do not cross-contaminate one food with another. Cross-contamination occurs when bacteria spread from a food to a surface, from a surface to another food, or from one food to another.

- Separate raw meat, poultry, seafood, and eggs from other foods in your grocery cart, grocery bags, and in your refrigerator. Be sure to use the plastic bags available in the meat and produce sections of the supermarket.

- Use one cutting board for fresh produce and a different one for raw meat, poultry, and seafood.

- Never place cooked food on a plate that previously held raw meat, poultry, seafood, or eggs.

- Do not allow juices from meat, seafood, poultry, or eggs to drip on other foods in the refrigerator. Use containers to keep these foods from touching other foods.

- Never reuse marinades that were used on raw food, unless you bring them to a boil first.

Cook Foods to Proper Temperature

Foods are safely cooked when they are heated for a long-enough time and at a high-enough temperature to kill the harmful bacteria that cause food-borne illness. The target temperature is different for different foods.

The only way to know for sure that meat is cooked to a safe temperature is to use a food thermometer. Make sure it reaches the temperature recommended for each specific food.

Refrigerate Foods Promptly

Cold temperatures slow the growth of harmful bacteria. So, refrigerate foods quickly. Do not overstuff the refrigerator, as cold air must circulate to help keep food safe.

- Keeping a constant refrigerator temperature of 40° F or below is one of the most effective ways to reduce the risk of food-borne illness. Use an appliance thermometer to be sure the temperature is consistently 40° F or below.

- The freezer temperature should be 0° F or below.

- Plan when you shop: Buy perishable foods such as dairy products, fresh meat, and hot, cooked foods at the end of your shopping trip. Refrigerate foods as soon as possibly to extend their storage life. Do not leave perishable foods out for more than two hours.

- If preparing picnic foods, be sure to include an ice pack to keep cold foods cold.

- Store leftovers properly.

Get Immunized

Getting immunizations is easy and low-cost—and most importantly, it saves lives. Make sure you and your children get the shots suggested by your doctor or health care provider at the proper time and keep records of all immunizations for the whole family. Also, ask your doctor about special programs that provide free shots for your child.

- Children should get their first immunizations before they are two months old. They should have additional doses four or more times before their second birthday.

- Adults need tetanus and diphtheria boosters every ten years. Shots are also often needed for protection from illnesses when traveling to other countries.

- Get your flu shot. The single best way to prevent the flu is to get vaccinated each fall.

Be Careful with Pets

Pets provide many benefits to people, including comfort and companionship. However, some animals can also pass diseases to humans. Keep these tips in mind to make sure your pet relationship is a happy and healthy one.

- Pets should be adopted from an animal shelter or purchased from a reputable pet store or breeder.

371

- All pets should be routinely cared for by a veterinarian. Follow the immunization schedule that the vet recommends.

- Obey local leash laws.

- Clean litter boxes daily. Pregnant women should not clean litter boxes.

- Do not allow children to play where animals go to the bathroom.

- Keep your child's sandbox covered when not in use.

Children and Pets

Babies and children under five are more likely to get diseases from animals, so keep these special guidelines in mind.

- Young children should not be allowed to kiss pets or to put their hands or other objects into their mouths after touching animals.

- Wash your child's hands thoroughly with soap and warm running water after contact with animals.

- Be particularly careful when visiting farms, petting zoos, and fairs.

Stopping the Spread of Germs at Work

Illnesses like the flu (influenza) and colds are caused by viruses that infect the nose, throat, and lungs. The flu and colds usually spread from person to person when an infected person coughs or sneezes.

Coughs and Sneezes

Cover your mouth and nose when you sneeze or cough. Cough or sneeze into a tissue and then throw it away. Cover your cough or sneeze if you do not have a tissue. Then, clean your hands, and do so every time you cough or sneeze.

Clean Your Hands Often

When available, wash your hands with soap and warm water rubbing your hands vigorously together and scrubbing all surfaces. Wash for 15 to 20 seconds. It is the soap combined with the scrubbing action that helps dislodge and remove germs.

When soap and water are not available, alcohol-based disposable hand wipes or gel sanitizer may be used. You can find them in most supermarkets and drugstores. If using a gel, rub the gel in your hands until they are dry. The gel doesn't need water to work; the alcohol in the gel kills germs that cause colds and the flu.

Avoid Touching Your Eyes, Nose, or Mouth

Germs are often spread when a person touches something that is contaminated with germs and then touches their eyes, nose, or mouth. Germs can live for a long time (some can live for two hours or more) on surfaces like doorknobs, desks, and tables.

Stay Home If You Are Sick

When you are sick or have flu symptoms, stay home, get plenty of rest, and check with a health care provider as needed. Your employer may need a doctor's note for an excused absence. Remember: Keeping your distance from others may protect them from getting sick. Common symptoms of the flu include:

- fever (usually high);
- headache;
- extreme tiredness;
- cough;
- sore throat;
- runny or stuffy nose;
- muscle aches; or
- nausea, vomiting, and diarrhea (much more common among children than adults).

Chapter 47

Chronic Illness and Depression

What is a chronic illness?

A chronic illness is one that lasts for a very long time and usually cannot be cured completely. Examples of chronic illnesses include diabetes, heart disease, arthritis, kidney disease, human immunodeficiency virus (HIV)/acquired immunodeficiency syndrome (AIDS), lupus, and multiple sclerosis. Many of these conditions can be improved through diet, exercise, and healthy living, in addition to medication.

Why is depression common in people who have a chronic illness?

Depression is one of the most common complications of chronic illness. It is estimated that up to one-third of individuals with a serious medical condition experience symptoms of depression. People diagnosed with chronic illnesses must adjust to the demands of the illness as well as to its treatment. The illness may affect a person's mobility and independence, and change the way a person lives, sees himself or herself, and relates to others. These requirements can be stressful and cause a certain amount of despair or sadness that is normal.

In some cases, having a chronic illness can trigger clinically significant depression, a potentially serious but treatable illness itself. The challenge for the doctor and the patient is to decide whether symptoms of depression are just a normal reaction to the stress of having a chronic medical condition, or so intense or disabling that they require additional specific antidepressant treatment.

Which long-term illnesses lead to depression?

Any chronic condition can trigger depression, but the risk increases with the severity of the illness and how much disruption it causes in one's life.

Depression caused by chronic illness can in turn aggravate the illness, causing a vicious cycle to develop. Depression is especially likely to occur when the illness is associated with pain, disability, or social isolation. Depression in turn can intensify pain, fatigue, and the self-doubt that can lead to avoidance of others.

The rate for depression occurring with other medical illnesses is quite high:

- heart attack: 40%–65%
- coronary artery disease (without heart attack): 18%–20%
- Parkinson disease: 40%
- multiple sclerosis: 40%
- stroke: 10%–27%
- cancer: 25%
- diabetes: 25%

What are the symptoms of depression?

Patients and their family members often overlook the symptoms of depression, assuming that feeling depressed is normal for someone struggling with a serious, chronic illness. Symptoms of depression such as fatigue, poor appetite, impaired concentration, and insomnia are also common features of chronic medical conditions, adding to the difficulty of deciding whether they are due to depression or to the underlying illness. When depression is present, it is extremely important to treat both the depression and the chronic medical illness at the same time.

Common symptoms of depression include:

- depressed mood or loss of interest or pleasure in daily activities;
- significant weight loss or weight gain;
- sleep disturbances—sleeping too much or not able to sleep;
- problems with concentration;
- apathy (lack of feeling or emotion);
- feelings of worthlessness or guilt;
- fatigue or loss of energy; and
- repeated thoughts of death or suicide.

What can be done to treat depression?

Early diagnosis and treatment for depression can reduce distress as well as the risk of suicide when it exists. Those with a chronic medical condition who get treatment for co-existing depression often experience an improvement in their overall medical condition, achieve a better quality of life, and find it easier to follow through with their treatment plan.

Sometimes improved treatment of the chronic medical condition will alleviate the symptoms of depression that it caused. When this is the case, specific treatment for depression is unnecessary. Some medications can cause depression; in these cases, the best thing to do is reduce or eliminate the offending agent. However, when depression becomes a separate problem, it should be treated on its own.

The success of antidepressant treatment—like any other treatment—cannot be guaranteed, but the majority of individuals treated for depression will recover. Recovery is often more rapid and complete when both antidepressant medication and psychotherapy (talk therapy) are combined. Many antidepressant medicines are available to treat depression. How these drugs work is not fully understood, but they affect brain chemicals that are believed to be involved in depression.

Psychotherapy, or therapy for short, actually refers to a variety of techniques used to treat depression. Psychotherapy involves talking to a licensed professional who helps the depressed person:

- Focus on the behaviors, emotions, and ideas that contribute to his or her depression.
- Understand and identify the life problems or events—such as a major illness, a death in the family, the loss of a job, or a divorce—

377

that contribute to depression and help them understand which aspects of those problems they may be able to solve or improve.

- Regain a sense of control and pleasure in life.

Tips for Coping with Chronic Illness

Depression, disability, and chronic illness form a vicious circle. Chronic illness can bring on bouts of depression, which, in turn, can lead to a rundown physical condition that interferes with successful treatment of the chronic condition.

The following are some tips to help you better cope with a chronic illness:

- Learn how to live with the physical effects of the illness.
- Learn how to deal with the treatments.
- Make sure there is clear communication with your doctors.
- Try to maintain emotional balance to cope with negative feelings.
- Try to maintain confidence and a positive self-image.
- Get help as soon as symptoms of depression appear.

Chapter 48

Assistive Technology

Assistive technology is any service or tool that helps the disabled or elderly do the activities they have always done but must now do differently. These tools are also sometimes called adaptive devices. Such technology may be something as simple as a walker to make moving around easier or an amplification device to make sounds easier to hear (for talking on the telephone or watching television, for instance). It could also include a magnifying glass that helps someone who has poor vision read the newspaper or a small motor scooter that makes it possible to travel over distances that are too far to walk. In short, anything that helps an individual continue to participate in daily activities is considered assistive technology.

There are many different categories of assistive devices and services available to help overcome disabilities. These include:

- **Adaptive switches:** Modified switches that can be used to adjust air conditioners, computers, telephone answering machines, power wheelchairs, and other types of equipment. These switches might be activated by the tongue or the voice.

- **Communication equipment:** Anything that enables a person to send and receive messages, such as a telephone amplifier.

- **Computer access:** Special software that helps access the internet or basic hardware, such as a modified keyboard or mouse, that makes the computer more user friendly.

Excerpted from "Assistive Technology," Administration on Aging, July, 2005.

- **Education:** Audio books or Braille writing tools for the blind come under this category, along with resources that allow people to get additional vocational training.

- **Home modifications:** Construction or remodeling work, such as building a ramp for wheelchair access, that allows an individual to overcome physical barriers and live more comfortably with a disability or recover from an accident or injury.

- **Tools for independent living:** Anything that empowers the individual to enjoy the normal activities of daily living without assistance from others such as a handicapped-accessible bathroom with grab bars in the bathtub.

- **Job-related items:** Devices or processes that a person needs to do his or her job better or easier. Examples might include a special type of chair or pillow for someone who works at a desk or a back brace for someone who does physical labor.

- **Mobility aids:** Items which help a person to get around more easily, such as a cane, walker, power wheelchair, wheelchair lift, or stair elevator.

- **Orthotic or prosthetic equipment:** A device that compensates for a missing or disabled body part. This could range from orthopedic shoe inserts for someone who has fallen arches to an artificial arm for someone whose limb has been amputated.

- **Recreational assistance:** New methods and tools to enable people who have disabilities to enjoy a wide range of fun activities. Examples include swimming lessons provided by recreational therapists or specially equipped skis for seniors who have lost a limb as a result of accident or illness.

- **Seating aids:** Any modifications to regular chairs, wheelchairs, or motor scooters that help a person stay upright or get up and down unaided or that help to reduce pressure on the skin. This could be something as simple as an extra pillow or as complex as a motorized seat.

- **Sensory enhancements:** Anything that makes it easier for those who are partially or fully blind or deaf to better appreciate the world around them.

- **Therapy:** Equipment or processes that help someone recover as much as possible from an illness or injury. Therapy might involve a combination of services and technology.

- **Transportation assistance:** Devices for individuals that make it easier for them to get into and out of their cars or trucks and drive more safely such as adjustable mirrors, seats, and steering wheels.

What are the benefits of assistive technology?

For many people, assistive technology makes the difference between being able to live independently and having to get long-term nursing or home-health care. For others, assistive technology is critical to the ability to perform simple activities of daily living such as bathing and going to the bathroom.

According to a 1993 study conducted by the National Council on Disability, 80 percent of the elderly persons who used assistive technology were able to reduce their dependence on others. In addition, half of those surveyed reduced their dependence on paid helpers, and half were able to avoid entering nursing homes. Assistive technology can also reduce the costs of care for the elderly and their families. Although families may need to make monthly payments for some pieces of equipment, for many, this cost is much less than the cost of home-health or nursing-home care.

How can I tell if assistive technology is right for me?

Needs must be carefully evaluated before deciding to purchase assistive technology. Using assistive technology may change the mix of services that a person requires or may affect the way that those services are provided. For this reason, the process of needs assessment and planning is important.

Usually, needs assessment has the most value when it is done by a team working with the person in the place where the assistive technology will be used. For example, an elderly person who has trouble communicating or is hard of hearing should consult with his or her doctor, an audiology specialist, a speech-language therapist, and family and friends. Together, these people can identify the problem precisely and determine a course of action to solve the problem.

By performing the needs assessment, defining goals, and determining what would help the individual communicate more easily in the home, the team can decide what assistive technology tools are appropriate. After that, the team can help select the most effective devices available at the lowest cost. A professional member of the team, such as the audiology specialist, can also arrange for any training that the senior and his or her family may require.

When considering all the options of assistive technology, it is often useful to look at the issue in terms of high-tech and low-tech solutions. Individuals must also remember to plan ahead and think about how their needs might change over time. High-tech devices tend to be more expensive but may be able to assist with many different needs. Low-tech equipment is usually cheaper but less adaptable for multiple purposes. Before buying any expensive piece of assistive technology, such as a computer, be sure to find out if it can be upgraded as improvements are introduced.

Whether you are conducting a needs assessment or trying to make a decision after such an assessment, it is always a good idea to ask the following questions about assistive technology:

- Does a more advanced device meet more than one of my needs?

- Does the manufacturer of the assistive technology have a preview policy that will let me try out a device and return it for credit if it does not work as expected?

- How are my needs likely to change over the next six months? How about over the next six years or longer?

- How up-to-date is this piece of assistive equipment? Is it likely to become obsolete in the immediate future?

- What are the tasks that I need help with, and how often do I need help with these tasks?

- What types of assistive technology are available to meet my needs?

- What, if any, types of assistive technology have I used before, and how did that equipment work?

- What type of assistive technology will give me the greatest personal independence?

- Will I always need help with this task? If so, can I adjust this device and continue to use it as my condition changes?

How can I pay for assistive technology?

Right now, no single private insurance plan or public program will pay for all types of assistive technology under any circumstances.

Medicare Part B: Medicare Part B will cover up to 80 percent of the cost of assistive technology if the items being purchased meet the definition of durable medical equipment. This is defined as devices that are primarily and customarily used to serve a medical purpose, and generally are not useful to a person in the absence of illness or injury. Contact Medicare to find out if the cost of a particular piece of assistive technology will be covered.

Medicare
Toll-Free: 800-MEDICARE (633-4227)
Toll-Free TTY/TDD: 877-486-2048
Website: http://www.medicare.gov

Medicaid: Depending on where you live, the state-run Medicaid program may pay for some assistive technology. Keep in mind, though, that even when Medicaid does cover part of the cost, the benefits usually do not provide the amount of financial aid needed to buy an expensive piece of equipment, such as a power wheelchair. Contact the Medicaid office in your state for details.

Veterans' benefits: People who are eligible for veterans' benefits should definitely look into whether they can receive assistance from the Department of Veterans Affairs (DVA). Many people consider the DVA to have a model payment system for assistive technology because the agency has a structure in place to pay for the large volume of equipment that it buys. The DVA also invests in training people in how to use assistive devices. For more information, contact DVA at:

VA Health Benefits Service Center
Toll-Free: 877-222-VETS (8387)
Website: http://www.vba.va.gov

Health insurance and payment: Private health insurance and out-of-pocket payment are two other options for purchasing assistive technology. The problem is that private health insurance does not cover the full price of expensive devices, such as power wheelchairs and motor scooters. Also, most private health insurance has a separate deductible for medical equipment beyond the required deductible for medical services.

Out-of-pocket payment is just that; you buy the assistive technology yourself. The internet is a helpful resource for finding reduced costs for medical equipment. Many internet companies will accept private insurance and assist in gathering necessary paperwork from health care providers. Just be careful to consider:

- Who sponsors the website? Can you easily identify the sponsor?

- Does contact information include mailing address, phone numbers, and e-mail?

- Is your privacy protected? Do they share information?

- Does the website have a secure server? This is important for protecting your credit card or bank account information.

Subsidies: Subsidy programs provide some types of assistive technology at a reduced cost or for free. Many businesses and not-for-profit groups have set up subsidy programs that include discounts, grants, or rebates to get consumers to try a specific product. The idea is that by offering this benefit, the program sponsors can encourage seniors and people with disabilities to use an item that they otherwise might not consider. Obviously, people should be careful about participating in subsidy programs that are run by businesses with commercial interests in the product or service because of the potential for fraud.

State programs: Most states have at least one agency that deals specifically with assistive technology issues. The Assistive Technology Act (Tech Act) provides funds to states for the development of statewide consumer information and training programs. A listing of state tech act programs is available at http://www.abledata.com.

Local assistance: Some area agencies on aging (AAA) have programs or link to services that assist older people obtain low-cost assistive technology. You can call the Eldercare Locator at 800-677-1116, or visit the website at http://www.eldercare.gov to locate your local AAA. In addition local civic groups, religious and veterans' organizations, and senior centers may be able to refer you to assistive technology resources.

Additional Information

DisabilityInfo.gov
http://www.disabilityinfo.gov

This site is designed to serve as a one-stop electronic link to an enormous range of useful information to people with disabilities and their families.

ABLEDATA

8630 Fenton St., Suite 930
Silver Spring, MD 20910
Toll-Free: 800-227-0216
TTY: 301-608-8912
Fax: 301-608-8958
Website: http://www.abledata.com
E-mail: abledata@verizon.net

ABLEDATA is a federally funded project whose primary mission is to provide information on assistive technology and rehabilitation equipment available from domestic and international sources to consumers, organizations, professionals, and caregivers within the United States.

Doodads, Gadgets, and Thingamajigs

Website: http://www.ndipat.org/publications/default.asp?ID=345

This publication provides information on the many uses of assistive technology. It also provides a list of possible resources.

Solutions: Assistive Technology for People with Hidden Disabilities

Website: http://www.uiowa.edu/infotech/Solutions.pdf

This resource guide provides information on adapted devices for people who have memory problems.

Chapter 49

Home Modifications for Independence and Safety

Home modifications are changes made to adapt living spaces to meet the needs of people with physical limitations so that they can continue to live independently and safely. These modifications may include adding assistive technology or making structural changes to a home. Modifications can range from something as simple as replacing cabinet doorknobs with pull handles to full-scale construction projects that require installing wheelchair ramps and widening doorways.

Other examples of home modifications include:

- grab bars in the bathroom (including by the bathtub, shower, and toilet);
- handheld, flexible shower heads;
- handrails on both sides of staircases and for outside steps;
- lever-operated faucets that are easy to turn on and off;
- sliding or revolving shelves for cabinets in the kitchen; and
- walk-in showers or bathtubs.

Benefits of Home Modifications

The main benefit of making home modifications is that they promote independence and prevent accidents. According to a recent AARP

Excerpted from "Home Modifications," Administration on Aging, July 2005.

housing survey, "83% of older Americans want to stay in their current homes for the rest of their lives," but other studies show that most homes are not designed to accommodate the needs of people over age 65.

Most older people live in homes that are more than 20 years old. As these buildings get older along with their residents, they may become harder to live in or maintain. A house that was perfectly suitable for a senior at age 55, for example, may have too many stairs or slippery surfaces for a person who is 70 or 80. Research by the national Centers for Disease Control and Prevention shows that home modifications and repairs may prevent 30% to 50% of all home accidents among seniors, including falls that take place in these older homes.

Planning Home Modifications

The best way to begin planning for home modifications is by defining the basic terms used and asking some simple questions. According to the Rehabilitation Engineering and Assistive Technology Society of North America (RESNA), home modifications should improve the following features of a home:

- **Accessibility:** Improving accessibility means making doorways wider, clearing spaces to make sure a wheelchair can pass through, lowering countertop heights for sinks and kitchen cabinets, installing grab bars, and placing light switches and electrical outlets at heights that can be reached easily. This remodeling must comply with the Fair Housing Amendments Act of 1988, the Americans with Disabilities Act accessibility guidelines, and American National Standards Institute regulations for accessibility. The work must also conform to state and local building codes. Some accessibility features include home modifications for people who may want to entertain disabled guests or who wish to plan ahead for the day when they may require some extra help in getting around their own homes. For example, installing a ramp to the front door of a house and remodeling the hallways and rooms to allow wheelchair access would make a home easier to visit for disabled family members or friends. Such changes may also give a head start on home modifications that may needed later in life.

- **Adaptability:** Adaptability features are changes that can be made quickly to accommodate the needs of seniors or disabled individuals without having to completely redesign the home or use different materials for essential fixtures. Examples include installing grab bars in bathroom walls and movable cabinets under the sink so that the space can be used by someone in a wheelchair.

- **Universal Design:** Universal design features are usually built into a home when the first blueprints or architectural plans are drawn. These features include appliances, fixtures, and floor plans that are easy for all people to use, flexible enough so that they can be adapted for special needs, sturdy and reliable, and functional with a minimum of effort and understanding of the mechanisms involved.

Before you make home modifications, you should evaluate your current and future needs by going through your home room by room and answering a series of questions to highlight where changes might be made. You can begin your survey by examining each area of your home and asking the following questions:

Appliances, Kitchen, and Bathroom

- Are cabinet doorknobs easy to use?
- Are stove controls easy to use and clearly marked?
- Are faucets easy to use?
- Are there grab bars where needed?
- Are all appliances and utensils conveniently and safely located?
- Can the oven and refrigerator be opened easily?
- Can you sit down while working?
- Can you get into and out of the bathtub or shower easily?
- Is the kitchen counter height and depth comfortable for you?
- Is the water temperature regulated to prevent scalding or burning?
- Would you benefit from having convenience items, such as a handheld shower head, a garbage disposal, or a trash compactor?

Closets and Storage Spaces

- Are your closets and storage areas conveniently located?
- Are your closet shelves too high?

- Can you reach items in the closet easily?
- Do you have enough storage space?
- Have you gotten the maximum use out of the storage space you have, including saving space with special closet shelf systems and other products?

Doors and Windows

- Are your doors and windows easy to open and close?
- Are your door locks sturdy and easy to operate?
- Are your doors wide enough to accommodate a walker or wheelchair?
- Do your doors have peepholes or viewing panels? If so, are they set at the correct height for you to use?
- Is there a step up or down at the entrance to your home? If so, is the door threshold too high or low for you to get in or out easily?
- Is there enough space for you to move around while opening or closing your doors?

Driveway and Garage

- Does your garage door have an automatic opener?
- Is your parking space always available?
- Is your parking space close to the entrance of your home?

Electrical Outlets, Switches, and Safety Devices

- Are light or power switches easy to turn on and off?
- Are electrical outlets easy to reach?
- Are the electrical outlets properly grounded to prevent shocks?
- Are your extension cords in good condition?
- Can you hear the doorbell in every part of the house?
- Do you have smoke detectors throughout your home?
- Do you have an alarm system?
- Is the telephone readily available for emergencies?
- Would you benefit from having an assistive device to make it easier to hear and talk on the telephone?

Floors

- Are all of the floors in your home on the same level?

- Are steps up and down marked in some way?

- Are all floor surfaces safe and covered with non-slip or non-skid materials?

- Do you have scatter rugs or doormats that could be hazardous?

Hallways, Steps, and Stairways

- Are hallways and stairs in good condition?

- Do all of your hallways and stairs have smooth, safe surfaces?

- Do your stairs have steps that are big enough for your whole foot?

- Do you have handrails on both sides of the stairway?

- Are your stair rails wide enough for you to grasp them securely?

- Would you benefit from building a ramp to replace the stairs or steps inside or outside of your home?

Lighting and Ventilation

- Do you have night lights where they are needed?

- Is the lighting in each room sufficient for the use of the room?

- Is the lighting bright enough to ensure safety?

- Is each room well-ventilated with good air circulation?

Paying for Home Modifications

Many minor home modifications and repairs can be done for about $150–$2,000. For bigger projects, some financing options may be available. For instance, many home remodeling contractors offer reduced rates and charge sliding-scale fees based on a senior's income and ability to pay or the homeowner may be able to obtain a modest loan to cover urgent needs. Other possible sources of public and private financial assistance include the following:

- Home modification and repair funds from Title III of the Older Americans Act: These funds are distributed by your local area agency on aging (AAA). To contact your local AAA, call the U.S. Administration on Aging Eldercare Locator (800-677-1116) or visit the Eldercare Locator website at http://www.eldercare.gov.

- Rebuilding Together, Inc., a national volunteer organization, through its local affiliates, is able to assist some low-income seniors with home modification efforts. To obtain more information contact your local area agency on aging or contact Rebuilding Together at 800-473-4229 or visit the website at http://www .rebuildingtogether.org.

- Investment capital from the U.S. Department of Energy's Low-Income Home Energy Assistance Program (LIHEAP) and the Weatherization Assistance Program (WAP)—Both of these programs are run by local energy and social services departments.

- Medicare and Medicaid funds: Although these programs usually cover only items that are used for medical purposes and ordered by a doctor, some types of home modifications may qualify. To find out if Medicare will help to cover the cost of a home modification ordered by a doctor, call 800-MEDICARE (800-633-4227 or TTY/ TDD 877-486-2048). You can also find answers to your questions by visiting the website at http://www.medicare.gov.

- Community development block grants: Many cities and towns make grant funds available through the local department of community development.

- Home equity conversion mortgages: Local banks may allow a homeowner to borrow money against the value of his or her home and pay for needed improvements. The homeowner then repays the loan as part or his or her regular mortgage.

In fact, your local AAA can tell you more about whether you are eligible for any of these forms of financial aid or refer you to the agency that can answer your questions.

Seniors may also choose to bypass public assistance programs and hire a contractor to do their home modifications or even do the job by themselves. Keep in mind these points if you want to have a professional contractor come into your home to work on a large project:

- Ask for a written agreement that includes only a small down payment and specifies exactly what work will be done and how much it will cost (with the balance of payment to be made when the job is finished).

- Check with your local Better Business Bureau and Chamber of Commerce to see if any complaints have been filed against the contractor.

- Make sure that the contractor has insurance and is licensed to do the work required.

- Talk with your family and friends to get recommendations based on their experiences with the contractors they have hired. This step may actually be the most important because contractors with a good reputation can usually be counted on to do a good job.

Additional Information

National Association of Home Builders (NAHB) Research Center, Inc.
400 Prince George's Blvd.
Upper Marlboro, MD 20774-8731
Toll-Free: 800-638-8556
Phone: 301-249-4000
Fax: 301-430-6180
Website: http://www.nahbrc.org

The NAHB National Center for Seniors' Housing Research offers the latest information about design features and products available through the home building industry. They are a repository for smart-aging residential design and are now training remodelers who are Certified Aging in Place Specialists in home environments that accommodate the needs of older persons with physical limitations and that assist family caregivers in their care.

National Resource Center on Supportive Housing and Home Modifications
Andrus Gerontology Center
University of Southern California
3715 McClintock Ave.
Los Angeles, CA 90089-0191
Phone: 213-740-1364
Fax: 213-740-7069
Website: http://www.homemods.org
E-mail: homemods@usc.edu

The center is a major clearinghouse for news on government-assisted housing, assisted-living policies, home modifications for older people, training and education courses, and technical assistance. It publishes fact sheets, guidebooks, and a newsletter. The center has a guide with useful information on home modification resources across the country and checklists to help you conduct a home review.

Rebuilding Together
1536 16th St., N.W.
Washington, DC 20036-1042
Toll-Free: 800-473-4229
Website: http://www.rebuildingtogether.org

Rebuilding Together is the nation's largest volunteer housing rehabilitation organization and the only national-level organization that focuses on the home repair and home improvement needs of lower-income homeowners. Through their partnership with the Administration on Aging, local affiliate chapters are working with area agencies and aging service providers to address the needs of low-income elderly.

Chapter 50

Transitional Care Planning

Transitional care planning helps the patient's care continue without interruption through different phases of their disease experience. Transition means passage from one phase to another. Transitional care planning is the bridge between two phases of care. As the patient's treatment goals change or the place of care changes, the patient may encounter problems during the transition. Patients will need to make decisions that balance disease status and treatment options with family needs, finances, employment, spiritual or religious beliefs, and quality of life. There may be practical problems such as finding an appropriate rehabilitation center, obtaining special equipment, or paying for needed care. There may be mental health problems such as depression or anxiety. Transitional care planning helps identify and manage these problems so the transition can go smoothly, without interruption of care. This can reduce stress on the patient and family and improve the patient's health outcome.

Transitional care planning may include support and education for the patient and family and referral to resources. Ideally, it involves a team approach by the patient's health care providers. It is important that there be close communication between members of the team and that this communication include the patient and family.

Excerpted from PDQ® Cancer Information Summary. National Cancer Institute; Bethesda, MD. Transitional Care Planning (PDQ®): Supportive Care - Patient. Updated 10/2007. Available at: http://cancer.gov. Accessed November 9, 2007.

Goals of care may change as the disease changes. Each type of chronic illness requires different care and the goals of a patient's treatment may change as his or her disease gets better or worse. For example, cancer care may include any of the following:

- **Active treatment:** Treatment given to cure the cancer.

- **Supportive care:** Care given to prevent or treat as early as possible the symptoms of the disease; side effects caused by treatment of the disease; and psychological, social, and spiritual problems related to the disease or its treatment.

- **Palliative therapy:** Treatment given to relieve symptoms and improve the patient's quality of life. Palliative therapy may be given along with other cancer treatments or when treatment is no longer curative, to make the patient comfortable at the end of life.

Transitional care planning can help the patient and family with medical, practical, and emotional issues that arise as they adjust to these different levels and goals of care.

A patient may receive care in several different settings during the course of the illness. Most of the care received by people with chronic illness is provided in places other than a hospital. The place where the patient receives treatment may change several times during the course of the illness. Patients may go from receiving care in a hospital or as an outpatient to receiving care at home, in a nursing home, at a rehabilitation center (a place for special training, such as help in regaining strength or movement), or from a hospice team for end-of-life care. When a patient moves from one place of care to another, the process of planning for the move is often called discharge planning. This may involve a case manager who acts on the patient's behalf when dealing with the hospital, visiting nurses, health care companies, rehabilitation facilities, nursing homes, and other groups that provide the care needed. The case manager is a link to resources and services in the community and can arrange for the provision of services, including patient and family education and referrals.

Transitional Care Planning Assessments

An assessment collects information that helps the health care team identify and manage problems a patient may have in adjusting to a change in care. Chronic illness affects more than the patient's physical condition. It also affects mental health, family life, employment, financial planning, social relationships, and faith. Many patients will encounter problems in one or more of these areas as they transfer from one level of care to another. For example, a patient's family may have problems obtaining special home equipment or learning to use special equipment. Another patient may have a difficult time accepting the change from anticancer care to symptom relief alone, such as that provided with some types of palliative or hospice care. Transitional care planning is unique to each patient and family. Assessments help identify patients who may have problems during the transition and help determine the kind of support they will need to make the change go smoothly. The assessments may include a complete medical history; a physical exam; a test of learning skills; tests to determine ability to perform activities of daily living; a mental health evaluation; a review of social support available to the patient; and referral to community resources as needed to assist with issues such as transportation, home care, healthy eating, and medication management.

Assessments are done many times during the patient's illness, as a routine part of care. Assessments are done when the patient moves from one facility to another, such as from hospital to home. They are also done at regular times during the course of the disease, usually at the time of diagnosis, after completing a course of treatment, when there is a relapse, when curative treatment stops, and when treatment is discontinued (end-of-life care begins). The patient may feel added emotional stress at these times. Regular assessments can identify these and other causes of distress in the patient, such as job loss or the death or illness of a patient's loved one or caretaker.

Because no one knows what the patient's needs will be in the future, assessments are done many times during the cancer experience as a routine part of care. This is helps ensure the patient receives the right services at the right times.

All members of the patient's health care team are involved in the assessment process. The following types of assessments may be done for transitional care planning:

Physical Assessment

A physical assessment will look at the patient's general health, treatment plan, and changes in disease status, including the following factors:

- type and stage of illness

- symptoms of the cancer
- side effects of treatment
- whether the patient smokes
- nutrition-related side effects and complications
- ability to perform activities of daily living

Family and Home Assessment

Factors such as the patient's age and living arrangements may affect how easily a change in level of care can be accomplished. The assessment will look at the following:

- age of the patient and family members
- living arrangements
- whether the patient has a spouse or children
- level of education of the patient and family
- language spoken in the home
- cultural beliefs and practices
- whether family and friends are able to help during treatment
- the age and floor plan of the home (Will medical equipment (such as a hospital bed, oxygen tank, or portable monitor) fit in the bedroom, if needed, and is wiring adequate? Can a person in a wheelchair move through the house easily?).

Mental Health Assessment

Change can be a stressful time for both the patient and family. The nature of the relationship between the patient and his or her family and others helps determine the kinds of services the family may need to cope with the transition. The following questions may be asked:

- How do the patient and family feel about the illness, the treatment, and the treatment goals? Sometimes patients develop serious problems such as depression or anxiety. Family members also may need help in dealing with their feelings. These problems are often treatable. The doctor or health care professional can make referrals to a support group, counselor, or mental health care worker.

- What beliefs and values are important to the patient and do they affect the patient's treatment decisions?

- How has the family coped with stress and crisis in the past? This may be helpful in predicting how they will react to the stress caused by the changes in the patient's treatment.

- Are there problems in the home that are unrelated to the cancer but may affect how well the patient and family can handle the change?

- Are there current or past mental health problems in the family?

- Has there been physical or sexual abuse in the patient's past?

- In the case of a patient considering home care, does the patient or any family member smoke or use drugs or alcohol? Smoking is not safe around oxygen equipment. Family members responsible for giving the patient medicines or other care must be clear-headed and not under the influence of any substance that could affect their ability to provide care in the prescribed way.

Social Assessment

Doctors and other health care professionals can provide referrals to supportive services available to the patient. A review of the kinds of social services already available to the patient will be done:

- What kind of support is available in the home and community? How will the patient travel to medical appointments or other places? Who can the patient call on for help if necessary? Where the patient lives may affect what services are available and how the patient can get to appointments. Referrals can be made to local providers of services such as home nursing, food and medication delivery, and transportation to and from treatment centers.

- Does the patient understand hospice care and palliative care and know about available programs in the community?

- Before home care is considered, the availability of in-home help must be determined. Is there someone at home who can help the patient or will outside help be needed?

- Will the primary caregiver have anyone to help with the caregiving duties and make it possible to take time off?

- How will the change affect the patient's ability to work?

- Does the patient have insurance coverage (group coverage from a job, Medicare, Medicaid, veteran's benefits, or other)?

- What are the patient's financial resources? How will the cost of care be paid?

Spiritual Assessment

Knowing the role that religion and spirituality play in the patient's life help the health care team understand how these beliefs may affect the patient's transition to a new level of care. A spiritual assessment may include the following questions:

- Does the patient consider himself or herself to be a spiritual person?

- What is the importance of religion to the patient?

- Is the cancer or its treatment causing spiritual distress?

- Is support available from the patient's religious group? Many patients find visits from members of their religious group valuable. A patient may want to talk to a spiritual advisor (for example, a priest, rabbi, or minister) during treatment.

Most hospitals, especially larger ones, employ hospital chaplains who are trained to work with medical patients and their families. Hospital chaplains are trained to be sensitive to a range of religious and spiritual beliefs and concerns.

Legal Assessment

Advance directives and other legal documents can help doctors and family members make decisions about treatment should the patient become unable to communicate his or her wishes. The patient may be asked if he or she has prepared any of the following documents:

- **Advance directive:** A general term for different types of documents that state what an individual's wishes are concerning certain medical treatments when the patient can no longer communicate those wishes. The patient may declare the wish to be given all possible treatments that are medically appropriate, only some treatments, or no treatment at all.

- **Health care proxy (HCP):** A document in which the patient identifies a person (called a proxy) to make medical decisions if the patient becomes unable to do so. The form may not need to be notarized, but it must be witnessed by two other people. The patient does not have to state specific decisions about individual treatments, only that the proxy may make medical decisions for him or her. HCP is also known as durable power of attorney for health care (DPOAHC) or medical power of attorney (MPOA).

- **Living will:** A living will is a legal document in which a person states that they want certain life-saving medical treatments to be either withheld or withdrawn under certain circumstances. A living will is a type of advance directive. Living wills are not legal in all states.

- **Durable power of attorney:** A document in which the patient names another person to make legal decisions for him or her.

- **Do not resuscitate (DNR) order:** A document in which the patient instructs doctors not to perform cardiopulmonary resuscitation (restart the heart) at the moment of death, so that the natural process of dying occurs. A DNR order may be medically appropriate when cardiopulmonary resuscitation is not likely to save the patient's life.

Transitional Care Options

Different types of care are available for different types of needs. Transitional care may include management of the patient's medical condition and rehabilitation, plus supportive services to ensure basic needs such as comfort, hygiene, safety, and nutrition. It may also include supportive services for educational, social, spiritual, and financial needs.

- Place of care may include the hospital, nursing home, rehabilitation unit, a home, or hospice in an inpatient setting specified by the hospice or in the patient's home.

- Caregivers may include doctors, nurses, dietitian, physical and occupational therapists, social worker, mental health professional, clergy, companions, and home health aides.

- Care may be provided through bereavement programs, community support groups, employment counseling agencies, home health agencies, home infusion agencies, hospice programs, legal aid organizations, and palliative care programs.

- Medication support may include pain and symptom management, chemotherapy, blood transfusions, medications that cause blood cells to grow and mature, antibiotics (drugs used to treat infections), treatments that help improve or restore lung function, and wound and skin care.

- Nutrition support may include normal meals or supplemental nutrition by mouth, tube feeding, or by delivery into a vein.

- Special equipment will depend on the patient's condition and may include medical appliances, assistive devices, pumps to deliver medication, or respirators.

Special Considerations

Caring for a patient at home can increase the physical and emotional burdens on the patient's caregivers. The stress and responsibility of in-home care can be hard on family relationships and should be carefully considered. Day-to-day routines may change for everyone. Many families have trouble getting used to the role changes that result. Patients and families may be referred to counseling to help them with these issues.

Pain control is a key factor in successful home care. Pain medications are given to help patients feel better and are often a part of cancer care. Controlling the patient's symptoms, especially pain, can make things easier on both the patient and the caregivers. It is important that the family and caregivers understand the use of pain control medications and other treatments that keep the patient comfortable.

If home care is to be considered, the following factors and others will be assessed:

- the kind of care to be given

- the decision-making skills required by the patient and caregiver

- whether equipment needed will fit in the home

- the family's ability and desire to provide the care, alone or with the aid of home care workers

This assessment will help determine if care at home is a workable option for the patient.

Advance directives need to move with the patient. During transitions in care, the patient's advance directives, health care proxy form, and durable power of attorney document need to be given to the appropriate caregivers. This step will ensure that the patient's wishes are known through all disease stages and places of care.

End-of-Life Decisions

Caring for a person with a chronic illness or disease such as cancer starts after symptoms begin and the diagnosis is made and continues until the patient is in remission, is cured, or has died. End-of-life decisions should be made soon after the diagnosis, before there is a need for them. These issues are not pleasant or easy to think about, but planning for them can help relieve the burden on family members to make major decisions for the patient at a time when they are likely to be emotionally upset.

A patient's views may reflect his or her philosophical, moral, religious, or spiritual background. If a person has certain feelings about end-of-life issues, these feelings should be made known so that they can be carried out. Since these are sensitive issues, they are often not discussed by patients, families, or doctors. People often feel that there will be plenty of time to talk later about the issues. Many times, though, when the end-of-life decisions are necessary, they must be made by people who do not know the patient's wishes. A patient should talk with the doctor and other caregivers about resuscitation decisions as early as possible (for example, when being admitted to the hospital); he or she may not be able to make these decisions later. Advance directives can ensure the patient's wishes are known ahead of time. These issues are important to discuss whether a patient is being cared for at home; in a hospital, nursing home, or hospice; or elsewhere.

Chapter 51

Palliative Care

Improving Quality of Life on the Way to Death: A Word to the Wise

It was the summer of her fourteenth year and an impressionable one at that. Her beloved grandfather was dying of bladder cancer. Distressed at the ineffectual way her family dealt with his illness and subsequent death, the young teen painfully learned how the effects of an incurable disease can bounce back and forth among family members and the patient. Dr. Ann Berger learned lessons that summer that propelled her through her subsequent training as a nurse, through medical school, and into her current position as the head of the pain and palliative care section at the National Institutes of Health (NIH)'s Warren Grant Magnuson Clinical Center.

Dr. Berger has a unique rapport with her patients, a sentiment reflected in her office, which displays a variety of floppy straw hats and a tea cart loaded with cups and saucers. The hats and tea cart are used when the patient or family members need their spirits lifted. Inspired by her colleague, Dr. Joann Lynn, a geriatrician, Dr. Berger steadfastly believes, "the end of life is really about living with a disease that is going to kill you — about 'good' living on the way to death." A recent study conducted at the University of Pittsburgh shows that people are beginning to value a good death as much as they do a long

"Palliative Care," by Marcia Doniger, *Word on Health*, August 2004, National Institutes of Health (NIH).

life. "People care a great deal about the quality of the death experience," the study concluded. "On average, interviewees would have been willing to trade seven months of healthy life to ensure a better quality of care in the final month of life."

The Need for Palliative Care

Palliative care aims to improve the quality of life for patients near the end of their lives. It involves not only medications to relieve pain, but also a team approach to provide comfort and support that involves family, friends and health care providers.

Dr. Berger and other advocates say that palliative care needs to expand beyond its traditional focus on terminally ill cancer patients. Those with a wide range of debilitating or life-threatening chronic illnesses such as diabetes, emphysema, multiple sclerosis and cardiovascular disease can also benefit from palliative care. For example, people with advanced heart disease can experience such severe shortness of breath they cannot walk to their next-door neighbor's house. They may become as severely depressed as a terminally ill patient, and thus may require this type of individualized treatment.

"Palliative care begins," Dr. Berger says, "at diagnosis, and should be administered throughout the course of the disease." Results of an epidemiological study led by Dr. June Lunney of NIH's National Institute of Nursing Research (NINR) echoes Dr. Berger's beliefs. "Because of the different ways people die, palliative care should start earlier for those who need it, and should involve health and social services that are adjusted to fit the anticipated pattern of death," Dr. Lunney reported.

NINR and another NIH component, the National Institute on Aging (NIA), examined four major pathways to death. The pathways range from people who died suddenly to those lingering, expected deaths associated with frailty in old age. The study concluded that palliative care should have a more extensive and far-reaching focus. Further, because of the different ways that people die, it should be flexible enough to accommodate those who need it earlier and adjusted to fit the anticipated patterns of decline.

Palliative care for Alzheimer patients, for example, can help both those with advanced Alzheimer disease and their families. This disease is marked by a progressive irreversible loss of mental ability, personality changes, and subsequent physical decline. If there is any merciful point in the progression of this disease, it is when the patient begins to forget what he or she has forgotten, and no longer has insight into his or her behavior. As the patient journeys through the various stages of illness, family members also experience a series of losses. While some families are able to tackle the issues that arise from terminal disease, others cannot even think about what will happen to their loved one.

The Future of Care

NIH, primarily through NINR, is currently supporting a broad portfolio of research into improving palliative care. For example, researchers are developing and testing models of palliative care to clarify when it should begin and how it should be structured. Other studies are looking at management of both the physical and psychological aspects of symptoms at the end of life. Researchers are trying to understand the importance and use of spirituality and other psychological influences to enhance quality of life at the end of life. Yet another research focus is to gain a better understanding of family support and the bereavement process.

At NIH's own medical center, while the doctor and patient are intensely immersed in curative medicine, they also recognize and respect the need for palliative care and acknowledge that although the physician's goal is curing disease, they must relieve and comfort always.

Advanced Medical Directives

It's hard to face losing a loved one, especially during the long, steady decline of a disease like Alzheimer disease. But, says Dr. Judith Salerno, deputy director of NIA, "If we start planning for illness before it occurs, we will take some stigma away from how we choose to live with the disease."

Many people complete an advance medical directive to state their wishes for end-of-life care, in case they become unable to make these decisions themselves. With this document, an individual can designate someone to take appropriate actions and make decisions, and guide family members in the event that they must choose, for example, whether or not to withdraw life support in a hopeless situation.

Dr. Virginia Tilden, in a study funded by NIH's National Institute of Nursing Research at the Oregon Health Sciences University, found that end-of-life decisions are especially difficult and stressful for family members in the absence of guidance from the patient. Having an advance directive in place helps family members and other caregivers lower their level of stress and achieve a sense of acceptance and calm from "doing the right thing."

Patients in the early stages of Alzheimer disease or facing a terminal illness should consider placing an advance directive in their records while they can still think and communicate clearly. However, only about 50% of Alzheimer disease patients have an advance directive. Without one, the health care team must often intervene to help family members arrive at a consensus, preserve the patient's dignity and quality of life, and begin the healing for those left behind. By providing a way for patients to express their wishes, advance directives can ease the stress and anxiety surrounding the sensitive decisions of end-of-life care.

Hospice Programs

Hospice care helps terminally ill patients and their families get through the hard times. Hospice care focuses on caring, not curing, and stresses quality of life: peace, comfort, and dignity. Patients' families are an important focus of hospice care, and these programs are designed to provide them with the assistance and support they need as well. You can find hospice programs in freestanding hospice centers, hospitals, nursing homes and other long-term care facilities.

Chapter 52

Tips for Caregivers of Individuals with Chronic Disease

First, Care for Yourself

On an airplane, an oxygen mask descends in front of you. What do you do? As we all know, the first rule is to put on your own oxygen mask before you assist anyone else. Only when we first help ourselves can we effectively help others. Caring for yourself is one of the most important—and one of the most often forgotten—things you can do as a caregiver. When your needs are taken care of, the person you care for will benefit, too.

Effects of Caregiving on Health and Well-Being

We hear this often: "My husband is the person with Alzheimer's, but now I'm the one in the hospital." Such a situation is all too common. Researchers know a lot about the effects of caregiving on health and well being. For example, if you are a caregiving spouse between the ages of 66 and 96 and are experiencing mental or emotional strain, you have a risk of dying that is 63 percent higher than that of people your age who are not caregivers.[1] The combination of loss, prolonged stress, the physical demands of caregiving, and the biological vulnerabilities that come with age place you at risk for significant health problems as well as an earlier death.

"Taking Care of YOU: Self-Care for Family Caregivers," reprinted with permission from the Family Caregiver Alliance, http://www.caregiver.org. © 2003 Family Caregiver Alliance. All rights reserved.

409

Older caregivers are not the only ones who put their health and well being at risk. If you are a baby boomer who has assumed a caregiver role for your parents while simultaneously juggling work and raising adolescent children, you face an increased risk for depression, chronic illness, and a possible decline in quality of life.

But despite these risks, family caregivers of any age are less likely than non-caregivers to practice preventive health care and self-care behavior. Regardless of age, sex, race, or ethnicity, caregivers report problems attending to their own health and well-being while managing caregiving responsibilities. They report:

- sleep deprivation;

- poor eating habits;

- failure to exercise;

- failure to stay in bed when ill; and

- postponement of or failure to make medical appointments.

Family caregivers are also at increased risk for excessive use of alcohol, tobacco, and other drugs, and for depression. Caregiving can be an emotional roller coaster. On the one hand, caring for your family member demonstrates love and commitment and can be a very rewarding personal experience. On the other hand, exhaustion, worry, inadequate resources, and continuous care demands are enormously stressful. Studies show that an estimated 46 percent to 59 percent of caregivers are clinically depressed.

Taking Responsibility for Your Own Care

You cannot stop the impact of a chronic or progressive illness or a debilitating injury on someone for whom you care. But, there is a great deal that you can do to take responsibility for your personal well being and to get your own needs met.

Identifying Personal Barriers

Many times, attitudes and beliefs form personal barriers that stand in the way of caring for yourself. Not taking care of yourself may be a lifelong pattern, with taking care of others an easier option. However, as a family caregiver you must ask yourself, "What good will I be to the person I care for if I become ill, or if I die?" Breaking old patterns and overcoming obstacles is not an easy proposition, but it can be done—regardless of your age or situation. The first task in removing personal barriers to self-care is to identify what is in your way. For example,

- Do you feel you have to prove that you are worthy of the care recipient's affection?

- Do you think you are being selfish if you put your needs first?

- Is it frightening to think of your own needs? What is the fear about?

- Do you have trouble asking for what you need? Do you feel inadequate if you ask for help? Why?

Sometimes caregivers have misconceptions that increase their stress and get in the way of good self-care. Here are some of the most commonly expressed:

- I am responsible for my parent's health.

- If I don't do it, no one will.

- If I do it right, I will get the love, attention, and respect I deserve.

"I never do anything right," or "There's no way I could find the time to exercise" are examples of negative self-talk, another possible barrier that can cause unnecessary anxiety. Instead, try positive statements: "I'm good at giving John a bath." "I can exercise for 15 minutes a day." Remember, your mind believes what you tell it.

Because we base our behavior on our thoughts and beliefs, attitudes and misconceptions like those noted can cause caregivers to continually attempt to do what cannot be done, to control what cannot be controlled. The result is feelings of continued failure and frustration and, often, an inclination to ignore your own needs. Ask yourself what might be getting in your way and keeping you from taking care of yourself.

Moving Forward

Once you've started to identify any personal barriers to good self-care, you can begin to change your behavior, moving forward one small step at a time. Following are some effective tools for self-care that can start you on your way.

1. Reducing Personal Stress

How we perceive and respond to an event is a significant factor in how we adjust and cope with it. The stress you feel is not only the result of your caregiving situation but also the result of your perception of it—whether you see the glass as half-full or half-empty. It is important to remember that you are not alone in your experiences.

Your level of stress is influenced by many factors, including the following:

- Whether your caregiving is voluntary. If you feel you had no choice in taking on the responsibilities, the chances are greater that you will experience strain, distress, and resentment.

- Your relationship with the care recipient. Sometimes people care for another with the hope of healing a relationship. If healing does not occur, you may feel regret and discouragement.

- Your coping abilities. How you coped with stress in the past predicts how you will cope now. Identify your current coping strengths so that you can build on them.

- Your caregiving situation. Some caregiving situations are more stressful than others. For example, caring for a person with dementia is often more stressful than caring for someone with a physical limitation.

- Whether support is available.

Steps to Managing Stress

1. Recognize warning signs early. These might include irritability, sleep problems, and forgetfulness. Know your own warning signs, and act to make changes. Don't wait until you are overwhelmed.

2. Identify sources of stress. Ask yourself, "What is causing stress for me?" Sources of stress might be too much to do, family disagreements, feelings of inadequacy, inability to say no.

3. Identify what you can and cannot change. Remember, we can only change ourselves; we cannot change another person. When you try to change things over which you have no control, you

will only increase your sense of frustration. Ask yourself, "What do I have some control over? What can I change?" Even a small change can make a big difference. The challenge faced as a caregiver is well expressed in words from the Serenity Prayer:

Grant me the serenity to
Accept the things I cannot change,
Courage to change the things I can,
And the wisdom to know the difference.

4. Take action. Taking some action to reduce stress gives us back a sense of control. Stress reducers can be simple activities like walking and other forms of exercise, gardening, meditation, having coffee with a friend. Identify some stress reducers that work for you.

2. Setting Goals

Setting goals or deciding what you would like to accomplish in the next three to six months is an important tool for taking care of yourself. Here are some sample goals you might set:

- Take a break from caregiving.
- Get help with caregiving tasks like bathing and preparing meals.
- Feel more healthy.

Goals are generally too big to work on all at once. We are more likely to reach a goal if we break it down into smaller action steps. Once you've set a goal, ask yourself, "What steps do I take to reach my goal?" Make an action plan by deciding which step you will take first, and when. Then get started.

Example: Goal and Action Steps

Goal: Feel more healthy.
Possible action steps:

1. Make an appointment for a physical check-up.

2. Take a half-hour break once during the week.

3. Walk three times a week for ten minutes.

413

3. Seeking Solutions

Seeking solutions to difficult situations is, of course, one of the most important tools in caregiving. Once you've identified a problem, taking action to solve it can change the situation and also change your attitude to a more positive one, giving you more confidence in your abilities.

Steps for Seeking Solutions

1. Identify the problem. Look at the situation with an open mind. The real problem might not be what first comes to mind. For example, you think that the problem is simply that you are tired all the time, when the more basic difficulty is your belief that "no one can care for John like I can." The problem? Thinking that you have to do everything yourself.

2. List possible solutions. One idea is to try a different perspective: "Even though someone else provides help to John in a different way than I do, it can be just as good." Ask a friend to help. Call Family Caregiver Alliance or the Eldercare Locator and ask about agencies in your area that could help provide care.

3. Select one solution from the list, then try it.

4. Evaluate the results. Ask yourself how well your choice worked.

5. Try a second solution. If your first idea didn't work, select another. But don't give up on the first; sometimes an idea just needs fine tuning.

6. Use other resources. Ask friends, family members, and professionals for suggestions.

7. If nothing seems to help, accept that the problem may not be solvable now. You can revisit it at another time.

Note: All too often, we jump from step one to step seven and then feel defeated and stuck. Concentrate on keeping an open mind while listing and experimenting with possible solutions.

4. Communicating Constructively

Being able to communicate constructively is one of a caregiver's most important tools. When you communicate in ways that are clear, assertive, and constructive, you will be heard and get the help and support you need.

Communication Guidelines

- Use "I" messages rather than "you" messages. Saying "I feel angry" rather than "You made me angry" enables you to express your feelings without blaming others or causing them to become defensive.

- Respect the rights and feelings of others. Do not say something that will violate another person's rights or intentionally hurt the person's feelings. Recognize that the other person has the right to express feelings.

- Be clear and specific. Speak directly to the person. Don't hint or hope the person will guess what you need. Other people are not mind readers. When you speak directly about what you need or feel, you are taking the risk that the other person might disagree or say no to your request, but that action also shows respect for the other person's opinion. When both parties speak directly, the chances of reaching understanding are greater.

- Be a good listener. Listening is the most important aspect of communication.

5. Asking For and Accepting Help

When people have asked if they can be of help to you, how often have you replied, "Thank you, but I'm fine." Many caregivers don't know how to marshal the goodwill of others and are reluctant to ask for help. You may not wish to burden others or admit that you can't handle everything yourself.

Be prepared with a mental list of ways that others could help you. For example, someone could take the person you care for on a 15-minute walk a couple of times a week. Your neighbor could pick up a few things for you at the grocery store. A relative could fill out some insurance papers. When you break down the jobs into very simple tasks, it is easier for people to help. And they do want to help. It is up to you to tell them how.

Help can come from community resources, family, friends, and professionals. Ask them. Don't wait until you are overwhelmed and exhausted or your health fails. Reaching out for help when you need it is a sign of personal strength.

Tips on How to Ask

- Consider the person's special abilities and interests. If you know a friend enjoys cooking but dislikes driving, your chances of getting help improve if you ask for help with meal preparation.

- Resist asking the same person repeatedly. Do you keep asking the same person because she has trouble saying no?

- Pick the best time to make a request. Timing is important. A person who is tired and stressed might not be available to help out. Wait for a better time.

- Prepare a list of things that need doing. The list might include errands, yard work, a visit with your loved one. Let the helper choose what she would like to do.

- Be prepared for hesitance or refusal. It can be upsetting for the caregiver when a person is unable or unwilling to help. But in the long run, it would do more harm to the relationship if the person helps only because he doesn't want to upset you. To the person who seems hesitant, simply say, "Why don't you think about it." Try not to take it personally when a request is turned down. The person is turning down the task, not you. Try not to let a refusal prevent you from asking for help again. The person who refused today may be happy to help at another time.

- Avoid weakening your request. "It's only a thought, but would you consider staying with Grandma while I went to church?" This request sounds like it's not very important to you. Use "I" statements to make specific requests: "I would like to go to church on Sunday. Would you stay with Grandma from 9 a.m. until noon?"

6. Talking to the Physician

In addition to taking on the household chores, shopping, transportation, and personal care, 37% of caregivers also administer medications, injections, and medical treatment to the person for whom they care. Some 77% of those caregivers report the need to ask for advice about the medications and medical treatments. The person they usually turn to is their physician.

But while caregivers will discuss their loved one's care with the physician, caregivers seldom talk about their own health, which is equally important. Building a partnership with a physician that

416

addresses the health needs of the care recipient and the caregiver is crucial. The responsibility of this partnership ideally is shared between you the caregiver, the physician, and other health care staff. However, it will often fall to you to be assertive, using good communication skills, to ensure that everyone's needs are met—including your own.

Tips on Communicating with Your Physician

- Prepare questions ahead of time. Make a list of your most important concerns and problems. Issues you might want to discuss with the physician are changes in symptoms, medications or general health of the care recipient, your own comfort in your caregiving situation, or specific help you need to provide care.

- Enlist the help of the nurse. Many caregiving questions relate more to nursing than to medicine. In particular, the nurse can answer questions about various tests and examinations, preparing for surgical procedures, providing personal care, and managing medications at home.

- Make sure your appointment meets your needs. For example, the first appointment in the morning or after lunch and the last appointment in the day are the best times to reduce your waiting time or accommodate numerous questions. When you schedule your appointment, be sure you convey clearly the reasons for your visit so that enough time is allowed.

- Call ahead. Before the appointment, check to see if the doctor is on schedule. Remind the receptionist of special needs when you arrive at the office.

- Take someone with you. A companion can ask questions you feel uncomfortable asking and can help you remember what the physician and nurse said.

- Use assertive communication and "I" messages. Enlist the medical care team as partners in care. Present what you need, what your concerns are, and how the doctor and/or nurse can help. Use specific, clear "I" statements like the following: "I need to know more about the diagnosis; I will feel better prepared for the future if I know what's in store for me." Or "I am feeling rundown. I'd like to make an appointment for myself and my husband next week."

7. Starting to Exercise

You may be reluctant to start exercising, even though you've heard it's one of the healthiest things you can do. Perhaps you think that physical exercise might harm you, or that it is only for people who are young and able to do things like jogging. Fortunately, research suggests that you can maintain or at least partly restore endurance, balance, strength, and flexibility through everyday physical activities like walking and gardening. Even household chores can improve your health. The key is to increase your physical activity by exercising and using your own muscle power.

Exercise promotes better sleep, reduces tension and depression, and increases energy and alertness. If finding time for exercise is a problem, incorporate it into your daily activity. Perhaps the care recipient can walk or do stretching exercise with you. If necessary, do frequent short exercises instead of those that require large blocks of time. Find activities you enjoy.

Walking, one of the best and easiest exercises, is a great way to get started. In addition to the physical benefits of walking, it helps to reduce psychological tension. Walking 20 minutes a day, three times a week, is very beneficial. If you can't get away for that long, try to walk for as long as you can on however many days you can. Work walking into your life. Walk around the mall, to the store, or a nearby park. Walk around the block with a friend.

8. Learning from Our Emotions

It is a strength to recognize when your emotions are controlling you (instead of you controlling your emotions). Our emotions are messages we need to listen to. They exist for a reason. However negative or painful, our feelings are useful tools for understanding what is happening to us.

Even feelings such as guilt, anger, and resentment contain important messages. Learn from them, and take appropriate action. For example, when you cannot enjoy activities you previously enjoyed, and your emotional pain overshadows all pleasure, it is time to seek treatment for depression—especially if you are having thoughts of suicide. Speaking with your physician is the first step.

Caregiving often involves a range of emotions. Some feelings are more comfortable than others. When you find that your emotions are intense, they might mean the following:

- You need to make a change in your caregiving situation.

418

- You are grieving a loss.

- You are experiencing increased stress.

- You need to be assertive and ask for what you need.

Summing Up

Remember, it is not selfish to focus on your own needs and desires when you are a caregiver—it's an important part of the job. You are responsible for your own self-care. Focus on the following self-care practices:

- Learn and use stress-reduction techniques.

- Attend to your own health care needs.

- Get proper rest and nutrition.

- Exercise regularly.

- Take time off without feeling guilty.

- Participate in pleasant, nurturing activities.

- Seek and accept the support of others.

- Seek supportive counseling when you need it, or talk to a trusted counselor or friend.

- Identify and acknowledge your feelings.

- Change the negative ways you view situations.

- Set goals.

Credits

1. Shultz, Richard and Beach, Scott (1999). Caregiving as A Risk for Mortality: The Caregiver Health Effects Study. *JAMA,* December 15, 1999–Vol. 282, No. 23.

Additional Information

Family Caregiver Alliance
National Center on Caregiving
180 Montgomery St., Suite 1100
San Francisco, CA 94104
Toll-Free: 800-445-8106

Phone: 415-434-3388
Fax: 415-434-3508
Website: http://www.caregiver.org
E-mail: info@caregiver.org

Family Caregiver Alliance (FCA) seeks to improve the quality of life for caregivers through education, services, research, and advocacy.

Administration on Aging
Department of Health and Human Services
Washington, DC 20201
Phone: 202-619-0724
Fax: 202-357-3555
Website: http://www.aoa.gov
E-mail: aoainfo@aoa.hhs.gov

Eldercare Locator
Toll-Free: 800-677-1116
Website: http://www.eldercare.gov

Part Six

Children and Chronic Disease

Chapter 53

Caring for a Seriously Ill Child

Taking care of a chronically ill child is one of the most draining and difficult tasks a parent can face. Beyond facing your child's physical challenges and medical needs, you will have to deal with the emotional needs your sick child may have and the emotional impact that the prolonged illness can have on the entire family.

Luckily, this tough balancing act doesn't have to be accomplished alone: support groups, social workers, and family friends often can lend a helping hand.

Explaining Long-Term Illness to Your Child

Honest communication is crucial to helping a child adjust to a serious medical condition. It's important for a child to know that he or she is sick and will be getting lots of medicine. The hospital and the medicine may feel frightening to your child, but they are part of what it takes to help your child feel better.

As you are explaining the illness and the treatment to your child, it's important to clearly and honestly answer your child's questions, and provide the information that he or she will need to know in a way he or she will understand and can respond. The aim is not to frighten your child, but to give your child the words to communicate information and concerns to medical professionals and others.

To maintain your child's trust, it's also important to accurately explain and prepare your child for any treatments—and possible discomfort that might go with along with those treatments. Avoid saying, "This won't hurt," if the procedure is likely to be painful. Instead, tell your child that a procedure may cause some discomfort, pain, pressure, or stinging, but then reassure your child that it will be temporary and that you'll be there to support him or her while, or after, it's done.

Many hospitals offer parents the choice of talking to their child about a long-term diagnosis alone, addressing the child with the doctor present, or including the entire medical team made up of doctors, social workers, and nurses. Your doctor or other medical professional may also be able to give you some advice on how to talk to your child about his or her illness.

Tackling Tough Emotions

Your child is going to have many feelings about the changes affecting his or her body, and should be encouraged and given opportunities to express any feelings, concerns, and fears. It's a good idea to ask your child what he or she is experiencing and listen to everything he or she has to say before bringing up your own feelings and explanations.

This kind of communication doesn't always have to be verbal. Music, drawing, or writing can often help a child living with a life-threatening disease to express his or her emotions and to escape through a fantasy world of his or her own design.

Your child may also need reminders that he or she is not responsible for the illness. It's common for kids to fear that they brought their sickness on by something they thought, said, or did. It is important to reassure your child that this is not the case, and to explain, in terms that he or she can understand, what caused the illness. (You may also want to reassure your child's siblings that nothing they said or did caused your child's illness.)

For many questions your child asks, there just aren't going to be easy answers. And you can't always promise that everything is going to be fine. But you can help your child feel better by listening to his or her feelings, making him or her understand that it's okay and it's completely understandable to have those feelings, and assuring your child that you and your family are going to be there to make him or her feel as comfortable as possible.

If a child asks "Why me?" it's okay to be honest, even if the answer is "I don't know." It's a good idea to follow this up by explaining that even though it's unknown why the illness occurred, the doctors do have treatment for it. (If that is the case.)

Your child may say, "It's not fair that I'm sick." Acknowledge that your child is right, that it's not fair. It's important for your child to feel like it's okay to feel angry about the illness.

Your child may ask: "Am I going to die?" How you answer is going to depend on your child's age and maturity level. It's important to discern, if possible, what specific fears or concerns your child may be having, and to address those concerns specifically. For example, your child may be actually worried about being in pain.

If it is reassuring to your child, you may refer to your religious, spiritual, and cultural beliefs about death. You may want to stay away from euphemisms for death such as "going to sleep." Saying that may cause your child and siblings to fear going to sleep. Regardless of your child's age, it's important that he or she know that there are going to be people who love him or her and who will be there for as long as they are needed, and that your child will be kept comfortable.

Just like any adult, your child is going to need some time to adjust to the diagnosis and the physical changes he or she may be experiencing, and it's likely that your child is going to feel sad, depressed, angry, afraid, or even denial. It's a good idea to think about getting some professional counseling help if you see signs that these feelings are starting to interfere with your child's ability to function, and your child begins to seem withdrawn, depressed, and show radical changes in eating and sleeping habits that aren't related to your child's physical illness.

Childhood Behavior

Although kids with chronic illnesses certainly require extra tender, loving, care (TLC), special medical requirements don't eliminate the routine needs of childhood. The foremost—and perhaps trickiest—task for worried parents is to treat a sick child as normally as possible. Despite the circumstances, this means setting limits on unacceptable behavior, sticking to a regular routine, and avoiding overindulgence. This may seem impossible, particularly if you are experiencing feelings of guilt or an intense need to protect your sick child. But, spoiling or coddling a child may only make it harder for him or her to readjust once he or she is ready to return to daily activities.

When your child leaves the hospital for home, normalcy remains the goal. Your child may want to visit or stay in touch with friends through visits, if possible, or through e-mail, the phone, or letters.

Dealing with Siblings

Family dynamics can be severely tested when a child is sick. Clinic visits, surgical procedures, and frequent checkups can throw big kinks into everyone's schedule, and take an emotional toll on the entire family. To ease these pressures, reach out for any help you can get to help keep the family routine as close to normal as possible. Friends and family members may be able to help handle errands, carpools, and meals. Siblings should continue to attend school and their usual recreational activities; the family should attempt to provide some predictability and time for everyone to be together.

Flexibility is key. The old "normal" may have been the entire family around the table for a home-cooked meal at 6:00, while the new "normal" may be take-out pizza on clinic nights.

Also, you may want to talk with your other kids' teachers or school counselors and let them know that a sibling in the family is ill. Those school personnel may be able to keep a look out for any behavioral changes or signs of stress among your children.

It is common for siblings of a chronically ill child to become angry, sullen, resentful, fearful, or withdrawn. They may pick fights or fall behind in schoolwork. In all cases, parents should pay close attention, so that the siblings don't feel shunted aside by the demands of the sick child.

It may also help your sick child's siblings to be included in the treatment process whenever possible. Depending on their ages and maturity level, visiting the hospital, meeting the nursing and physician staffs, or accompanying their sick sibling to the clinic for treatments can also help make the situation less frightening and more understandable.

What they imagine about the illness and hospital visits are often a lot worse than the reality. When they come to the hospital, hopefully they'll develop a more realistic picture and see that, while unpleasant things may be part of the treatment, there are also people who care about their sibling and try to minimize discomfort.

Lightening Your Load

Although no magic potion exists to reduce the stress involved in caring for a child with a long-term illness, there are ways to ease the strain.

- Break problems into manageable parts. If your child's treatment is expected to be given over an extended time, view it in more manageable time blocks. Planning a week or a month at a time may be less overwhelming.

- Attend to your own needs. Get appropriate rest and food. To the extent possible, pay attention to your relationship with your spouse, hobbies, and friendships.

- Depend on friends. Let them carpool siblings to soccer or theater practice. Permit others—relatives, friends—to share responsibilities of caring for your child. Remember that you can't do it all.

- Ask for help in managing the financial implications of your child's illness.

- Recognize that everyone handles stress differently. If you and your spouse have distinct worrying styles, talk about them and try to accommodate them. Don't pretend that they don't exist.

- Develop collaborative working relationships with health care professionals. Realize you are all part of the team. Ask questions and learn all you can about your child's illness.

- Consult other parents in support groups at your care center or hospital. They can offer information and understanding.

- Explore support groups for parents who have children with the same or similar illness.

- Keep a journal.

- Utilize support staff offered at the treating hospital.

Chapter 54

Managing Home Health Care for Children with Chronic Illness

Kids need intensive health care at home after they have been in the hospital for many different reasons. Medical equipment and devices can:

- function as a monitor;
- provide foods and oxygen when kids can't eat or breathe on their own;
- perform some of the vital functions of the kidneys, heart, and lungs.

In each case, it's vital that parents, siblings, and other family members learn about the medical devices and equipment that the kids they love depend on.

During the transition from the hospital to home health care, families will have a support network to lean on, including a team of medical professionals—doctors, nurses, therapists, home health aides, and equipment suppliers. At many hospitals, a staff social worker can help coordinate this team. The social worker also may be able to help arrange home nursing and respiratory services, public health nurse support, medical follow-up, and emotional support.

The process of getting comfortable with your child's home health care begins at the hospital. Learn from the medical staff by closely observing how they take care of your child, and how they operate and maintain the necessary equipment. Be sure to ask questions about anything you don't understand. Consider talking with families whose children require similar medical equipment or levels of care.

Planning Ahead

Family caregivers should be prepared for and well-informed about the care a child requires. Caregivers will need to know how each machine works, how to troubleshoot, and how to perform preventive maintenance and any backup procedures.

Here are some factors to consider as you prepare for home health care:

- You may need to make changes to your home to make it accessible for a walker or wheelchair.

- The child's room will need the proper equipment, sufficient electrical outlets, and a backup power supply from a battery or generator. (Some insurance companies may provide reimbursement.)

- It can be helpful if a bathroom or source of water is near the child's room for bathing.

- Keep a list of emergency numbers by the phone.

- Emergency medical assistance and transportation should be nearby. Inform your local ambulance company of your child's medical condition before any situation comes up where you need one.

- Devise a plan on how you'll handle all types of emergencies, such as natural disasters, to handle getting the child and any life-sustaining equipment out of harm's way.

Family members should learn how to use and maintain all medical equipment. They also should:

- understand the child's medical condition;

- know how to detect problems;

- know what to do in emergencies;

- learn cardiopulmonary resuscitation (CPR);

- know what to do if other emergencies arise—such as handling dislodged equipment;

- understand which situations are emergencies that require medical care.

The specific skills needed will depend on your child's condition. The nurses and doctors can help you understand what you may need to know, and may even have training dolls to help you practice different procedures.

Home Health Care Assistance

The hospital social worker can help families arrange for nurses and aides to come into the home to assist with care, if necessary. They also can help determine any special qualifications home-care workers might need to have.

In general, home caregivers should understand how to:

- spot the slightest change in the child's behavior or appearance and communicate those changes to other caregivers;
- administer medications;
- monitor medication schedules;
- assist with exercise and other therapies.

You may want to prepare notes on your child's status and require each nursing shift to do the same. That way, early signs of trouble can be recognized and medical help summoned quickly. Consider keeping a patient journal near your child's bed so that nurses and family members can communicate about various issues.

Types of Medical Equipment

Multitudes of medical equipment can be required for different medical conditions, but there is some commonly used equipment for when kids need assistance to breathe, eat, and perform vital bodily functions, like voiding (urinating and defecating). Everyone involved in caregiving should know how to use and maintain the equipment and what to do if something goes wrong.

Breathing

- **Tracheostomy:** A tracheostomy, often referred to as just a "trach" (say: "trake"), is a procedure in which a tube is inserted directly into the airway through an opening made in the neck,

431

often done when a child cannot be weaned off of a ventilator. Breathing equipment may be attached to the tube. The term "trach" can refer to both the procedure and the piece of equipment itself. All caregivers will have to remove, change, and clean the tube on a regular basis.

- **Ventilator:** The ventilator, which attaches to the tracheostomy, performs mechanical breathing for the child. Valves on the ventilator are set to combine air and oxygen (if needed) to meet the child's needs. All caregivers must learn how and when to adjust the settings on the machine.

- **Manual resuscitation bag:** This breathing device is used as a backup for a ventilator or in an emergency. It allows a caregiver to provide breaths for the patient by squeezing a bag. It should be on hand in case the ventilator fails.

- **Suction machine:** If a child can't cough to clear the airway, a suction machine may be needed. Suctioning is done via a tiny tube inserted into the airway (or trach opening). A variety of factors, such as the child's condition and the humidity level in the home, will determine how often suctioning needs to be done. Anyone providing care should learn how to use the suctioning machine. Both a bedside and a portable machine may be needed.

- **Pulse oximeter:** This small monitoring device measures heart rate and the amount of oxygen in the blood. It can be attached to a finger or toe. A wire leading to a monitor shows the readings and sounds an alarm if they're abnormal. All caregivers need to know what the child's normal readings are and how to recognize a false alarm, which may occur if the device isn't properly attached or the child is moving the finger or toe.

Feeding

Sometimes kids cannot swallow food or need nutrition assistance. To get this nutrition into the body, some systems use the child's gastrointestinal (GI) tract (these are called enteral feeds) and some go directly into the bloodstream (these are called parenteral feeds).

The health care team will provide specific information about how to handle different situations involving the equipment, such as displacement or clogging of tubes.

- **Nasogastric tube (NG tube):** An NG tube is inserted through the nose and down the throat into the stomach. It is used to provide formula when children need help getting nourishment for a short period of time, such as a few weeks. Some medications also can be given through an NG tube.

- **Feeding tube:** When longer-term support is needed, a tube can be placed through the skin into the GI tract. A feeding pump sends formula into the tubes and controls the rate and amount given. Some medications also can be given through these tubes. Two commonly used tubes are:

  - gastrostomy tube (G-tube) goes directly into the stomach;
  - jejunostomy tube goes directly into the small intestine.

- **Parenteral feeds:** When the GI tract isn't working properly, nutrition can be given directly into the bloodstream. This can be done using a central line, which is inserted through a large vessel in the chest, neck, or groin. The central line, and the area surrounding where it enters the body, must be kept very clean to prevent infection. Formula cannot be given directly through a central line; a special mixture of nutrients must be given, based on the child's needs. Parenteral feeds require an intravenous (IV) pump to control the rate and amount of nutrition given.

Voiding

- **Diapers:** Older kids with conditions that make them unable to control their excretions may urinate and defecate uncontrollably. These kids may need to wear diapers made especially for bigger children. It is important for parents or caregivers to change the diapers frequently so that a child is not wearing a soiled diaper for an extended period of time. That can be uncomfortable and lead to skin infections.

- **Catheter:** Children who need help urinating may have a tube that goes through their urethra into the bladder, called a catheter. This tube may stay in and continuously drain into a bag or may be inserted several times a day to empty the bladder. Sometimes, through surgery, a special pathway is made through the skin into the bladder for easier catheterization. Whenever a catheter is placed, it must be done according to the doctor's instructions so that bacteria do not get into the bladder and cause an infection.

- **Colostomy bag:** A colostomy is an operation in which the colon is rerouted to empty through an artificial opening, bypassing the anus. Instead, wastes are eliminated directly into a pouch worn over a surgical opening on the abdomen. This bag must be changed frequently.

Support for Parents

It's important to be able to reach out for help and support, whether it's from the medical professionals involved in your child's care, or friends, family, or peers in similar situations.

The medical care responsibilities of home health care can feel overwhelming. And the demands of home care can easily make parents feel isolated.

Whether you need emotional support or help managing the household duties, don't hesitate to consult your doctor or hospital about resources in your community.

Chapter 55

Questions and Answers about the Pediatric Intensive Care Unit

It can be frightening whenever kids are in the hospital—maybe even more so when they're admitted to the pediatric intensive care unit (PICU). But a basic understanding of the people and equipment in the PICU can help you feel less scared and better prepared to help your child recover.

What's the PICU?

The PICU is the section of the hospital that provides sick children with the highest level of medical care. It differs from other parts of the hospital, like the general medical floors, in that the PICU allows intensive nursing care and monitoring of bodily functions and conditions (heart rate, breathing, and blood pressure, for example). The PICU also allows medical staff to provide therapies that might not be available in other parts of the hospital. Some of these more intensive therapies include ventilators, or breathing machines, and certain medications that can be given only under close medical supervision.

"When Your Child's in the Pediatric Intensive Care Unit" was provided by KidsHealth, one of the largest resources online for medically reviewed information written for teens, kids, and parents. For more articles like this one, visit www.KidsHealth.org, or www.TeensHealth.org. © 2007 The Nemours Foundation.

Who's sent to the PICU?

Any child who's seriously ill and needs intensive care and whose medical needs can't be met on the hospital's main medical floors goes to the PICU.

Kids in the PICU might include those with severe breathing problems from asthma, serious infections, certain heart defects, some complications of diabetes, or those involved in a serious automobile accident or near-drowning. Some kids may have been stable enough to initially be cared for on the hospital's main medical floor, but may be transferred to the PICU if they become more acutely ill. Following major surgery, many children are cared for in the PICU for several days.

Kids are admitted to the PICU when they're at their sickest. How long they'll be in the PICU depends on their condition—some kids might stay a single day; others might need to stay for weeks or even months. As always, ask the doctor or nurse caring for your child if you have any questions.

Who takes care of kids in the PICU?

One of the biggest advantages of the PICU is that it has many highly skilled people to closely care for your child. But not knowing who everyone is and what they do can be confusing and a little overwhelming at first. Most people will introduce themselves and indicate how they're involved in your child's care, but if they don't, feel free to ask. At all times, you should feel comfortable asking the doctors and nurses questions about your child and the care being given.

The nurses who work in the PICU are experienced in caring for the sickest children in the hospital. They're the people most intimately involved with the minute-to-minute care of the kids. The PICU also tends to have a higher nurse-to-patient ratio than other parts of the hospital (in other words, each nurse cares for fewer patients, which gives them more time with your child).

Numerous physicians may care for your child, but the attending intensivist is the leader in the PICU. A pediatric intensivist is a doctor who did a three-year residency in pediatrics after medical school, followed by additional years of subspecialty fellowship training in intensive care. Also on the PICU team are residents (doctors who've completed medical school and are training to be pediatricians) and PICU fellows (pediatricians training to be attending intensivists).

Many other subspecialists, such as cardiologists (heart doctors) or neurosurgeons (brain surgeons), may be involved, depending on your child's needs. Respiratory therapists are experienced with ventilators and other breathing equipment, and are often involved in the care of PICU patients. In addition, physical therapists, occupational therapists, nutritionists, and pharmacists may play a role in your child's care.

You may also meet social workers who help families cope with the emotional burdens of having a critically ill child. They can help to arrange housing for families (through organizations like Ronald McDonald House), assist with insurance issues, or coordinate discharge planning when your child is ready to go home.

You may also want to ask whether the hospital has child life specialists. Trained in fields like development, education, psychology, and counseling, they can help your child understand and manage being in the hospital by, for example, listening if your child needs to talk, calming fears about what's happening, or providing distractions like books and games.

The medical team meets every day, usually in the morning, to discuss each patient's case in detail; these discussions are known as rounds. You may see a group of doctors, nurses, and others walking from patient to patient, planning the medical care for each child. By understanding everyone's role and how each contributes, you may find the group of people caring for your child less intimidating.

What should kids expect while in the PICU?

Possibly the most alarming aspect of the intensive care environment is the medical equipment that may be attached to your child. The machines have alarms and display panels, and the noise and lights can be overwhelming.

Your child's stay in the PICU might include:

- **IVs:** Almost all kids in the PICU have an intravenous catheter (or IV for short) for fluids and medications—usually in the hands or arms, but sometimes in the feet, legs, or even scalp. An IV is a thin, flexible tube inserted into the vein with a small needle. Once in the vein, the needle is removed, leaving just the soft plastic tubing. Some situations require larger IVs that can be used to deliver greater volumes of fluids and medications. These special IVs are known as central lines because they're inserted into the larger, more central veins of the chest, neck, or groin, as opposed to the hands and feet. Arterial lines are very similar to IVs, but they're placed in arteries, not veins, and are not generally used to administer medication but to monitor blood pressure and oxygen levels in the blood.

- **Medications:** Most medicines can be administered anywhere in the hospital, but certain ones that can have dangerous side effects are only administered to children who are closely monitored in the PICU. Instead of being given every few hours, some are given continuously, several IV drops at a time, and are known as drips. Doctors may use these medications—like epinephrine, dopamine, and morphine, for example—to help with heart function, blood pressure, or pain relief.

- **Monitors:** Children are always attached to monitors while in the PICU. The monitors are secured to the body with chest leads, which are small painless stickers connected to wires. The chest leads can count the child's heart rate and breathing rate. Many kids are also connected to a pulse oximetry machine (or pulse ox) to check blood oxygen levels. Also painless, the pulse ox machine is attached to the fingers or toes like a small bandage and emits a soft red light. Unless blood pressure is being directly monitored through an arterial catheter, the child will usually have a blood pressure cuff in place as well.

- **Tests:** Doctors may order a variety of tests to obtain more information, including tests on the child's blood and urine, and sometimes on the cerebrospinal fluid, which surrounds the brain and spinal cord. Additionally, images or pictures of different parts of the body may be taken through x-rays, ultrasound, computed tomography (also called a CT or CAT scan), and magnetic resonance imaging (MRI).

- **Ventilators:** Kids in the PICU sometimes need extra help to breathe. This may mean getting some extra oxygen from a mask on the face or tubing in the nose. But sometimes, a child needs to be connected to the ventilator (or breathing machine). This is done via an endotracheal tube (a plastic tube placed into the windpipe through the mouth or nose) or a tracheostomy (a plastic tube inserted directly through the skin into the windpipe) connected to the ventilator on the other end. There are many different kinds of ventilators—different situations call for different machines—but they all serve the same basic purpose: to help your child breathe.

What should parents of kids in the PICU do?

In the PICU, all of your child's physical needs will be met by the staff. You, as a parent, are there to provide emotional support, love, and a familiar voice or touch. However, you shouldn't feel as if you have to stay at your child's bedside every minute of the day. Getting away from the commotion of the PICU briefly or even leaving the hospital grounds can help you gather your thoughts.

Staying around the clock with a child who's in the PICU for more than a few days can be both physically and emotionally draining. Although some hospitals allow parents to spend the night with their child, many do not. Often, hospitals encourage parents to go home, get a good night's rest in their own bed, and return to the PICU refreshed in the morning, which can help them be even more of a comfort to their child.

If the hospital does allow you to spend the night, the decision whether to stay in your child's room is a personal one. Either way, the PICU staff will support you and reassure you that your child will be well cared for. Whatever you do, make sure you get enough rest to be able to support your child throughout the PICU stay.

What happens when kids leave the PICU?

While some patients are sent home directly from the PICU, most are transferred to the regular floor of the hospital for further, less intense monitoring and follow-up care. Still, discharge from the PICU is a significant milestone on the road to recovery. It means that a child no longer needs such an intensive level of monitoring, therapy, and nursing care.

But leaving the PICU might also cause some anxiety. It's not unusual for parents of children who were in the PICU to think, "He was so sick, and now he's better. But shouldn't he stay here until he's completely back to normal?" Although certainly understandable, this shouldn't be a concern. The doctors and nurses in the PICU won't transfer kids before they're ready and stable, and the team on the hospital's regular floor will have the resources necessary to continue guiding your child's recovery.

Caring for a critically ill child is always stressful and difficult. But with a basic understanding of the people and things in the PICU, the stress on the family can be minimized—leaving you better able to support your child and plan for when the entire family is home together again.

Chapter 56

Civil Rights of Students with Hidden Disabilities

Section 504 of the Rehabilitation Act of 1973 protects the rights of persons with handicaps in programs and activities that receive federal financial assistance. Section 504 protects the rights not only of individuals with visible disabilities but also those with disabilities that may not be apparent.

Section 504 provides that: "No otherwise qualified individual with handicaps in the United States . . . shall, solely by reason of her or his handicap, be excluded from the participation in, be denied the benefits of, or be subjected to discrimination under any program or activity receiving federal financial assistance...."

The U.S. Department of Education (ED) enforces Section 504 in programs and activities that receive financial assistance from ED. Recipients of this assistance include public school districts, institutions of higher education, and other state and local education agencies. ED maintains an Office for Civil Rights (OCR), with ten regional offices and a headquarters office in Washington, DC, to enforce Section 504 and other civil rights laws that pertain to recipients of ED funds.

Disabilities Covered under Section 504

The ED Section 504 regulation defines an "individual with handicaps" as any person who (1) has a physical or mental impairment

"The Civil Rights of Students with Hidden Disabilities Under Section 504 of the Rehabilitation Act of 1973," U.S. Department of Education, March 14, 2005.

which substantially limits one or more major life activities, (2) has a record of such an impairment, or (3) is regarded as having such an impairment. The regulation further defines a physical or mental impairment as:

- any physiological disorder or condition, cosmetic disfigurement, or anatomical loss affecting one or more of the following body systems: neurological, musculoskeletal, special sense organs, respiratory (including speech organs), cardiovascular, reproductive, digestive, genitourinary, hemic and lymphatic, skin, and endocrine; or

- any mental or psychological disorder, such as mental retardation, organic brain syndrome, emotional or mental illness, and specific learning disabilities.

The definition does not set forth a list of specific diseases and conditions that constitute physical or mental impairments because of the difficulty of ensuring the comprehensiveness of any such list.

The key factor in determining whether a person is considered an individual with handicaps covered by Section 504 is whether the physical or mental impairment results in a substantial limitation of one or more major life activities. Major life activities, as defined in the regulation, include functions such as caring for one's self, performing manual tasks, walking, seeing, hearing, speaking, breathing, learning, and working.

The impairment must have a material effect on one's ability to perform a major life activity. For example, an individual who has a physical or mental impairment would not be considered a person with handicaps if the condition does not in any way limit the individual, or only results in some minor limitation. However, in some cases Section 504 also protects individuals who do not have a handicapping condition but are treated as though they do because they have a history of, or have been misclassified as having, a mental or physical impairment that substantially limits one or more major life activities. For example, if you have a history of a handicapping condition but no longer have the condition, or have been incorrectly classified as having such a condition, you too are protected from discrimination under Section 504. Frequently occurring examples of the first group are persons with histories of mental or emotional illness, heart disease, or cancer; of the second group, persons who have been misclassified as mentally retarded. Persons who are not disabled may be covered by Section 504 also if they are treated as if they are handicapped, for example, if they are infected with the human immunodeficiency virus (HIV).

What Are Hidden Disabilities?

Hidden disabilities are physical or mental impairments that are not readily apparent to others. They include such conditions and diseases as specific learning disabilities, diabetes, epilepsy, and allergy. A disability such as a limp, paralysis, total blindness or deafness is usually obvious to others. But hidden disabilities such as low vision, poor hearing, heart disease, or chronic illness may not be obvious. A chronic illness involves a recurring and long-term disability such as diabetes, heart disease, kidney and liver disease, high blood pressure, or ulcers.

Approximately four million students with disabilities are enrolled in public elementary and secondary schools in the United States. Of these 43% are students classified as learning disabled, 8% as emotionally disturbed, and 1% as other health impaired. These hidden disabilities often cannot be readily known without the administration of appropriate diagnostic tests.

The Responsibilities of the U.S. Department of Education Recipients in Preschool, Elementary, Secondary, and Adult Education

For coverage under Section 504, an individual with handicaps must be qualified for service by the school or institution receiving ED funds. For example, the ED Section 504 regulation defines a "qualified handicapped person" with respect to public preschool, elementary, secondary, or adult education services, as a person with a handicap who is:

- of an age during which persons without handicaps are provided such services;

- of any age during which it is mandatory under state law to provide such services to persons with handicaps; or

- a person for whom a state is required to provide a free appropriate public education under the Individuals with Disabilities Education Act (IDEA).

Under the Section 504 regulation, a recipient that operates a public elementary or secondary education program has a number of responsibilities toward qualified handicapped persons in its jurisdiction. These recipients must:

- undertake annually to identify and locate all handicapped children not being served;

- provide a free appropriate public education to each student with handicaps, regardless of the nature or severity of the handicap (This means providing regular or special education and related aids and services designed to meet the individual educational needs of handicapped persons as adequately as the needs of non-handicapped persons are met.);

- ensure that each student with handicaps is educated with non-handicapped students to the maximum extent appropriate to the needs of the handicapped person;

- establish nondiscriminatory evaluation and placement procedures to avoid the inappropriate education that may result from the misclassification or misplacement of students;

- establish procedural safeguards to enable parents and guardians to participate meaningfully in decisions regarding the evaluation and placement of their children; and

- afford handicapped children an equal opportunity to participate in nonacademic and extracurricular services and activities.

A recipient that operates a preschool education or day care program, or an adult education program may not exclude qualified handicapped persons and must take into account the needs of qualified handicapped persons in determining the aid, benefits, or services to be provided under those programs and activities.

Students with hidden disabilities frequently are not properly diagnosed. For example, a student with an undiagnosed hearing impairment may be unable to understand much of what a teacher says; a student with a learning disability may be unable to process oral or written information routinely; or a student with an emotional problem may be unable to concentrate in a regular classroom setting. As a result, these students, regardless of their intelligence, will be unable to fully demonstrate their ability or attain educational benefits equal to that of non-handicapped students. They may be perceived by teachers and fellow students as slow, lazy, or as discipline problems.

Whether a child is already in school or not, if his or her parents feel the child needs special education or related services, they should get in touch with the local superintendent of schools. For example, a parent who believes his or her child has a hearing impairment or is having difficulty understanding a teacher, may request to have the child evaluated so that the child may receive appropriate education. A child with behavior problems, or one who is doing poorly academically, may have an undiagnosed hidden disability. A parent has the right to request that the school determine whether the child is handicapped and whether special education or related services are needed to provide the child an appropriate education. Once it is determined that a child needs special education or related services, the recipient school system must arrange to provide appropriate services.

The Responsibilities of Department of Education Recipients in Postsecondary Education

The ED Section 504 regulation defines a qualified individual with handicaps for postsecondary education programs as a person with a handicap who meets the academic and technical standards requisite for admission to, or participation in, the college's education program or activity.

A college has no obligation to identify students with handicaps. In fact, Section 504 prohibits a postsecondary education recipient from making a preadmission inquiry as to whether an applicant for admission is a handicapped person. However, a postsecondary institution is required to inform applicants and other interested parties of the availability of auxiliary aids, services, and academic adjustments, and the name of the person designated to coordinate the college's efforts to carry out the requirements of Section 504. After admission (including the period between admission and enrollment), the college may make confidential inquiries as to whether a person has a handicap for the purpose of determining whether certain academic adjustments or auxiliary aids or services may be needed.

Many students with hidden disabilities, seeking college degrees, were provided with special education services during their elementary and secondary school years. It is especially important for these students to understand that postsecondary institutions also have responsibilities to protect the rights of students with disabilities. In elementary and secondary school, their school district was responsible for identifying, evaluating, and providing individualized special education and related services to meet their needs. At the postsecondary level, however, there are some important differences. The key provisions of Section 504 at the postsecondary level are highlighted below.

At the postsecondary level it is the student's responsibility to make his or her handicapping condition known and to request academic adjustments. This should be done in a timely manner. A student may choose to make his or her needs known to the Section 504 coordinator, to an appropriate dean, to a faculty advisor, or to each professor on an individual basis.

A student who requests academic adjustments or auxiliary aids because of a handicapping condition may be requested by the institution to provide documentation of the handicap and the need for the services requested. This may be especially important to an institution attempting to understand the nature and extent of a hidden disability.

The requested documentation may include the results of medical, psychological, or emotional diagnostic tests, or other professional evaluations to verify the need for academic adjustments or auxiliary aids.

How can the needs of students with hidden disabilities be addressed?

The following examples illustrate how schools can address the needs of their students with hidden disabilities.

- A student with a long-term, debilitating medical problem such as cancer, kidney disease, or diabetes may be given special consideration to accommodate the student's needs. For example, a student with cancer may need a class schedule that allows for rest and recuperation following chemotherapy.

- A student with a learning disability that affects the ability to demonstrate knowledge on a standardized test or in certain testing situations may require modified test arrangements, such as oral testing or different testing formats.

- A student with a learning disability or impaired vision that affects the ability to take notes in class may need a note taker or tape recorder.

- A student with a chronic medical problem such as kidney or liver disease may have difficulty in walking distances or climbing stairs. Under Section 504, this student may require special parking space, sufficient time between classes, or other considerations, to conserve the student's energy for academic pursuits.

- A student with diabetes, which adversely affects the body's ability to manufacture insulin, may need a class schedule that will accommodate the student's special needs.

- An emotionally or mentally ill student may need an adjusted class schedule to allow time for regular counseling or therapy.

- A student with epilepsy who has no control over seizures, and whose seizures are stimulated by stress or tension, may need accommodation for such stressful activities as lengthy academic testing or competitive endeavors in physical education.

- A student with arthritis may have persistent pain, tenderness, or swelling in one or more joints. A student experiencing arthritic pain may require a modified physical education program.

These are just a few examples of how the needs of students with hidden disabilities may be addressed.

Additional Information

Office for Civil Rights (OCR)
U.S. Department of Health and Human Services (HHS)
200 Independence Ave., S.W.
Room 509F, HHH Building
Washington, DC 20201
Toll-Free: 800-368-1019
Website: http://www.hhs.gov/ocr
E-mail: OCRMail@hhs.gov

Chapter 57

Students with Chronic Illnesses: Guidance for Families, Schools, and Students

Chronic illnesses affect at least 10–15 percent of American children. Responding to the needs of students with chronic conditions, such as asthma, allergies, diabetes, and epilepsy (also known as seizure disorders), in the school setting requires a comprehensive, coordinated, and systematic approach. Students with chronic health conditions can function to their maximum potential if their needs are met. The benefits to students can include better attendance, improved alertness and physical stamina, fewer symptoms, fewer restrictions on participation in physical activities and special activities, such as field trips, and fewer medical emergencies. Schools can work together with parents, students, health care providers, and the community to provide a safe and supportive educational environment for students with chronic illnesses and to ensure that students with chronic illnesses have the same educational opportunities as do other students.

Family's Responsibilities

- Notify the school of the student's health management needs and diagnosis when appropriate. Notify schools as early as possible and whenever the student's health needs change.

- Provide a written description of the student's health needs at school, including authorizations for medication administration

National Heart, Lung, and Blood Institute (NHLBI), 2002. Reviewed in November, 2007 by Dr. David A. Cooke, M.D., Diplomate, American Board of Internal Medicine.

and emergency treatment, signed by the student's health care provider.

- Participate in the development of a school plan to implement the student's health needs:

  - Meet with the school team to develop a plan to accommodate the student's needs in all school settings.

  - Authorize appropriate exchange of information between school health program staff and the student's personal health care providers.

  - Communicate significant changes in the student's needs or health status promptly to appropriate school staff.

- Provide an adequate supply of student's medication, in pharmacy-labeled containers, and other supplies to the designated school staff, and replace medications and supplies as needed. This supply should remain at school.

- Provide the school a means of contacting you or another responsible person at all times in case of an emergency or medical problem.

- Educate the student to develop age-appropriate self-care skills.

- Promote good general health, personal care, nutrition, and physical activity.

School District's Responsibilities

- Develop and implement districtwide guidelines and protocols applicable to chronic illnesses generally and specific protocols for asthma, allergies, diabetes, epilepsy (seizure disorders), and other common chronic illnesses of students.

- Guidelines should include safe, coordinated practices (as age and skill level appropriate) that enable the student to successfully manage his or her health in the classroom and at all school-related activities.

- Protocols should be consistent with established standards of care for students with chronic illnesses and federal laws that provide protection to students with disabilities, including ensuring confidentiality of student health care information and appropriate information sharing.

- Protocols should address education of all members of the school environment about chronic illnesses, including a component addressing the promotion of acceptance and the elimination of stigma surrounding chronic illnesses.

- Develop, coordinate, and implement necessary training programs for staff that will be responsible for chronic illness care tasks at school and school-related activities.

- Monitor schools for compliance with chronic illness care protocols.

- Meet with parents, school personnel, and health care providers to address issues of concern about the provision of care to students with chronic illnesses by school district staff.

School's Responsibilities

- Identify students with chronic conditions, and review their health records as submitted by families and health care providers.

- Arrange a meeting to discuss health accommodations and educational aids and services that the student may need and to develop a 504 Plan, individualized education program (IEP), or other school plan, as appropriate. The participants should include the family, student (if appropriate), school health staff, 504/IEP coordinator (as applicable), individuals trained to assist the student, and the teacher who has primary responsibility for the student. Health care provider input may be provided in person or in writing.

- Provide nondiscriminatory opportunities to students with disabilities. Be knowledgeable about and ensure compliance with applicable federal laws, including Americans with Disabilities Act (ADA), Individuals with Disabilities Education Act (IDEA), Section 504, and Family Educational Rights and Privacy Act of 1974 (FERPA). Be knowledgeable about any state or local laws or district policies that affect the implementation of students' rights under federal law.

- Clarify the roles and obligations of specific school staff, and provide education and communication systems necessary to ensure that students' health and educational needs are met in a safe and coordinated manner.

451

- Implement strategies that reduce disruption in the student's school activities, including physical education, recess, offsite events, extracurricular activities, and field trips.

- Communicate with families regularly and as authorized with the student's health care providers.

- Ensure that the student receives prescribed medications in a safe, reliable, and effective manner and has access to needed medication at all times during the school day and at school-related activities.

- Be prepared to handle health needs and emergencies and to ensure that there is a staff member available who is properly trained to administer medications or other immediate care during the school day and at all school-related activities, regardless of time or location.

- Ensure that all staff who interact with the student on a regular basis receive appropriate guidance and training on routine needs, precautions, and emergency actions.

- Provide appropriate health education to students and staff.

- Provide a safe and healthy school environment.

- Ensure that case management is provided as needed.

- Ensure proper record keeping, including appropriate measures to both protect confidentiality and to share information.

- Promote a supportive learning environment that views students with chronic illnesses the same as other students except to respond to health needs.

- Promote good general health, personal care, nutrition, and physical activity.

Student's Responsibilities

- Notify an adult about concerns and needs in managing his or her symptoms or the school environment.

- Participate in the care and management of his or her health as appropriate to his or her developmental level.

452

Chapter 58

Finding a Camp for a Child with Chronic Health Needs

Ah, summer camp, the mosquitoes, the swim races, the friendships, the bug juice, the postcards home. What child wouldn't benefit from the fun and structured freedom camps provide?

Kids with special needs are no exception. But the prospect can seem daunting to parents and kids alike—how can you be sure that your child will get the attention he or she needs? Will your child be able to participate fully? What about the other kids? Will your child make friends? Will they understand your child's special needs?

The good news is that there are more camp choices now than at any other time for kids with special needs. From highly specialized camps to regular camps that accommodate kids with special needs, there are options for every child. With careful consideration of what will benefit your child most, along with thorough research, you should be able to find the right camp for your child.

What Are the Different Types of Camps?

When it comes to camps, kids with special needs have as many choices as other children. The Americans with Disabilities Act (ADA) requires all camps to make reasonable accommodations (such as the installation of wheelchair-accessible ramps) so that kids with special

"Finding a Camp for Your Child with Special Needs" was provided by KidsHealth, one of the largest resources online for medically reviewed health information written for teens, kids, and parents. For more articles like this one, visit www.KidsHealth.org, or www.TeensHealth.org. © 2004 The Nemours Foundation.

needs can attend. So, camps that had never had a child with special needs attend before may now be on your list of possibilities.

Inclusionary (or mainstream) camps do just what their name implies: They include kids with special needs in their groups of children with regular needs. These camps may have started out serving only a general population of kids, but they've gradually changed as the needs of the families they serve have changed.

There are also camps designed just for kids with special needs, including kids who have learning or behavioral problems, kids with specific chronic illnesses, and kids with mental or physical impairments. Many of these camps accept kids with a variety of needs, but some camps only accept kids with specific problems (such as camps for kids with diabetes, cancer, speech or hearing impairment, cystic fibrosis, cerebral palsy, epilepsy, etc.).

Within all of these categories, you'll have even more choices to consider in terms of duration, philosophy, and cost. There are nonprofit and for-profit camps, religious camps, camps run by national organizations, private camps, day camps, camps that run weekend sessions, and sleep-over camps that accept kids for the entire summer.

What Are the Benefits of Camp?

The benefits of camp for kids with special needs are often the same as they would be for any child:

- increased confidence and independence
- activity and exercise
- the opportunity to interact with other kids, develop friendships, and build relationships
- positive role modeling by adults
- a chance for parents to have a likely much-needed break

Independence is another benefit that camp can provide. For example, an overnight mainstream camp can give a special-needs child the chance to be without parents, doctors, or physical therapists for a week. This allows children to do more things for themselves and learn how to ask friends to help.

Learning that their peers or other adults can help them is also valuable for kids with special needs. Children can learn to be assertive in problem-solving and communicating needs.

In addition, camp provides the physical benefits of increased activity as well. Many kids with disabilities or chronic illnesses are sedentary and don't often participate in the sports or recreational activities that their peers do. They therefore miss out on the social and health benefits that exercise brings. Camp provides a variety of activities such as swimming, wheelchair racing, dancing, tennis, or golf. These give immediate health benefits in terms of improved cardiovascular fitness and also provide recreational options that can carry over into adult life.

In addition, many camps combine learning environments with these physical activities, giving kids with behavioral or learning problems the chance to develop, or catch up on, needed skills during the summer.

Starting Your Camp Search

A good way to begin looking for a camp is to make several lists that establish the basics you're looking for: a list of goals, a list of caretaking priorities, and a list of other considerations (such as cost).

You'll also need to figure out which type of camp might best suit your child:

- inclusionary (or mainstream) camp
- camp for kids with a specific special need
- camp for kids with many different kinds of special needs

When trying to find the right camp, consider whether your child has ever been away from home, for the weekend or even longer, and what experiences might have helped prepare him or her for camp. This will help you to decide not only the type of camp, but whether your child is ready for a day camp or a sleep-over (residential) camp.

Involving kids in the camp search will help to ensure that they get the most out of the camp selected. So, ask kids the following:

- What do you want to get out of summer camp?
- What are your preferences?
- Do you want to go to a coed camp, or just be around kids of the same gender?
- Are there any activities you really want to try?
- Would you be more comfortable going to a camp with kids who do or don't have special needs?

- Are you comfortable being away from home? If so, for how long?

- Do you have classmates or friends who have gone to a summer camp? If so, which ones? And did they like it?

If it turns out that the idea of camp is a bit overwhelming for both you and your child, you want might to try starting small, like weekend sessions at a special-needs camp.

Doing Your Research

Whatever type of camp you're leaning toward, it's important to do your research. And there are plenty of places to get information on camps these days. The American Camp Association (ACA), for example, has an online listing (www.acacamps.org) of special-needs camps that's broken down by the types of camps, cost, length of stay, state/region, and campers' ages. The site is also loaded with general as well as age-appropriate advice for parents of would-be campers.

You can also call local chapters of major disability organizations to find out what camps are available in your area. Many organizations publish lists of camps and can connect you with camp directors and former campers.

In addition, you might be able to find a special-needs camp fair in your area. Check the calendar listings in your local newspapers and monthly parenting magazines. Many of these are held in January or February, which means that you need to start your camp search early.

Of course, part of your research will involve figuring out what you can afford. The cost of camps varies widely, with some high-end special-needs camps costing thousands of dollars for multiple-week sessions.

Although you can help fund your child's camp experience by applying for scholarships, experts say you should make sure to do so from December through March, because the money is gone by April or May. You can contact charitable organizations and fraternal organizations (such as the Lions, Kiwanis, and Rotary Clubs, all of which sponsor special-needs camps). And depending on your child's specific special need, he or she may be eligible for financial aid from your state. Other sources of scholarships include religious or ethnic charities.

One thing to bear in mind, though: You usually first need to find a camp that's willing to take your child—most of these organizations send the scholarship money to the camp in the child's name, not to the parents directly.

Questions to Ask

So, how do you narrow down your choices and pick the camp that's right for your child? Some basic and special-needs-specific questions you'll need to have answered include:

- How long are the sessions?

- What's the cost? Are scholarships available?

- Is it coed, girls-only, or boys-only?

- What's the age range of campers?

- Where is it located—and how far away from your home is it?

- What's the staff-to-camper ratio?

- How old are most of the counselors?

- What type of certification do the counselors have?

- What's the turnover rate? Do kids and staff come back?

- What's the camp's philosophy? Does it fit with your goals for your child?

- What's the camp's transportation system like?

- If physical accessibility is an issue, what's the layout of the camp? What provisions has the camp made (or can it make) for wheelchairs or crutches?

- If your child needs a special diet, can the camp provide appropriate meals? If not, can you provide food for your child?

- Do staff members have a background working with kids with special needs?

- Do the counselors have first-aid training?

- What kind of medical staff is available in the infirmary and during what hours? Can the staff administer any medications your child needs?

- If your child has behavior problems, what's the training and experience of the available staff to help? And how does the camp staff handle behavioral problems?

- What's the procedure if your child develops a complication related to his or her medical problems? How far is the nearest hospital? If your child needs specialized treatment, is it available at that hospital?

Although you can get some of this information through phone calls, e-mails, brochures, and websites, experts recommend visiting the camp. You can talk to the director, visit the site, and get a comprehensive picture of where your child will be.

Probably the only way to get a true feel for the camp is for you and your child to visit it together. This is especially important if your child is going to a regular (inclusionary or mainstream) camp where they haven't dealt with many children with special needs, because it gives you the opportunity to point out changes they might need to make and to gauge the reaction of the camp's staff to your requests.

If you can't visit a camp, interview the director and some staff members to get a feel for the place. Ask them to describe the physical layout and the kinds of activities your child will do. You should also ask to speak with other families whose children have attended the camp to see what their experiences were like. In fact, word of mouth is one of the most effective ways to find out what you need to know about each camp.

As you're trying to figure out which camp is best, just remember that whatever the special need, there's likely a camp out there to suit your child. With some research and understanding between you, your child, and the camp director, your camper-to-be will likely be well on the way to having an unforgettable summer.

Additional Information

American Camp Association
5000 SR 67 N.
Martinsville, IN 46151-7902
Phone: 765-342-8456
Fax: 765-342-2065
Website: http://www.acacamps.org

Part Seven

Legal, Financial, and Insurance Issues That Impact Disease Management

Chapter 59

Americans with Disabilities Act

Barriers to employment, transportation, public accommodations, public services, and telecommunications have imposed staggering economic and social costs on American society and have undermined our well-intentioned efforts to educate, rehabilitate, and employ individuals with disabilities. By breaking down these barriers, the Americans with Disabilities Act (ADA) will enable society to benefit from the skills and talents of individuals with disabilities, will allow us all to gain from their increased purchasing power and ability to use it, and will lead to fuller, more productive lives for all Americans.

The Americans with Disabilities Act gives civil rights protections to individuals with disabilities similar to those provided to individuals on the basis of race, color, sex, national origin, age, and religion. It guarantees equal opportunity for individuals with disabilities in public accommodations, employment, transportation, state and local government services, and telecommunications.

Employment

What employers are covered by title I of the ADA, and when is the coverage effective?

The title I employment provisions apply to private employers, state and local governments, employment agencies, and labor unions.

Excerpts from "Americans with Disabilities Act: Questions and Answers," U.S. Department of Justice, June 2006.

Employers with 25 or more employees were covered as of July 26, 1992. Employers with 15 or more employees were covered two years later, beginning July 26, 1994.

What practices and activities are covered by the employment nondiscrimination requirements?

The ADA prohibits discrimination in all employment practices, including job application procedures, hiring, firing, advancement, compensation, training, and other terms, conditions, and privileges of employment. It applies to recruitment, advertising, tenure, layoff, leave, fringe benefits, and all other employment-related activities.

Who is protected from employment discrimination?

Employment discrimination is prohibited against "qualified individuals with disabilities." This includes applicants for employment and employees. An individual is considered to have a disability if she or he has a physical or mental impairment that substantially limits one or more major life activities, has a record of such an impairment, or is regarded as having such an impairment. Persons discriminated against because they have a known association or relationship with an individual with a disability also are protected.

The first part of the definition makes clear that the ADA applies to persons who have impairments and that these must substantially limit major life activities such as seeing, hearing, speaking, walking, breathing, performing manual tasks, learning, caring for oneself, and working. An individual with epilepsy, paralysis, human immunodeficiency virus (HIV) infection, acquired immunodeficiency syndrome (AIDS), a substantial hearing or visual impairment, mental retardation, or a specific learning disability is covered, but an individual with a minor, non-chronic condition of short duration, such as a sprain, broken limb, or the flu, generally would not be covered.

The second part of the definition protecting individuals with a record of a disability would cover, for example, a person who has recovered from cancer or mental illness.

The third part of the definition protects individuals who are regarded as having a substantially limiting impairment, even though they may not have such an impairment. For example, this provision would protect a qualified individual with a severe facial disfigurement from being denied employment because an employer feared the negative reactions of customers or co-workers.

Who is a "qualified individual with a disability?"

A qualified individual with a disability is a person who meets legitimate skill, experience, education, or other requirements of an employment position that she or he holds or seeks, and who can perform the essential functions of the position with or without reasonable accommodation. Requiring the ability to perform essential functions assures that an individual with a disability will not be considered unqualified simply because of inability to perform marginal or incidental job functions. If the individual is qualified to perform essential job functions except for limitations caused by a disability, the employer must consider whether the individual could perform these functions with a reasonable accommodation. If a written job description has been prepared in advance of advertising or interviewing applicants for a job, this will be considered as evidence, although not conclusive evidence, of the essential functions of the job.

Does an employer have to give preference to a qualified applicant with a disability over other applicants?

No. An employer is free to select the most qualified applicant available and to make decisions based on reasons unrelated to a disability.

What limitations does the ADA impose on medical examinations and inquiries about disability?

An employer may not ask or require a job applicant to take a medical examination before making a job offer. It cannot make any pre-employment inquiry about a disability or the nature or severity of a disability. An employer may, however, ask questions about the ability to perform specific job functions and may, with certain limitations, ask an individual with a disability to describe or demonstrate how she or he would perform these functions.

An employer may condition a job offer on the satisfactory result of a post-offer medical examination or medical inquiry if this is required of all entering employees in the same job category. A post-offer examination or inquiry does not have to be job-related and consistent with business necessity.

However, if an individual is not hired because a post-offer medical examination or inquiry reveals a disability, the reason(s) for not hiring must be job-related and consistent with business necessity. The employer also must show that no reasonable accommodation was available that would enable the individual to perform the essential job functions, or that accommodation would impose an undue hardship. A post-offer medical examination may disqualify an individual if the employer can demonstrate that the individual would pose a direct threat in the workplace (for example, a significant risk of substantial harm to the health or safety of the individual or others) that cannot be eliminated or reduced below the direct threat level through reasonable accommodation. Such a disqualification is job-related and consistent with business necessity. A post-offer medical examination may not disqualify an individual with a disability who is currently able to perform essential job functions because of speculation that the disability may cause a risk of future injury.

After a person starts work, a medical examination or inquiry of an employee must be job-related and consistent with business necessity. Employers may conduct employee medical examinations where there is evidence of a job performance or safety problem, examinations required by other federal laws, examinations to determine current fitness to perform a particular job, and voluntary examinations that are part of employee health programs.

Information from all medical examinations and inquiries must be kept apart from general personnel files as a separate, confidential medical record, available only under limited conditions.

Tests for illegal use of drugs are not medical examinations under the ADA and are not subject to the restrictions of such examinations.

When can an employer ask an applicant to "self-identify" as having a disability?

Federal contractors and subcontractors who are covered by the affirmative action requirements of section 503 of the Rehabilitation Act of 1973 may invite individuals with disabilities to identify themselves on a job application form or by other pre-employment inquiry, to satisfy the section 503 affirmative action requirements. Employers who request such information must observe section 503 requirements regarding the manner in which such information is requested and used, and the procedures for maintaining such information as a separate, confidential record, apart from regular personnel records.

A pre-employment inquiry about a disability is allowed if required by another federal law or regulation such as those applicable to disabled veterans and veterans of the Vietnam era. Pre-employment inquiries about disabilities may be necessary under such laws to identify applicants or clients with disabilities in order to provide them with required special services.

What is "reasonable accommodation?"

Reasonable accommodation is any modification or adjustment to a job or the work environment that will enable a qualified applicant or employee with a disability to participate in the application process or to perform essential job functions. Reasonable accommodation also includes adjustments to assure that a qualified individual with a disability has rights and privileges in employment equal to those of employees without disabilities.

What are some of the accommodations applicants and employees may need?

Examples of reasonable accommodation include making existing facilities used by employees readily accessible to and usable by an individual with a disability; restructuring a job; modifying work schedules; acquiring or modifying equipment; providing qualified readers or interpreters; or appropriately modifying examinations, training, or other programs. Reasonable accommodation also may include reassigning a current employee to a vacant position for which the individual is qualified, if the person is unable to do the original job because of a disability even with an accommodation. However, there is no obligation to find a position for an applicant who is not qualified for the position sought. Employers are not required to lower quality or quantity standards as an accommodation; nor are they obligated to provide personal use items such as glasses or hearing aids.

The decision as to the appropriate accommodation must be based on the particular facts of each case. In selecting the particular type of reasonable accommodation to provide, the principal test is that of effectiveness, for example, whether the accommodation will provide an opportunity for a person with a disability to achieve the same level of performance and to enjoy benefits equal to those of an average, similarly situated person without a disability. However, the accommodation does not have to ensure equal results or provide exactly the same benefits.

When is an employer required to make a reasonable accommodation?

An employer is only required to accommodate a known disability of a qualified applicant or employee. The requirement generally will be triggered by a request from an individual with a disability, who frequently will be able to suggest an appropriate accommodation. Accommodations must be made on an individual basis, because the nature and extent of a disabling condition and the requirements of a job will vary in each case.

What are the limitations on the obligation to make a reasonable accommodation?

The individual with a disability requiring the accommodation must be otherwise qualified, and the disability must be known to the employer. In addition, an employer is not required to make an accommodation if it would impose an "undue hardship" on the operation of the employer's business. Undue hardship is defined as an "action requiring significant difficulty or expense" when considered in light of a number of factors. These factors include the nature and cost of the accommodation in relation to the size, resources, nature, and structure of the employer's operation. Undue hardship is determined on a case-by-case basis.

If a particular accommodation would be an undue hardship, the employer must try to identify another accommodation that will not pose such a hardship. Also, if the cost of an accommodation would impose an undue hardship on the employer, the individual with a disability should be given the option of paying that portion of the cost which would constitute an undue hardship or providing the accommodation.

Can an employer be required to reallocate an essential function of a job to another employee as a reasonable accommodation?

No. An employer is not required to reallocate essential functions of a job as a reasonable accommodation.

Can an employer maintain existing production/performance standards for an employee with a disability?

An employer can hold employees with disabilities to the same standards of production and performance as other similarly situated employees without disabilities for performing essential job functions, with or without reasonable accommodation. An employer also can hold employees with disabilities to the same standards of production/performance as other employees regarding marginal functions unless the disability affects the person's ability to perform those marginal functions.

Can an employer consider health and safety when deciding whether to hire an applicant or retain an employee with a disability?

Yes. The ADA permits employers to establish qualification standards that will exclude individuals who pose a direct threat—for example, a significant risk of substantial harm—to the health or safety of the individual or of others, if that risk cannot be eliminated or reduced below the level of a direct threat by reasonable accommodation.

Is testing for the illegal use of drugs permissible under the ADA?

Yes. A test for the illegal use of drugs is not considered a medical examination under the ADA; therefore, employers may conduct such testing of applicants or employees and make employment decisions based on the results. The ADA does not encourage, prohibit, or authorize drug tests.

If the results of a drug test reveal the presence of a lawfully prescribed drug or other medical information, such information must be treated as a confidential medical record.

What is discrimination based on relationship or association under the ADA?

The ADA prohibits discrimination based on relationship or association in order to protect individuals from actions based on unfounded assumptions that their relationship to a person with a disability would affect their job performance, and from actions caused by bias or misinformation concerning certain disabilities. For example, this provision would protect a person whose spouse has a disability from being denied employment because of an employer's unfounded assumption that the applicant would use excessive leave to care for the spouse. It also would protect an individual who does volunteer work for people with AIDS from a discriminatory employment action motivated by that relationship or association.

Public Accommodations

What are public accommodations?

A public accommodation is a private entity that owns, operates, leases, or leases to, a place of public accommodation. Places of public

467

accommodation include a wide range of entities, such as restaurants, hotels, theaters, doctors' offices, pharmacies, retail stores, museums, libraries, parks, private schools, and day care centers. Private clubs and religious organizations are exempt from the ADA title III requirements for public accommodations.

Additional Information

U.S. Department of Justice
Civil Rights Division
950 Pennsylvania Ave., N.W.
Disability Rights Section–NYAV
Washington, DC 20530
Toll-Free: 800-514-0301
Toll-Free TTY: 800-514-0383
Website: http://www.ada.gov

U.S. Equal Employment Opportunity Commission (EEOC)
1801 L Street, N.W.
Washington, DC 20507
Toll-Free: 800-669-4000
Toll-Free TTY: 800-669-6820
Website: http://www.eeoc.gov

Chapter 60

Family and Medical Leave Act

How much leave am I entitled to under the Family and Medical Leave Act (FMLA)?

If you are an eligible employee, you are entitled to 12 weeks of leave for certain family and medical reasons during a 12-month period.

How is the 12-month period calculated under FMLA?

Employers may select one of four options for determining the 12-month period:

- the calendar year

- any fixed 12-month leave year such as a fiscal year, a year required by state law, or a year starting on the employee's anniversary date

- the 12-month period measured forward from the date any employee's first FMLA leave begins

- a rolling 12-month period measured backward from the date an employee uses FMLA leave

---

"Family and Medical Leave Act Advisor: Frequently Asked Questions and Answers," U.S. Department of Labor, 2007.

Does the law guarantee paid time off?

No. The FMLA only requires unpaid leave. However, the law permits an employee to elect, or the employer to require the employee, to use accrued paid leave, such as vacation or sick leave, for some or all of the FMLA leave period. When paid leave is substituted for unpaid FMLA leave, it may be counted against the 12-week FMLA leave entitlement if the employee is properly notified of the designation when the leave begins.

Does workers' compensation leave count against an employee's FMLA leave entitlement?

It can. FMLA leave and workers' compensation leave can run together, provided the reason for the absence is due to a qualifying serious illness or injury and the employer properly notifies the employee in writing that the leave will be counted as FMLA leave.

Can the employer count leave taken due to pregnancy complications against the 12 weeks of FMLA leave for the birth and care of my child?

Yes. An eligible employee is entitled to a total of 12 weeks of FMLA leave in a 12-month period. If the employee has to use some of that leave for another reason, including a difficult pregnancy, it may be counted as part of the 12-week FMLA leave entitlement.

Can the employer count time on maternity leave or pregnancy disability as FMLA leave?

Yes. Pregnancy disability leave or maternity leave for the birth of a child would be considered qualifying FMLA leave for a serious health condition and may be counted in the 12 weeks of leave so long as the employer properly notifies the employee in writing of the designation.

If an employer fails to tell employees that the leave is FMLA leave, can the employer count the time they have already been off against the 12 weeks of FMLA leave?

In most situations, the employer cannot count leave as FMLA leave retroactively. Remember, the employee must be notified in writing that an absence is being designated as FMLA leave. If the employer was not aware of the reason for the leave, leave may be designated as

FMLA leave retroactively only while the leave is in progress or within two business days of the employee's return to work.

Who is considered an immediate family member for purposes of taking FMLA leave?

An employee's spouse, children (son or daughter), and parents are immediate family members for purposes of FMLA. The term parent does not include a parent in-law. The terms son or daughter do not include individuals age 18 or over unless they are incapable of self-care because of mental or physical disability that limits one or more of the major life activities as those terms are defined in regulations issued by the Equal Employment Opportunity Commission (EEOC) under the Americans with Disabilities Act (ADA).

May I take FMLA leave for visits to a physical therapist, if my doctor prescribes the therapy?

Yes. FMLA permits you to take leave to receive "continuing treatment by a health care provider," which can include recurring absences for therapy treatments such as those ordered by a doctor for physical therapy after a hospital stay or for treatment of severe arthritis.

Which employees are eligible to take FMLA leave?

Employees are eligible to take FMLA leave if they have worked for their employer for at least 12 months, and have worked for at least 1,250 hours over the previous 12 months, and work at a location where at least 50 employees are employed by the employer within 75 miles.

Do the 12 months of service with the employer have to be continuous or consecutive?

No. The 12 months do not have to be continuous or consecutive; all time worked for the employer is counted.

Do the 1,250 hours include paid leave time or other absences from work?

No. The 1,250 hours include only those hours actually worked for the employer. Paid leave and unpaid leave, including FMLA leave, are not included.

How do I determine if I have worked 1,250 hours in a 12-month period?

Your individual record of hours worked would be used to determine whether 1,250 hours had been worked in the 12 months prior to the commencement of FMLA leave. As a rule of thumb, the following may be helpful for estimating whether this test for eligibility has been met:

- 24 hours worked in each of the 52 weeks of the year; or

- over 104 hours worked in each of the 12 months of the year; or

- 40 hours worked per week for more than 31 weeks (over seven months) of the year.

Do I have to give my employer my medical records for leave due to a serious health condition?

No. You do not have to provide medical records. The employer may, however, request that, for any leave taken due to a serious health condition, you provide a medical certification confirming that a serious health condition exists.

Can my employer require me to return to work before I exhaust my leave?

Subject to certain limitations, your employer may deny the continuation of FMLA leave due to a serious health condition if you fail to fulfill any obligations to provide supporting medical certification. The employer may not, however, require you to return to work early by offering you a light duty assignment.

Are there any restrictions on how I spend my time while on leave?

Employers with established policies regarding outside employment while on paid or unpaid leave may uniformly apply those policies to employees on FMLA leave. Otherwise, the employer may not restrict your activities. The protections of FMLA will not, however, cover situations where the reason for leave no longer exists, where the employee has not provided required notices or certifications, or where the employee has misrepresented the reason for leave.

Can my employer make inquiries about my leave during my absence?

Yes, but only to you. Your employer may ask you questions to confirm whether the leave needed or being taken qualifies for FMLA purposes, and may require periodic reports on your status and intent to return to work after leave. Also, if the employer wishes to obtain another opinion, you may be required to obtain additional medical certification at the employer's expense, or rectification during a period of FMLA leave. The employer may have a health care provider representing the employer contact your health care provider, with your permission, to clarify information in the medical certification or to confirm that it was provided by the health care provider. The inquiry may not seek additional information regarding your health condition or that of a family member.

Can my employer refuse to grant me FMLA leave?

If you are an eligible employee who has met FMLA notice and certification requirements (and you have not exhausted your FMLA leave entitlement for the year), you may not be denied FMLA leave.

Will I lose my job if I take FMLA leave?

Generally, no. It is unlawful for any employer to interfere with or restrain or deny the exercise of any right provided under this law. Employers cannot use the taking of FMLA leave as a negative factor in employment actions, such as hiring, promotions, or disciplinary actions; nor can FMLA leave be counted under no fault attendance policies. Under limited circumstances, an employer may deny reinstatement to work—but not the use of FMLA leave—to certain highly-paid, salaried (key) employees.

Are there other circumstances in which my employer can deny me FMLA leave or reinstatement to my job?

In addition to denying reinstatement in certain circumstances to key employees, employers are not required to continue FMLA benefits or reinstate employees who would have been laid off or otherwise had their employment terminated had they continued to work during the FMLA leave period as, for example, due to a general layoff.

473

Employees who give unequivocal notice that they do not intend to return to work lose their entitlement to FMLA leave.

Employees who are unable to return to work and have exhausted their 12 weeks of FMLA leave in the designated 12 month period no longer have FMLA protections of leave or job restoration

Under certain circumstances, employers who advise employees experiencing a serious health condition that they will require a medical certificate of fitness for duty to return to work may deny reinstatement to an employee who fails to provide the certification, or may delay reinstatement until the certification is submitted.

Can my employer fire me for complaining about a violation of FMLA?

No. Nor can the employer take any other adverse employment action on this basis. It is unlawful for any employer to discharge or otherwise discriminate against an employee for opposing a practice made unlawful under FMLA.

Does an employer have to pay bonuses to employees who have been on FMLA leave?

The FMLA requires that employees be restored to the same or an equivalent position. If an employee was eligible for a bonus before taking FMLA leave, the employee would be eligible for the bonus upon returning to work. The FMLA leave may not be counted against the employee. For example, if an employer offers a perfect attendance bonus, and the employee has not missed any time prior to taking FMLA leave, the employee would still be eligible for the bonus upon returning from FMLA leave.

On the other hand, FMLA does not require that employees on FMLA leave be allowed to accrue benefits or seniority. For example, an employee on FMLA leave might not have sufficient sales to qualify for a bonus. The employer is not required to make any special accommodation for this employee because of FMLA. The employer must, of course, treat an employee who has used FMLA leave at least as well as other employees on paid and unpaid leave (as appropriate) are treated.

Under what circumstances is leave designated as FMLA leave and counted against the employee's total entitlement?

In all circumstances, it is the employer's responsibility to designate leave taken for an FMLA reason as FMLA leave. The designation must be based upon information furnished by the employee. Leave may not be designated as FMLA leave after the leave has been completed and the employee has returned to work, except if:

- the employer is awaiting receipt of the medical certification to confirm the existence of a serious health condition;

- the employer was unaware that leave was for an FMLA reason, and subsequently acquires information from the employee such as when the employee requests additional or extensions of leave; or

- the employer was unaware that the leave was for an FMLA reason, and the employee notifies the employer within two days after return to work that the leave was FMLA leave.

Can my employer count FMLA leave I take against a no fault absentee policy?

No.

Additional Information

U.S. Department of Labor
Frances Perkins Building
200 Constitution Ave., N.W.
Washington, DC 20210
Toll-Free: 866-487-2365
Toll-Free TTY: 877-889-5627
Website: http://www.dol.gov

Chapter 61

Advance Directives

Alternative names: Power of attorney; do not resuscitate (DNR); living will

Definition

Advanced care directives are specific instructions, prepared in advance, that are intended to direct a person's medical care if he or she becomes unable to do so in the future.

Information

Advanced care directives allow patients to make their own decisions regarding the care they would prefer to receive if they develop a terminal illness or a life-threatening injury. Advanced care directives can also designate someone the patient trusts to make decisions about medical care, if the patient becomes unable to make (or communicate) these decisions.

Federal law requires hospitals, nursing homes, and other institutions that receive Medicare or Medicaid funds to provide written information regarding advanced care directives to all patients upon admission.

Advanced care directives can reduce:

* personal worry;

- futile, costly, specialized interventions that a patient may not want;

- overall health care costs;

- feelings of helplessness and guilt for family; and

- legal concerns for everyone involved.

However, advanced care directives cannot predict what situations may arise in the future or what new modes of care may be available for situations considered nearly hopeless today.

Examples of Advance Directives

Verbal instructions: These are any decisions regarding care that are communicated verbally by an individual to health care providers and family members.

Organ donation: This may be accomplished by completing an organ donation card and carrying it in your wallet. A second card may be placed with important papers (such as a living will, insurance papers, and so on). Most hospitals or other major health care centers have organ donor information available.

Many states offer people who are applying for new or renewed driver's license the opportunity to make a decision regarding organ donation and have it recorded on the driver's license.

Living will: This is a written, legal document that conveys the wishes of a person in the event of terminal illness. This document can speak for a patient who is unable to communicate. A living will may indicate specific care or treatment the person does or does not want performed under specific circumstances. This may include specific procedures, care, or treatments such as the following:

- cardiopulmonary resuscitation (CPR) (if cardiac or respiratory arrest occurs)

- artificial nutrition through intravenous or tube feedings

- prolonged maintenance on a respirator (if unable to breathe adequately alone)

- blood cultures, spinal fluid evaluations, and other diagnostic tests

- blood transfusions

State laws vary regarding living wills. Information specific to individual states usually may be obtained from the State Bar Association, State Medical Association, State Nursing Association, and most hospitals or medical centers.

A living will is not to be confused with a last will and testament that distributes assets after a person's death.

Special medical power of attorney: A legal document that allows an individual to appoint someone else (proxy) to make medical or health care decisions, in the event the individual becomes unable to make or communicate such decisions personally.

Note: This document provides for power to make medically related decisions only and does not give any individual power to make legal or financial decisions.

DNR (do not resuscitate) order: This states that CPR is not to be performed if your breathing stops or your heart stops beating. The order may be written by the person's doctor after discussing the issue with the person (if possible), the proxy, or family.

Recommendations

- In the event you choose to write up a living will or special medical power of attorney, know specific state laws that may apply. Write the document to be consistent with your state's laws.

- If you have a living will or special medical power of attorney, provide copies for your family members and health care providers. Carry a copy with you in a wallet, glove compartment of car, or similar location. If you have a planned admission to a hospital, take copies for the hospital to include in your medical chart and tell all medical personnel involved with your case about the documents.

- Consider the possibilities of the future, and plan ahead. Studies have shown that although the majority of people believe having some form of advance directives is a good idea, most people have not actually developed advance directives for themselves. Many people state that they want their families to make health care decisions. However, less than half of these people have ever discussed the issue and their specific desires with family members.

- These decisions can be changed at any time. However, if a living will is changed, everyone involved—including family or proxies and all health care providers—must be informed and new copies of instructions made and distributed.

Summary

The process of creating advanced care directives may be difficult. It requires you to think about your priorities regarding quality of life and your death. Treatment options, and their possible influence on your quality of life, need to be fully understood and considered. Know the potential implications of choosing or refusing specific forms of care.

Discuss your wishes regarding advanced care directives with your health care providers, family members, and friends. Review your wishes from time to time to remind everyone.

Chapter 62

Understanding Hospital Bills

How much do I really owe?

After your insurance company has reviewed your hospital bill and paid or denied their portion (a process that can take several months), the hospital will bill you for your part of the bill. Your hospital bill will show charges for whatever your insurance does not pay. Most insurance plans require patients to pay part of their hospital bill. If you have questions about your insurance, please contact your insurance company.

Who will bill my insurance?

Hospitals will bill your insurance company if you have given them the correct insurance information.

What if I cannot pay?

Hospitals have ways to help their patients. If you need help, please call the hospital billing office. Among the ways hospitals can help are:

- **Hospital financial assistance:** Hospitals provide free or reduced price care if you qualify based on your income. Financial assistance can help with hospital bills for inpatient or outpatient

"Understanding Hospital Bills—Frequently Asked Questions," © 2006 Washington State Hospital Association. Reprinted with permission.

care. Hospitals will help you find out if you qualify for financial assistance and help is offered to people with and without insurance.

- **Insurance programs:** Hospitals can help you apply for public insurance programs such as Medicaid and Basic Health. These programs may help you with your current bill and will help you pay for health needs in the future.

- **Payment plans:** If you need to pay your bill over time, hospitals can usually help you set up an appropriate payment plan.

People with health insurance sometimes get negotiated discounts so they are not required to pay full charges. Are there special discounts for people who do not have insurance?

Yes. Most hospitals have generous charity care and financial assistance policies for people with and without insurance. If you have concerns in this area, ask the staff in the hospital's billing office for an explanation.

Why does hospital care cost so much?

The answer is complex. As with any business, hospitals must attempt to cover their expenses by charging for their services. But with hospitals the cost of providing services includes many necessary and costly items that do not readily come to mind when most of us think about our care. We take it for granted that the hospital is there 24 hours a day, 7 days a week. Likewise, we have come to expect that hospitals will have all of the latest technology that could possibly be needed for our care. And we expect that the people caring for us are highly trained, highly skilled professionals. Finally, although we seldom think about it, the health care world is unique in that those who can pay for the services they use are asked to help pay for the care of others who cannot or will not pay.

Who do I call for help?

If you have questions about your bill, you should contact the billing office at the hospital where you received your care. If you do not have the direct number for the hospital billing office, call the hospital's main switchboard and ask for the billing office.

Why did I receive a separate lab, doctor, or ambulance bill?

Many doctors, ambulance companies, and labs are separate businesses with their own billing and account procedures. State law requires a hospital to provide patients with a list of the groups that regularly provide care for patients at that hospital and from whom the patient may receive a bill. Ask your hospital's billing office for this list.

Why did I receive a bill from a doctor I did not see?

Hospitals often consult with specialized doctors as part of caring for patients. Often these specialists are sent items such as lab tests or x-rays for their expert review. You will receive a bill directly from those doctors for their work.

What if my hospitalization is the result of an accident?

If you had a non-work related accident, the hospital will ask you for information about other insurance, like car insurance. If your accident or illness is work-related, the hospital will bill your employer's workers' compensation program. You must fill out the paperwork they need.

Chapter 63

Financial Management during Crisis

Every parent knows that raising a child is one of life's most fulfilling challenges. But if your child has a chronic illness, condition, or disability, your role takes on an even greater purpose. You are more than a loving parent—you have become your child's primary health advocate.

Although the emotional price of raising a seriously ill child can be devastating, it's only part of the picture. Even during this difficult time, you have to consider the financial implications of your child's illness. Some parents become overwhelmed by medical expenses or are blind-sided by unexpected bills and additional fees. Even wealthier families can find themselves on the brink of financial free fall because of accumulating medical expenses.

Even so, maintaining your family's financial health is not impossible. With organization and careful planning, you can learn to manage your money during a medical crisis.

Costs of Health Care

The costs of long-term health care can be staggering, and families don't always heed them until they're hit with the first bill or explanation of benefits that they don't understand. "When you're faced with

---

This information was provided by TeensHealth, one of the largest resources online for medically reviewed health information written for teens, kids, and parents. For more articles like this one, visit www.TeensHealth.org, or www.KidsHealth .org. © 2005 The Nemours Foundation.

485

a child with as many medical complications as our son, we were just worried about having him breathe every day and the last thing we thought about were the bills," explains Carol, whose son Dylan has spina bifida.

Some parents may think that insurance will cover all or most of their child's medical expenses—or that being able to afford their child's health care needs won't be a problem. But each medical service comes with its own price tag, and parents are often shocked to learn that hospital care, surgical procedures, doctor visits, and laboratory tests are separate services with separate bills. "Financially, it was a disaster coming. Her first hospital bill, not including surgery and anesthesia, was $308,000," says Kellie, whose daughter has a serious disability. Even the typical 10% co-pay can consume a family's financial reserves.

Some parents may overlook costs that are indirectly related to their child's care—costs that can quickly add up. These include missed time at work, child care for siblings, increased utility bills, custom transportation, and home renovations, such as ramps for wheelchair accessibility.

There are ways to handle these costs, but you need information to negotiate your way through the health care system.

Understanding the Health Care System

The best way to make sense of bills and prevent financial problems is to take a proactive stance. Learn all you can about your health plan.

Just as you want to know as much as possible about your child's health, you should learn as much as you can about your insurance policy. Which doctors participate in your plan? What services are covered? Learn the meaning of insurance language:

co-pay: The part or percentage of the bill you are responsible for.

deductible: The amount you must pay before your insurance company will pay for services.

referral: Your insurance company may require your child's primary care doctor to refer your child to another doctor or specialist before your insurance company will pay for services performed by another doctor.

pre-certification: You may have to let your insurance company know in advance about any medical tests or treatments the doctor has ordered.

486

If you do not pre-certify before receiving treatment, the procedure may not be covered.

network provider: Any doctor, hospital, or other provider of medical services who has agreed to participate in your insurance company's network and to offer their services at negotiated rates; also called a participating provider.

pre-existing condition: An injury or illness that existed prior to the effective date of your current insurance policy and therefore may not be fully covered.

usual, customary, and reasonable: Refers to the amount usually charged by health care providers for services and treatments in the area where you live.

Understanding your health plan's design and its policies can ultimately save you thousands of dollars.

You may find it useful to get a written copy of your policy from the insurer. Although you may have an enrollment information book from your employer, the actual policy provides specific details about your coverage. If your insurance company has a website, you should check it out for additional information.

Policies and bills can be confusing, but help is available. These simple steps can help you avoid problems:

- Locate the resources available within your child's hospital, such as a financial counselor or hospital business office, for answers to your questions about medical expenses.

- Ask the hospital to have a case manager assigned to your child. If the hospital has none on staff, ask your insurance company.

- Make your child's health care providers aware of your plan's benefits and limitations. They can become your partners in coordinating care with your health plan.

- Negotiate fees with the doctors, clinics, and hospital, and set up realistic payment plans.

- Organize. Keep a journal and files to record doctor visits and any services performed (including lab work, x-rays, CT scans, etc.) and the fees for these services so that detailed information about your child's health care is easily accessible. This may seem like a lot of work, but it will be extremely helpful when dealing with your insurance company.

- Know your rights as a health consumer. If your insurance company denies coverage for certain expenses, appeal the decision. The doctors can sometimes write letters or help you appeal to the insurance company to get certain services covered.

- Contact your state's department of insurance if you encounter problems with your health care coverage—especially if you've already appealed denied or inadequate coverage.

Warning Signs of Financial Trouble

Families may struggle to meet new expenses, particularly if one parent must stop working to care for a child. Regular monthly bills may be put aside or ignored. Debt begins to grow, and a family that has maintained a comfortable lifestyle can find itself headed for trouble.

If the following questions seem all too familiar, it's time to seek help:

- Do you spend more than you earn?

- Are you using credit for everyday purchases?

- Do you make only minimum payments on bills or skip payments entirely?

- Are your savings inadequate or nonexistent?

- Do you use cash advances on credit cards to pay other expenses?

- Are you getting calls from collection agencies?

- Have you received notices about utility disconnection?

Procrastination can be your worst enemy. Ignoring financial obligations now can lead to even greater problems later, like bankruptcy, loss of assets, and a bad credit record—all of which can affect the entire family. Instead of putting things off, communicate your problem as early as possible to the appropriate person or office.

Negotiating Payments

It's vital that you stay in regular contact with the people on the other end of your bills. As soon as possible, call doctors' offices, billing departments, hospital business offices, creditors, and lending institutions to explain the change in your family's situation. Most people are willing to work with you, but they won't know that you need help unless you tell them.

Some offices may ask you to "put it in writing." Most doctors or hospital social workers are happy to write a letter on your behalf, explaining why more time is needed to pay a bill or to appeal an insurance company decision.

Creditors can be lenient—arranging payment schedules, accepting partial payments, and so on—but they need to hear from you. Even if you can only make a portion of a payment, it will show an attempt to keep up your side of the obligation.

Parents who have gone through this process advise that you:

- Notify the appropriate offices as soon as you can.

- Keep in touch with your creditors.

- Remember to record the names and phone numbers of the people you are dealing with.

- Document the date, time, and results of your phone communications.

- Pay something—even a small amount—on each bill each month as a gesture of good faith.

Where to Get Help

Few people get through a catastrophic illness without needing help of some kind. You may find it difficult to put aside your pride and ask for help, but family and friends usually take genuine pleasure in helping out.

Make use of your case manager, particularly in deciphering bills and making sense of paperwork. Remember to update your case manager with new information and stay in frequent contact. Hospital business offices can be valuable too, by interpreting bills, estimating costs, or contacting your insurance company on your behalf.

Compare notes with other families who have dealt with catastrophic health issues. Their efforts may save you time and energy, and many parents appreciate the support of those who have experienced similar problems.

Short- and long-term financial assistance is also available from various sources, including private as well as government agencies. You may be surprised by the services available and the enthusiasm with which others embrace your needs.

Explore these private organizations:

- charitable foundations
- disease- or disability-related organizations
- civic or social welfare associations
- churches and community groups

Although not all provide financial aid, they may be able to direct you to other sources and services.

Government organizations can also assist in the medical and related care of your child. You don't need to be at poverty level to qualify; you may, in fact, be eligible for programs you never knew existed. Two such government programs that supplement the health insurance of a chronically or seriously ill child are Medicaid and Supplemental Security Income (SSI). As you research various avenues of assistance, ask your case manager about these and other options.

You can also take advantage of free financial advice and support offered by national agencies like the Consolidated Credit Counseling Service (CCCS). The CCCS provides certified financial counselors who help families examine their financial picture and overcome debt. They can negotiate with creditors on your behalf for lower payments, reduced interest rates, and forgiveness of late charges or penalties. You may choose to enroll in their formal debt management program, in which case you would send one payment per month to the CCCS office, which then prorates and disburses your payments to creditors.

The bottom line, though, is that even as you seek financial assistance, you will need to reduce your expenses.

Reducing Your Expenses

To ensure financial stability, you must learn to cut your expenses by making lifestyle changes. When you have a sick child, your priorities will shift. Going out to dinner a few times a month may no longer be in your budget; paying the electric bill has to be.

You may find it helpful to compare monthly costs against your income, then eliminate any expenses that aren't completely necessary. Other tips:

- Avoid impulse purchases.

- Eliminate "luxuries" such as cable television (TV).

- Switch to generic prescriptions whenever possible.

- Buy groceries in bulk and take advantage of coupons and store specials.

- Use cash instead of credit whenever possible.

By making a conscious decision to reduce spending, acting early, asking questions, and learning how to find and accept help, you can protect your family's future.

Chapter 64

Medicaid and Hill-Burton Free and Reduced-Cost Health Care

Overview of Medicaid

Good health is important to everyone. If you can't afford to pay for medical care right now, Medicaid can make it possible for you to get the care that you need so that you can get healthy—and stay healthy.

Medicaid is available only to certain low-income individuals and families who fit into an eligibility group that is recognized by federal and state law. Medicaid does not pay money to you; instead, it sends payments directly to your health care providers. Depending on your state's rules, you may also be asked to pay a small part of the cost (co-payment) for some medical services. Medicaid is a state administered program and each state sets its own guidelines regarding eligibility and services.

Many groups of people are covered by Medicaid. Even within these groups, though, certain requirements must be met. These may include your age, whether you are pregnant, disabled, blind, or aged; your income and resources (like bank accounts, real property, or other items that can be sold for cash); and whether you are a U.S. citizen or a lawfully admitted immigrant. The rules for counting your income and resources vary from state to state and from group to group. There are special rules for those who live in nursing homes and for disabled children living at home.

This chapter includes text from "Overview," April 2006, and "Medicaid at a Glance 2005," from the Centers for Medicare and Medicaid Services (CMS); and text from "Hill-Burton Free and Reduced Cost Health Care," and "Community Health Centers," October 2006, Health Resources and Services Administration (HRSA).

Your child may be eligible for coverage if he or she is a U.S. citizen or a lawfully admitted immigrant, even if you are not (however, there is a five-year limit that applies to lawful permanent residents). Eligibility for children is based on the child's status, not the parent's. Also, if someone else's child lives with you, the child may be eligible even if you are not because your income and resources will not count for the child.

In general, you should apply for Medicaid if your income is low and you match one of the descriptions of the eligibility groups. (Even if you are not sure whether you qualify, if you or someone in your family needs health care, you should apply for Medicaid and have a qualified caseworker in your state evaluate your situation.)

When does eligibility start?

Coverage may start retroactive to any or all of the three months prior to application, if the individual would have been eligible during the retroactive period. Coverage generally stops at the end of the month in which a person's circumstances change. Most states have additional state-only programs to provide medical assistance for specified poor persons who do not qualify for the Medicaid program. No federal funds are provided for state-only programs.

What is not covered?

Medicaid does not provide medical assistance for all poor persons. Even under the broadest provisions of the federal statute (except for emergency services for certain persons), the Medicaid program does not provide health care services, even for very poor persons, unless they are in one of the designated eligibility groups. Low income is only one test for Medicaid eligibility; assets and resources are also tested against established thresholds. Categorically needy persons who are eligible for Medicaid may or may not also receive cash assistance from the Temporary Assistance for Needy Families (TANF) program or from the Supplemental Security Income (SSI) program. Medically needy persons who would be categorically eligible except for income or assets may become eligible for Medicaid solely because of excessive medical expenses.

Medicaid At-a-Glance: Key Eligibility Groups

States are required to include certain types of individuals or eligibility groups under their Medicaid plans and they may include others.

States' eligibility groups will be considered one of the following: categorically needy, medically needy, or special groups. Following are brief descriptions of some of the key eligibility groups included under states' plans. These descriptions do not include all groups. Contact your state for more information on all Medicaid groups in your state.

Categorically Needy

Families who meet states' Aid to Families with Dependent Children (AFDC) eligibility requirements in effect on July 16, 1996 include:

- pregnant women and children under age six whose family income is at or below 133% of the federal poverty level;

- children ages 6–19 with family income up to 100% of the federal poverty level;

- caretakers (relatives or legal guardians who take care of children under age 18 [or 19 if still in high school]);

- supplemental security income (SSI) recipients (or, in certain states, aged, blind, and disabled people who meet requirements that are more restrictive than those of the SSI program); and

- individuals and couples who are living in medical institutions and who have monthly income up to 300% of the SSI income standard (federal benefit rate).

The medically needy have too much money (and in some cases resources, like savings) to be eligible as categorically needy. If a state has a medically needy program, it must include pregnant women through a 60-day postpartum period, children under age 18, certain newborns for one year, and certain protected blind persons.

States may also, at the state's option, provide Medicaid to:

- children under age 21, 20, 19, or under age 19 who are full-time students—if a state doesn't want to cover all of these children, it can limit eligibility to reasonable groups of these children;

- caretaker relatives (relatives or legal guardians who live with and take care of children);

- aged persons (age 65 and older);

- blind persons (blindness is determined using the SSI program standards or state standards);

- disabled persons (disability is determined using the SSI program standards or state standards); and

- persons who would be eligible if not enrolled in a health maintenance organization.

Special Groups

- Medicare beneficiaries: Medicaid pays Medicare premiums, deductibles, and coinsurance for qualified medicare beneficiaries (QMB)—individuals whose income is at or below 100% of the federal poverty level and whose resources are at or below twice the standard allowed under SSI. There are additional groups for whom Medicare related expenses are paid by Medicaid—Medicare beneficiaries with income greater than 100% but less than 135% of the federal poverty level.

- Qualified working disabled individuals: Medicaid can pay Medicare part A premiums for certain disabled individuals who lose Medicare coverage because of work. These individuals have income below 200% of the federal poverty level and resources that are no more than twice the standard allowed under SSI.

- States may also improve access to employment, training, and placement of people with disabilities who want to work through expanded Medicaid eligibility. Eligibility can be extended to working disabled people between ages 16 and 65 who have income and resources greater than that allowed under the SSI program. States can extend eligibility even more to include working individuals who become ineligible for the group described because their medical conditions improve. States may require such individuals to share in the cost of their medical care.

- There are two eligibility groups related to specific medical conditions that states may include under their Medicaid plans. One is a time-limited eligibility group for women who have breast or cervical cancer; the other is for people with tuberculosis (TB) who are uninsured. Women with breast or cervical cancer receive all plan services; TB patients receive only services related to the treatment of TB.

Long-Term Care

- All states provide community long-term care services for individuals who are Medicaid eligible and qualify for institutional care. Most states use eligibility requirements for such individuals that are more liberal than those normally used in the community.

Hill-Burton Free and Reduced Cost Health Care

In 1946, Congress passed a law that gave hospitals, nursing homes, and other health facilities grants and loans for construction and modernization. In return, they agreed to provide a reasonable volume of services to persons unable to pay and to make their services available to all persons residing in the facility's area. The program stopped providing funds in 1997, but about 300 health care facilities nationwide are still obligated to provide free or reduced-cost care.

Steps to Apply for Hill-Burton Free or Reduced-Cost Care

1. Find the Hill-Burton obligated facility nearest you from the list of Hill-Burton obligated facilities.

2. Go to the facility's admissions or business office and ask for a copy of the Hill-Burton Individual Notice. The Individual Notice will tell you what income level makes you eligible for free or reduced-cost care, what services might be covered, and exactly where in the facility to apply.

3. Go to the office listed in the Individual Notice and say you want to apply for Hill-Burton free or reduced-cost care. You may need to fill out a form.

4. Gather any other required documents (such as a pay stub to prove income eligibility) and take or send them to the obligated facility.

5. If you are asked to apply for Medicaid, Medicare, or some other financial assistance program, you must do so.

6. When you return the completed application, ask for a Determination of Eligibility. Check the Individual Notice to see how much time the facility has before it must tell you whether or not you will receive free or reduced-cost care.

More about Hill-Burton Free or Reduced-Cost Care

You are eligible to apply for Hill-Burton free care if your income is at or below the current U.S. Health and Human Services (HHS) poverty guidelines. You may be eligible for Hill-Burton reduced-cost care if your income is as much as two times (triple for nursing home care) the HHS poverty guidelines.

Care at a Hill-Burton obligated facility is not automatically free or reduced-cost. You must apply at the admissions or business office at the obligated facility and be found eligible to receive free or reduced-cost care. You may apply before or after you receive care—you may even apply after a bill has been sent to a collection agency. Some Hill-Burton facilities may use different eligibility standards and procedures.

Hill-Burton facilities must post a sign in their admissions and business offices and emergency room that says: "Notice—Medical care for those who cannot afford to pay." They must provide you with a written individual notice that lists the types of services eligible for Hill-Burton free or reduced-cost care, what income level qualifies for free or reduced-cost care, and how long the facility may take in determining an applicant's eligibility. Only facility costs are covered, not your private doctors' bills. Facilities may require you to provide documentation that verifies your eligibility, such as proof of income.

Hill-Burton facilities must provide a specific amount of free or reduced cost care each year, but can stop once they have given that amount. Obligated facilities publish an allocation plan in the local newspaper each year. The allocation plan includes the income criteria and the types of services it intends to provide at no cost or below cost. It also specifies the amount of free or reduced cost services it will provide for the year.

When you apply for Hill-Burton care, the obligated facility must provide you with a written statement that tells you what free or reduced-cost care services you will get or why you have been denied.

The facility may deny your request if:

- your income is more than the income specified in the allocation plan;

- the facility has given out its required amount of free care as specified in its allocation plan;

- the services you requested or received are not covered in the facility's allocation plan;

- the services you requested or received are to be paid by a governmental program such as Medicare or Medicaid or insurance;

- the facility asked you to apply for Medicare or Medicaid or other governmental program, and you did not; or

- you did not give the facility proof of your income, such as a pay stub.

You may file a complaint with the U.S. Department of Health and Human Services if you believe you have been unfairly denied Hill-Burton free or reduced-cost care. Your complaint must be in writing and can be a letter that simply states the facts and dates concerning the complaint. You may call your local legal aid services for help in filing a complaint. Send complaints to:

Director, Division of Facilities Compliance and Recovery
5600 Fishers Lane
Room 10–105
Rockville, MD 20857

Health Center Program

Health centers provide health care regardless of your ability to pay and even if you have no health insurance. Find the health center closest to you. Phone the health center for more information or to make an appointment.

Health Centers refer to all the diverse public and non-profit organizations and programs that receive federal funding under section 330 of the Public Health Service (PHS) Act, as amended by the Health Centers Consolidated Act of 1996 (P.L. 104–299) and the Safety Net Amendments of 2002. They include community health centers, migrant health centers, health care for the homeless health centers, and primary care public housing health centers.

Health centers are characterized by five essential elements that differentiate them from other providers:

1. They must be located in or serve a high need community, for example, medically underserved areas or medically underserved populations.

2. They must provide comprehensive primary care services as well as supportive services such as translation and transportation services that promote access to health care.

3. Their services must be available to all residents of their service areas, with fees adjusted upon patients' ability to pay.

4. They must be governed by a community board with a majority of members being health center patients.

5. They must meet other performance and accountability requirements regarding their administrative, clinical, and financial operations.

Additional Information

Bureau of Primary Health Care
5600 Fishers Lane, 17–89
Rockville, MD 20854
Phone: 301-594-4110
Website: http://bphc.hrsa.gov
E-mail: comments@hrsa.gov

Centers for Medicare and Medicaid (CMS)
7500 Security Blvd.
Baltimore, MD 21244-1850
Toll-Free: 877-267-2323
Toll Free TTY: 866-226-1819
Phone: 410-786-3000
TTY: 410-786-0727
Website: http://cms.hhs.gov

Chapter 65

Health Care Benefit Laws: Health Insurance Portability and Accountability Act (HIPAA) and Consolidated Omnibus Budget Reconciliation Act (COBRA)

Perhaps you have heard of HIPAA—the Health Insurance Portability and Accountability Act—during a visit to your doctor's office. The doctor's staff may have handed you a HIPAA privacy notice advising you of protections for your personal health information. But HIPAA covers a lot more than privacy.

For many people, health coverage is an important benefit of their jobs. At the time HIPAA was passed, a lot of people were afraid to switch jobs because they might lose the insurance coverage they needed for their families. This chapter will explain how HIPAA's protections make it easier to change employers without losing health coverage for your (and your family's) medical conditions.

HIPAA's umbrella of protection:

- limits the ability of a new employer plan to exclude coverage for preexisting conditions;

- provides additional opportunities to enroll in a group health plan if you lose other coverage or experience certain life events;

Excerpted from "Your Health Plan and HIPAA—Making the Law Work for You," U.S. Department of Labor, September 2006.

- prohibits discrimination against employees and their dependent family members based on any health factors they may have, including prior medical conditions, previous claims experience, and genetic information; and

- guarantees that certain individuals will have access to, and can renew, individual health insurance policies.

HIPAA is complemented by state laws that, while similar to HIPAA, may offer more generous protections. You may want to contact your state insurance commissioner's office to ask about the law where you live. A good place to start is the website of the National Association of Insurance Commissioners (contact information is listed at the end of this chapter).

This chapter focuses on HIPAA's coverage as it applies to private-sector group health plans only. State and local government employees should contact the Centers for Medicare and Medicaid Services at the U.S. Department of Health and Human Services about whether they have comparable protections.

Preexisting Conditions, Job Changes, and General Protections

One of the most important protections under HIPAA is that it helps those with preexisting conditions get health coverage. In the past, some employers' group health plans limited, or even denied, coverage if a new employee had such a condition before enrolling in the plan. Under HIPAA, that is not allowed. If the plan generally provides coverage but denies benefits to you because you had a condition before your coverage began, then HIPAA applies.

Under HIPAA, a plan is allowed to look back only six months for a condition that was present before the start of coverage in a group health plan. Specifically, the law says that a preexisting condition exclusion can be imposed on a condition only if medical advice, diagnosis, care, or treatment was recommended or received during the six months prior to your enrollment date in the plan. As an example, you may have had arthritis for many years before you came to your current job. If you did not have medical advice, diagnosis, care, or treatment—recommended or received—in the six months before you enrolled in the plan, then the prior condition cannot be subject to a preexisting condition exclusion. If you did receive medical advice, diagnosis, care, or treatment within the past six months, then the plan may impose a preexisting condition exclusion for that condition (arthritis). In addition, HIPAA prohibits plans from applying a preexisting condition exclusion to pregnancy, genetic information, and certain children.

If you have a preexisting condition that can be excluded from your plan coverage, then there is a limit to the preexisting condition exclusion period that can be applied. HIPAA limits the preexisting condition exclusion period for most people to 12 months (18 months if you enroll late), although some plans may have a shorter time period or none at all. In addition, some people with a history of prior health coverage will be able to reduce the exclusion period even further using creditable coverage. Remember, a preexisting condition exclusion relates only to benefits for your (and your family's) preexisting conditions. If you enroll, you will receive coverage for the plan's other benefits during that time.

Although HIPAA adds protections and makes it easier to switch jobs without fear of losing health coverage for a preexisting condition, the law has limitations. For instance, HIPAA does not:

- require that employers offer health coverage;

- guarantee that any conditions you now have (or have had in the past) are covered by your new employer's health plan; or

- prohibit an employer from imposing a preexisting condition exclusion period if you have been treated for a condition during the past six months (creditable coverage to reduce or eliminate the exclusion might apply).

Using Prior Health Coverage to Reduce the Length of any Preexisting Condition Exclusion

If you change jobs or begin new health coverage, and you or a dependent family member have a preexisting condition, you may be able to reduce or eliminate this maximum preexisting condition exclusion period if you can show creditable coverage.

- Most health coverage can be used as creditable coverage, including participation in a group health plan, COBRA continuation coverage, Medicare and Medicaid, as well as coverage through an individual health insurance policy.

- However, you should try to avoid a significant break in coverage (63 days) if you want to be able to count your previous coverage.

If you have a break shorter than 63 days, coverage you had before that break is creditable coverage and can be used to offset a preexisting condition exclusion period.

- Days spent in a waiting period for coverage cannot be used as credit. But, they also are not counted toward the significant break (63 days) you are trying to avoid.

How do I avoid a 63-day significant break in health coverage?

There are several ways:

- If a spouse has coverage in a health plan that allows family members to join, you may want to enroll.

- If your last coverage was in a group health plan, you may want to sign up for COBRA continuation coverage. While you (and your family members, if they were also part of your prior plan) will have to pay for this temporary coverage, COBRA can prevent or reduce a break in coverage.

- You can buy an individual health insurance policy if you think you would otherwise have a break of 63 days or more.

Some states have high-risk pools for people who cannot otherwise get health benefits. Your state insurance commissioner's office can tell you if such a pool exists where you live.

Note: HIPAA allows for short breaks when you are counting back to accumulate creditable coverage. For example, you have a break in coverage of 30 days, followed by more coverage, and then followed by another 30-day break. Both periods of health coverage can be counted as you add up the time spent in prior health plans. As long as any break is no longer than 63 days, you will not have a significant break. You can continue to count back coverage to accumulate 12 (or 18 for late enrollees) months of total coverage.

Getting and Using Certificates to Show Prior Health Plan Coverage

Your group health plan, HMO, or health insurance company should provide you with a certificate of creditable coverage, a document that shows your prior periods of coverage in a health plan:

- before you lose your present coverage—if you know you will be leaving a job, you can request a certificate, free of charge;

- after coverage ends—you should receive a certificate automatically upon loss of coverage, even if you are also eligible for COBRA continuation coverage (If you don't get one, or if you need a new one, you can request a certificate, free of charge, up to 24 months after prior coverage ends.);

- when COBRA coverage ends—you should also automatically receive a certificate when COBRA continuation coverage ends.

With your permission, another person can request a certificate of creditable coverage on your behalf.

What information will be on the certificate?

In addition to standard identification information, the certificate will include the dates on which your prior health plan coverage began and ended. The certificate also should have contact information so that old and new plans can be in touch if necessary. Finally, there should be information about your HIPAA rights.

When must my employer provide the certificate?

- If you're eligible for COBRA, the certificate must be provided no later than your COBRA election notice (generally 44 days after a qualifying event).

- For all other automatic certificates, generally you should receive it within a reasonable amount of time after coverage ends.

- The plan should provide a requested certificate as early as possible.

Also, be aware that health plans must issue certificates, even if they do not exclude coverage for preexisting conditions. While an employee may not need a certificate in a current job, she might if a future employer's plan has a preexisting condition exclusion.

What steps should I take if I didn't get a certificate or I lose it? How can I show that I had prior coverage?

If your new plan imposes a preexisting condition exclusion, your claims processing will go smoother if you don't delay. There is an alternate way to show that you had creditable coverage—you can present evidence of your prior health coverage to your new health plan. Evidence can include:

- pay stubs that reflect a deduction for health coverage premiums;

- copies of premium payments or other documents showing evidence of coverage;

- explanation of benefit forms; and

- verification by a doctor or your former health plan.

In addition to providing these documents, an individual may be asked to attest to the period of creditable coverage and cooperate with the new plan's reasonable efforts to verify creditable coverage. You should still get in touch with the plan's administrator to request a certificate for your records. The administrator's contact information is usually included in the plan brochure you received when you signed up for health coverage.

Are health plans required to issue certificates of creditable coverage to dependents?

Yes. A plan must make every reasonable effort to collect dependent information and then issue certificates to dependents if they are also covered. However, if an employee and a dependent have the same coverage, only one certificate reflecting both individuals may be issued.

What are the next steps after I get my certificate?

First, check it for accuracy. Does it reflect the amount of time you had prior coverage? Does it include the contact information of the issuer in case your old and new plans need to communicate? Is your personal data correct? Second, either give it to your new employer (after you make a copy for yourself) or file it away in a safe place.

Taking Advantage of Special Enrollment Opportunities

Special enrollment allows individuals who previously declined health coverage to enroll for coverage. Special enrollment rights arise regardless of a plan's open enrollment period. There are two types of special enrollment—upon loss of eligibility for other coverage and upon certain life events. Under the first, employees and dependents who decline coverage due to other health coverage and then lose eligibility or lose employer contributions have special enrollment rights. For instance, an employee turns down health benefits for herself and her family because the family already has coverage through her spouse's plan. Coverage under the spouse's plan ceases. That employee then can request enrollment in her own company's plan for herself and her dependents. Under the second, employees, spouses, and new dependents are permitted to special enroll because of marriage, birth, adoption, or placement for adoption. For both types, the employee must request enrollment within 30 days of the loss of coverage or life event triggering the special enrollment.

HIPAA's Protections from Discrimination

Under HIPAA, you and your family members cannot be denied eligibility or benefits based on certain health factors when enrolling in a health plan. In addition, you may not be charged more than similarly situated individuals based on any health factors.

The health factors are:

* health status;
* medical conditions, including physical and mental illnesses;
* claims experience;
* receipt of health care;
* medical history;
* genetic information;
* evidence of insurability; and
* disability.

Conditions arising from acts of domestic violence as well as participation in activities like motorcycling, snowmobiling, all-terrain vehicle riding, horseback riding, and skiing are considered evidence of insurability. Therefore, a plan cannot use them to deny you enrollment or charge you more for coverage. (However, benefit exclusions known as source of injury exclusions could affect your benefits.)

Can my plan require me to take a physical exam or fill out a health care questionnaire in order to enroll?

Yes, as long as it does not use individual health information to restrict enrollment or charge you more.

My group health plan required me to complete a detailed health history questionnaire and then subtracted "health points" for prior or current health conditions. To enroll in the plan, an employee had to score 70 out of 100 total points. I scored only 50 and was denied a chance to enroll. Can the plan do this?

No. In this case the plan used health information to exclude you from enrolling in the plan. This practice is discriminatory, and it is prohibited.

My group health plan booklet states that if a dependent is confined to a hospital or other medical facility at the time he is eligible to enroll in the plan, that person's eligibility is postponed until he is discharged. Is this permitted?

No. A group health plan may not delay an individual's eligibility, benefits, or effective date of coverage based on confinement to a hospital or medical facility at the time he becomes eligible. Additionally, a health plan may not increase that person's premium because he was in a hospital or medical facility.

How do you determine "similarly situated individuals"?

HIPAA states that plans may distinguish among employees only on bona fide employment-based classifications consistent with the employer's usual business practice. For example, part-time and full-time employees, employees working in different geographic locations, and employees with different dates of hire or lengths of service can be treated as different groups of similarly situated individuals.

A plan may draw a distinction between employees and their dependents. Plans can also make distinctions between beneficiaries themselves if the distinction is not based on a health factor. For example, a plan can distinguish between spouses and dependent children, or between dependent children based on their age or student status.

Can my health plan deny benefits for an injury based on how I got it?

Maybe. A plan can deny benefits based on an injury's source, unless an injury is the result of a medical condition or an act of domestic violence. Therefore, a plan cannot exclude coverage for self-inflicted wounds, including those resulting from attempted suicide, if they are otherwise covered by the plan and result from a medical condition (such as depression).

However, a plan may exclude coverage for injuries that do not result from a medical condition or from domestic violence. For example, a plan generally can exclude coverage for injuries in connection with an activity like bungee jumping. While the bungee jumper may have to pay for treatment for those injuries, her plan cannot exclude her from coverage for the plan's other benefits.

My group health plan says that dependents are generally eligible for coverage only until they reach age 25. However, this age restriction does not apply to disabled dependents, who seem to be covered past age 25. Does HIPAA permit a policy favoring disabled dependents?

Yes. A plan can treat an individual with an adverse health factor (such as a disability) more favorably by offering extended coverage.

HIPAA and Wellness Programs

More and more employers are establishing wellness programs that encourage employees to work out, stop smoking, and generally adopt healthier lifestyles. HIPAA encourages group health plans to adopt wellness programs but also includes protections for employees and dependents from impermissible discrimination based on a health factor.

Can a plan charge a lower premium for nonsmokers than it does for smokers?

For wellness programs that would allow the plan to offer a reward based on an individual's ability to meet a standard relevant to a health factor (such as smoking/nicotine addiction), Department of Labor guidance suggests that:

- the premium differential should be limited;

- the program should be designed to promote good health or prevent disease;

- individuals should have a chance to qualify for the nonsmoker's premium discount at least once a year;

- the program should accommodate those for whom it is unreasonably difficult to quit using tobacco (for example, due to nicotine addiction) by providing a reasonable alternative standard (such as a discount in return for attending educational classes or for trying a nicotine patch); and

- plan materials describing the wellness program should disclose the availability of a reasonable alternative standard to qualify for the lower premium.

Note: As of the print date of this information (September, 2006), these guidelines are merely suggested. Contact EBSA at 1-866-444-EBSA (3272) or http://askebsa.dol.gov for more information on the status of this guidance.

More Coverage under HIPAA's Umbrella

Flexibility in State Laws

State laws may complement HIPAA by allowing more protections than the federal law. However, these state laws only apply if your plan provides benefits through an insurance company or HMO (an insured plan). To determine if your plan offers insured coverage, consult your summary plan description (SPD) or contact your plan administrator.

The list below summarizes those areas where state laws can complement HIPAA's preexisting condition and special enrollment provisions:

- States may reduce the number of months a plan can look back to determine a preexisting condition. For instance, a state's law may have a look-back period of three months instead of the six in the federal law. The look-back period begins on the day you enroll in a plan.

- States may decrease the number of months a new employee or dependent may be subject to a preexisting condition exclusion period. For example, state laws may limit the exclusion period to six months rather than twelve. They may also reduce the maximum 18-month exclusion period for late enrollees.

- States may increase the number of days that constitute a significant break in coverage. For instance, instead of 63 days, a state may allow someone to have a break of 120 days between periods of health coverage.

- States may increase the number of days (30 under federal law) parents have to enroll newborns, adopted children, and children placed for adoption without a preexisting condition being excluded.

- Under federal law, certain preexisting conditions cannot be excluded from coverage (pregnancy; newborns, adopted children, and children placed for adoption within 30 days; and genetic information in the absence of a diagnosis). States may add to this list. For example, a state may add cancer, so that plans cannot exclude it from coverage, even if you received treatment during the six months before enrolling in a new plan.

- States may require additional circumstances that entitle you to special enrollment periods beyond those in the federal law.

- States may reduce an HMO's affiliation period prior to enrollment (similar to a group health plan's waiting period) to fewer than two months (three months for late enrollees).

In other areas of HIPAA, such as protections from discrimination, state laws may also supplement HIPAA's protections if the coverage is through an insured plan.

Using COBRA to Extend Your Health Coverage

COBRA is a law that can help if you lose your job or if your hours are reduced to the point where the employer no longer provides you with health coverage. COBRA can provide a temporary extension of your health coverage—as long as you and your family members, if eligible, belonged to the previous employer's health plan and generally the employer had 20 or more employees. Usually, you pay the entire cost of coverage (both your share and the employer's, plus a two percent administrative fee). As long as the prior plan exists, COBRA coverage lasts up to 18 months for most people, although it can continue as long as 36 months in some cases.

There are several ways to use COBRA in conjunction with HIPAA:

- COBRA coverage can help you avoid a significant break between periods of health plan coverage. For example, if you expect to have a six-month interruption between jobs and health plans, you can purchase COBRA coverage during that time.

- COBRA coverage can be counted as creditable coverage—as long as there is no significant break after your COBRA coverage ends. Creditable coverage can be used to offset any preexisting condition exclusion period you or a family member might have.

- COBRA continuation coverage can be used as a bridge to ensure that you remain covered during a waiting period or a preexisting condition exclusion period.

- If you have COBRA and become covered under other group health plan coverage that is not subject to a preexisting condition exclusion period, your COBRA coverage can be cut off.

- Once you are no longer eligible for COBRA coverage, you will get a special enrollment opportunity for any other coverage for which you are eligible. However, if you voluntarily stop COBRA coverage or stop paying your COBRA premiums, that will not trigger a special enrollment right based on loss of eligibility for coverage.

Tips

- Your COBRA plan and other available health coverage may be different in terms of their cost, scope of benefits, or level of coverage.

- COBRA can be used instead of, or in addition to, your new health coverage, if you are subject to a preexisting condition exclusion period. When deciding whether to choose COBRA, consider the length of your preexisting condition exclusion period, whether you are likely to need treatment for your preexisting condition during this time, and the costs of and benefits of COBRA coverage.

- Whether you elect COBRA coverage is an individual decision. Taking into account this information, you can make a decision that is best for the health of you and your family.

Changing from Group Health Coverage to an Individual Insurance Policy

HIPAA also protects those who are otherwise unable to get group health insurance. The law guarantees access to individual insurance policies and state high-risk pools for eligible individuals. They must meet all of the following criteria:

- had coverage for at least 18 months, most recently in a group health plan, without a significant break;

- lost group coverage but not because of fraud or nonpayment of premiums; and

- are not eligible for COBRA coverage; or if COBRA coverage was offered under federal or state law, elected and exhausted it.

The opportunity to buy an individual policy is the same whether a person quits a job, was fired, or was laid off. Ask your state insurance commissioner's office about high-risk pools and individual insurance policies.

Additional Information

National Association of Insurance Commissioners
Executive Headquarters
2301 McGee St., Suite 800
Kansas City, MO 64108-2662
Toll-Free: 866-470-6242
Phone: 816-842-3600
Fax: 816-783-8175
Website: http://www.naic.org

U.S. Department of Labor (DOL)
Frances Perkins Building
200 Constitution Ave., N.W.
Washington, DC 20210
Toll-Free: 866-444-3272
Toll-Free TTY: 877-889-5627
Phone: 202-693-8664
TTY: 202-501-3911
Website: http://www.dol.gov

DOL Employee Benefits Security Administration (EBSA)
Toll-Free: 866-444-3272
E-Fast Help Line: 866-463-3278
Website: http://www.dol.gov/ebsa

Call EBSA or visit http://askebsa.dol.gov if you believe you are the subject of discrimination due to a health factor.

Chapter 66

Eligibility for Medicare Coverage of Home Health Care

Who is eligible to get Medicare covered home health care and what services are covered?

If you have Medicare, you can use your home health care benefits if you meet all the following conditions.

1. Your doctor must decide that you need medical care at home, and make a plan for your care at home.

2. You must need at least one of the following: intermittent skilled nursing care, or physical therapy, or speech-language therapy, or continue to need occupational therapy.

3. The home health agency caring for you must be approved by the Medicare program (Medicare-certified).

4. You must be homebound, or normally unable to leave home unassisted. To be homebound means that leaving home takes considerable and taxing effort. A person may leave home for medical treatment or short, infrequent absences for non-medical reasons, such as a trip to the barber or to attend religious service. A need for adult day care does not keep you from getting home health care.

"Who is eligible to get Medicare covered home health care and what services are covered?" U.S. Department of Health and Human Services (HHS), September 2006.

If you meet all four of the listed conditions for home health care, Medicare will cover:

- Skilled nursing care on a part-time or intermittent basis which includes services and care that can only be performed safely and correctly by a licensed nurse (either a registered nurse or a licensed practical nurse).

- Home health aide services on a part-time or intermittent basis. A home health aide does not have a nursing license. The aide provides services that give additional support to the nurse. These services include help with personal care such as bathing, using the bathroom, or dressing. These types of services don't need the skills of a licensed nurse. Medicare doesn't cover home health aide services unless you are also getting skilled care such as nursing care or other therapy. The home health aide services must be part of the home care for your illness or injury.

- Physical therapy, speech-language therapy, and occupational therapy for as long as your doctor says you need it including:

  1. Physical therapy including exercise to regain movement and strength in a body area, and training on how to use special equipment or do daily activities, like how to get in and out of a wheelchair or bathtub.

  2. Speech-language therapy (pathology services) including exercise to regain and strengthen speech skills.

  3. Occupational therapy to help you become able to do usual daily activities by yourself. You might learn new ways to eat, put on clothes, comb your hair, and new ways to do other usual daily activities. You may continue to receive occupational therapy even if you no longer need other skilled care if ordered by your doctor.

- Medical social services to help you with social and emotional concerns related to your illness. This might include counseling or help in finding resources in your community.

- Certain medical supplies like wound dressings, but not prescription drugs or biologicals.

- Durable medical equipment such as a wheelchair or walker.

- FDA (Food and Drug Administration)-approved injectable osteoporosis drugs in certain circumstances.

Currently, Medicare does not cover (does not pay) for the following:

- 24-hour-a-day care at home

- meals delivered to your home

- homemaker services like shopping, cleaning, and laundry

- personal care given by home health aides like bathing, dressing, and using the bathroom when this is the only care you need

Most of the time, your doctor, a social worker, or a hospital discharge planner will help arrange for Medicare-covered home health. However, you have a say in which home health care agency you use.

Additional Information

Centers for Medicare and Medicaid Services (CMS)
7500 Security Blvd.
Baltimore, MD 21244-1850
Toll-Free: 877-267-2323
Toll Free TTY: 866-226-1819
Phone: 410-786-3000
TTY: 410-786-0727
Website: http://cms.hhs.gov

Chapter 67

Purchasing Health Insurance as an Individual

You should take shopping for health insurance as seriously as you might take shopping for a new home or car. When buying a house or a car, you look it over closely and then shop around to make sure your money will be well spent. The same should be true when you're purchasing a health insurance policy. If you don't shop carefully, you could end up spending a lot of money on a policy that won't cover you when you're sick and need it the most.

Here are some tips to help you make the most informed decision for you and your family when purchasing health insurance.

Before Leaving a Group Plan

If you are leaving a plan offered by your employer, be sure to check whether you are eligible for COBRA (Consolidated Omnibus Budget Reconciliation Act) continuation coverage. (COBRA is a law that requires employers to allow former workers and their dependents to remain in the company's health plan. This law applies to some, but not all, employers.) Although COBRA coverage may be expensive, you should think carefully before turning it down: If you don't opt for COBRA, you may find it impossible to purchase an individual plan, or you could face a preexisting condition exclusion.

Also, when deciding whether you want to go with COBRA coverage, you need to act quickly. You only have 60 days from the time you lose the plan offered by your employer to choose COBRA, and if you go without coverage for more than 63 days, you could face a preexisting condition exclusion. Your employer's human resources department may be able to help you weigh your options.

Special Rights

If your only option is to purchase coverage in the individual market, you may have special rights under a federal law called HIPAA (the Health Insurance Portability and Accountability Act) to buy certain kinds of health coverage and be free from preexisting condition exclusions. These rights may apply if you meet the following conditions:

- you've had at least 18 months of group coverage,

- you've used up any COBRA continuation coverage for which you are eligible, and

- you haven't had any gaps in coverage longer than 63 days.

Contact your state insurance department to find out what plans you have a right to enroll in under HIPAA.

Be a Smart Shopper

- To help you find the right policy for the right price, you may want to talk with a licensed health insurance agent (you can find agents listed in the phone book). Make sure to consult only reputable insurance companies and agents. Check with your state's insurance department to be sure that the company and the agent are licensed to do business in your state.

- Fraudulent health plans do exist, and frequently the coverage they offer sounds too good to be true. Call your state's health insurance department to make sure the plan you are considering is offered by a licensed carrier.

- Take the time to fully understand the policy you are thinking about buying. Pay close attention to the fine print.

- Make sure you feel comfortable with the company, the agent, and the product.

- Compare prices across several plans. The internet can be very helpful in this regard. And while not all information on the internet is reliable, you can use reputable websites such as eHealthInsurance.com. Remember that the premiums you see when you do a search are the lowest premiums someone might pay for the plans. Your premiums, which will depend on factors such as your age and your medical history, may be much higher.

- When you are considering purchasing a policy, find out if there's a limit on how much your premiums could go up if you decide to renew the policy. Be sure to ask both your agent and the state insurance department about such premium increases.

- Check on the cancellation terms of the policy. Unless it is temporary and only covers you for a certain amount of time (for example, six months), your policy should have guaranteed renewability and should not be cancelled if you get sick. However, your premiums may increase each year as your health changes and as you grow older.

- Make sure you are purchasing health insurance and not discount health benefits. These discount plans are not insurance policies—they provide only discounts on the cost of health care services or access to network providers for discounted fees.

- Catastrophic insurance policies have high deductibles ($5,000–$25,000) and low monthly premiums. If you are considering buying a policy like this, make sure you have enough money saved to pay for routine medical care. You will have to spend money out of your own pocket on such care until you reach your plan's deductible amount.

Other Important Tips

- When you decide to purchase a policy, always make the check payable to the actual insurance company and never to the agent.

- Be sure to get copies of all documents that influenced your decision to purchase the policy.

- Make sure to get all promises in writing.

Important Questions to Ask when Considering Buying a Policy

1. When will the policy become effective?

2. When can I expect to receive my insurance cards, and how do I use my benefits in the interim?

3. When is my premium payment due? How often can my premium rate change?

4. What medical services are covered and specifically excluded from coverage?

5. Are there any preexisting condition exclusions?

6. How much do I have to pay for medical services (deductible, co-payments, and coinsurance)? Do these out-of-pocket charges differ if I get treated by a participating or non-participating provider?

7. After I reach my deductible, how much will I have to pay each time I get treatment?

8. How long does it take the plan to pay claims?

9. Are there any limits on the number of annual or lifetime visits or any dollar limits for specific types of benefits (for example, physical therapy, chiropractic, mental health and substance abuse treatment)?

10. Is there an annual maximum out-of-pocket amount that I must pay? Once I've paid that amount, will the plan cover 100 percent of my claims?

11. Are my current doctors a part of the insurance plan's network? If not, will the insurance company cover any costs related to my treatment with out-of-network providers?

12. May I see a copy of the list of prescription drugs covered by the plan (called the drug formulary)? How often can this formulary change?

13. What are my rights and responsibilities under the terms of the policy?

14. What happens when you disagree with the insurance company? For example, what if they refuse to pay for a service?

15. If I change my mind about purchasing the policy, how long do I have to cancel and still be eligible for a refund? How do I obtain a refund?

Types of Health Insurance

Make sure that you understand all of your insurance product options. Here are some common types of health insurance:

- **Indemnity or fee-for-service:** With this kind of coverage, you can visit the provider of your choice. Your insurance company will pay a percentage of the billed amount, and you are responsible for the balance of the bill.

- **Health maintenance organization (HMO):** This is the most restrictive type of plan. All treatment must be coordinated through your primary care physician, and you will usually need a referral from your primary care physician to visit a specialist. An HMO is likely to have the lowest out-of-pocket costs.

- **Preferred provider organization (PPO):** In this kind of plan, you must visit a provider who participates in your insurance plan's network, but you do not have to see a primary care physician before you see a specialist. This kind of plan will likely have somewhat higher out-of-pocket costs than an HMO, but it also provides more options.

- **Point of service (POS):** This plan is a hybrid of an indemnity plan and an HMO plan. You can visit doctors in the plan's HMO-like network and pay very little. You can also visit doctors outside of the plan's network if you are willing to pay a greater portion of the bill. A POS plan provides a broader array of options than an HMO, but at a higher price.

An ombudsman or consumer health assistance program may be able to assist you with questions you have about shopping for private insurance. Not every state has an ombudsman program for private insurance.

Additional Information

Families USA
201 New York Ave. N.W., Suite 1100
Washington, DC 20005
Phone: 202-628-3030
Fax: 202-347-2417
Website: http://www.familiesusa.org
E-mail: info@familiesusa.org

Chapter 68

High Deductible Health Insurance and Health Savings Accounts

Health Savings Accounts

A health savings account (HSA) is an account that you can put money into to save for future medical expenses. There are certain advantages to putting money into these accounts, including favorable tax treatment. HSAs were signed into law by President Bush on December 8, 2003.

Who Can Have an HSA?

Any adult can contribute to an HSA if they:

- have coverage under an HSA-qualified high deductible health plan (HDHP);

- have no other first-dollar medical coverage (other types of insurance like specific injury insurance or accident, disability, dental care, vision care, or long-term care insurance are permitted);

- are not enrolled in Medicare; or

- cannot be claimed as a dependent on someone else's tax return.

This chapter includes text from "Health Savings Accounts," U.S. Department of the Treasury, November 2006; and excerpts from "Consumer-Directed Health Plans: Early Enrollee Experiences with Health Savings Accounts and Eligible Health Plans," U.S. Government Accountability Office (GAO), August 2006.

Contributions to your HSA can be made by you, your employer, or both. However, the total contributions are limited annually. If you make a contribution, you can deduct the contributions (even if you do not itemize deductions) when completing your federal income tax return.

Contributions to the account must stop once you are enrolled in Medicare. However, you can keep the money in your account and use it to pay for medical expenses tax-free.

High Deductible Health Plans (HDHP)

You must have coverage under an HSA-qualified high deductible health plan (HDHP) to open and contribute to an HSA. Generally, this is health insurance that does not cover first dollar medical expenses. Federal law requires that the health insurance deductible be at least:

- $1,100*—self-only coverage
- $2,200*—family coverage

In addition, annual out-of-pocket expenses under the plan (including deductibles, co-pays, and co-insurance) cannot exceed:

- $5,500*—self-only coverage
- $11,000*—family coverage

* 2007 amounts; adjusted annually for inflation

In general, the deductible must apply to all medical expenses (including prescriptions) covered by the plan. However, plans can pay for preventive care services on a first-dollar basis (with or without a co-pay). Preventive care can include routine pre-natal and well-child care, child and adult immunizations, annual physicals, mammograms, pap smears, etc.

Finding HDHP Coverage

Any company that sells health insurance coverage in your state may offer HDHP policies. Although Treasury cannot recommend any specific names of companies selling these policies, you should be able to find a qualified policy by contacting your current insurance company, an agent or broker licensed to sell health insurance in your state, or your state insurance department.

HSA Contributions

You can make a contribution to your HSA each year that you are eligible. For 2007, you can contribute up to $2,850 if you have self-only coverage and $5,650 if you have family coverage. Individuals age 55 and older can also make additional contributions. The maximum annual catch-up contribution is $800 in 2007, $900 in 2008, and $1,000 in 2009 and after.

Determining Your Contribution

Your eligibility to contribute to an HSA is determined by the effective date of your HDHP coverage. If you do not have HDHP coverage for the entire year, you will not be able to make the maximum contribution. All contributions (including catch-up contributions) must be pro-rated. Your annual contribution depends on the number of months of HDHP coverage you have during the year (count only the months where you have HDHP coverage on the first day of the month). For years after 2006 a special rule allows you to contribute the maximum amount for the year as long as you have coverage for December. However, if you fail to remain covered for 2008, the extra contribution above the pro-rated amount is included in income and subject to an additional 10 percent tax. Contributions can be made as late as April 15 of the following year.

Using Your HSA

You can use the money in the account to pay for any qualified medical expense permitted under federal tax law. This includes most medical care and services, and dental and vision care, and also includes over-the-counter drugs such as aspirin.

You can generally not use the money to pay for medical insurance premiums, except under specific circumstances, including:

- any health plan coverage while receiving federal or state unemployment benefits;

- COBRA continuation coverage after leaving employment with a company that offers health insurance coverage;

- qualified long-term care insurance;

- Medicare premiums and out-of-pocket expenses, including deductibles, co-pays, and coinsurance for:

    - part A (hospital and inpatient services),

527

- part B (physician and outpatient services),
- part C (Medicare HMO and PPO plans),
- part D (prescription drugs).

You can use the money in the account to pay for medical expenses of yourself, your spouse, or your dependent children. You can pay for expenses of your spouse and dependent children even if they are not covered by your HDHP.

Any amounts used for purposes other than to pay for qualified medical expenses are taxable as income and subject to an additional 10% tax penalty. Examples include:

- medical expenses that are not considered qualified medical expenses under federal tax law (for example, cosmetic surgery);
- other types of health insurance unless specifically described above;
- Medicare supplement insurance premiums; or
- expenses that are not medical- or health-related.

After you turn age 65, the 10% additional tax penalty no longer applies. If you become disabled and/or enroll in Medicare, the account can be used for other purposes without paying the additional 10% penalty.

Advantages of an HSA

Security: Your high deductible insurance and HSA protect you against high or unexpected medical bills.

Affordability: You should be able to lower your health insurance premiums by switching to health insurance coverage with a higher deductible.

Flexibility: You can use the funds in your account to pay for current medical expenses, including expenses that your insurance may not cover, or save the money in your account for future needs, such as:

- health insurance or medical expenses if unemployed;
- medical expenses after retirement (before Medicare);
- out-of-pocket expenses when covered by Medicare; or
- long-term care expenses and insurance.

Savings: You can save the money in your account for future medical expenses and grow your account through investment earnings.

Control: You make all the decisions about:

- how much money to put into the account;
- whether to save the account for future expenses or pay current medical expenses;
- which medical expenses to pay from the account;
- which company will hold the account;
- whether to invest any of the money in the account; and
- which investments to make.

Portability: Accounts are completely portable, meaning you can keep your HSA even if you:

- change jobs;
- change your medical coverage;
- become unemployed;
- move to another state; or
- change your marital status.

Ownership: Funds remain in the account from year to year, just like an IRA. There are no use it or lose it rules for an HSA.

Tax Savings: An HSA provides you triple tax savings:

1. Tax deductions when you contribute to your account.
2. Tax-free earnings through investment.
3. Tax-free withdrawals for qualified medical expenses.

What Happens to My HSA When I Die?

If your spouse becomes the owner of the account, your spouse can use it as if it were their own HSA. If you are not married, the account will no longer be treated as an HSA upon your death. The account will pass to your beneficiary or become part of your estate (and be subject to any applicable taxes).

Opening Your Health Savings Account

Banks, credit unions, insurance companies, and other financial institutions are permitted to be trustees or custodians of these accounts. Other financial institutions that handle individual retirement accounts (IRA) or Archer medical savings accounts (MSA) are also automatically qualified to establish HSA.

Early Enrollee Experience with Health Savings Accounts and Eligible Health Plans

The financial features of HSA-eligible plans differ from those of traditional plans, but both plan types cover similar health care services. HSA-eligible plans had lower premiums, higher deductibles, and higher out-of-pocket spending limits than traditional plans in 2005. It was estimated that HSA-eligible plan enrollees would incur higher annual costs than preferred provider organization (PPO) plan enrollees for extensive use of health care, but would incur lower annual costs than PPO enrollees for low to moderate use of health care.

Other findings about HSA plans include:

- HSA-eligible plan enrollees generally had higher incomes than comparison groups.

- Employer groups indicated that the average age of HSA-eligible plan enrollees, excluding retirees, was 2–6 years lower than that of other groups of enrollees.

- Just over half of HSA-eligible plan enrollees and about two-thirds of employers contributed to HSAs and account holders used HSA funds to pay for medical care and to accumulate savings.

- HSA-eligible plan enrollees who participated in focus groups at the three employers reviewed, generally reported positive experiences with their plan, but most would not recommend these plans to all consumers.

Concluding Observations

When individuals are given a choice between HSA-eligible and traditional plans—as in the individual market and with employers offering multiple health plans—HSA-eligible plans may attract healthier individuals who use less health care or, as we found, higher-income individuals with the means to pay higher deductibles and the desire to accrue tax-free savings.

Few of the HSA-eligible plan enrollees who participated in the focus groups researched cost before obtaining health care services. According to proponents, an increase in such health care consumerism is central to cost reductions that may occur under the plans.

HSA-eligible plans may not be appropriate for everyone and satisfaction may be lower when employees are not given a choice or when employer contributions to premiums or accounts do not sufficiently offset the greater costs faced by the enrollees.

Additional Information

U.S. Department of the Treasury
Toll-Free for Individuals: 800-829-1040
Toll-Free for Businesses: 800-829-4933
Website: http://www.treas.gov

Chapter 69

Medical Discount Plans and Cards—Service or Scam?

With health care costs increasing so rapidly, there is an ever-increasing demand for ways in which Americans can access medical treatment services less expensively. To help meet this demand, a wide variety of discount cards for health care and related products and services are currently being marketed to American health care consumers.

Legitimate health care discount card plans are not the same thing as insurance coverage, but they do offer consumers reduced costs on certain health care products and services when they are purchased through designated quality providers. Many mainstream health insurance plans offer valid discount cards for certain non-covered services, such as prescription drugs, dental or vision care. Medicare also has its authorized prescription drug discount cards for seniors, and many legitimate health care assistance programs also include discount cards for participants.

In addition to discount cards that are designed to accompany traditional private insurance coverage or government assistance programs to provide price reductions on non-covered services, there is a growing number of medical discount plans that are being marketed to people without any insurance coverage to help them pay for routine health care expenses, like doctor visits. Many of these plans are

This chapter includes: "Medical Discount Plans—Red Flags for Consumers and Health Insurance Producers," © 2007 National Association of Health Underwriters. Reprinted with permission. And, text from "Medical Discount Plans: They're Not Health Insurance," Federal Trade Commission (FTC), October 2005.

marketed as nothing more than a discount card, and utilize a valid network of providers and negotiate true discounted service rates for their customers. Unfortunately, there are also many discount plans in the marketplace that have been found to be either fraudulent, misleading, or not really a good value for consumers.

The National Association of Health Underwriters (NAHU), a trade association made up of approximately 20,000 employee benefit specialist and licensed health insurance producers, has developed this list of "red flags" for consumers and producers alike to use when performing their due diligence checks of the various medical discount plans. This list is designed to help evaluate both whether or not the plan is legitimate, and also if it is actually a good value for the consumer.

Watch Out For

- Discount plans that are presented to you through unsolicited phone calls, faxes, or e-mail

- High administrative fees, hidden fees, or a fee each time you access your benefits

- Plans that claim to provide discounts with an extraordinary number of providers, for example, "discounts with 50 percent of all U.S. doctors," or "over 250,000 providers participate in our network"

- Plans that offer to give discounts on excessive types of services, such as pet care, concierge services, legal services, vitamins, helicopter service, etc.

- Special "limited time" discounts if you sign up immediately

- Plans that require advance notice of any utilization of the discount, for example, seven days notice prior to a doctor visit, or 30 days notice prior to hospitalization

- Discounts that are only available on certain drugs or products, for example, if the discount only works for certain name-brand drugs, what you need might not be covered or the generic version might be cheaper even without discount

- No insurance license required to sell the product

- Language that is intended to discourage the buyer from purchasing private health insurance and signing up for the discount plan instead, for example, "most individual health insurance plans do not cover X, Y, or Z—with our discount plan, you can save thousands on those services"

- Discount advertised as "up to" a specified percentage

- The use of general terms like "affordable coverage," or insurance terms like "no preexisting condition requirements," "guaranteed issue," and "deductible" that are designed to make the product sound like insurance coverage, but really it is not insurance

- No clearly displayed list of prices, fees, and rules for usage

- Non-refundable fees for participation

- Plans that ask for detailed medical information or unnecessary personal financial information. (If they are not insuring you, but simply providing a discount, then the plan has no need for this data to assess risk. So what are they doing with this personal information?)

- Plans that claim affiliation with associations or entities that sound official, but really might not be, for example, "we are affiliated with an Alliance of Healthcare Providers"

- Plans that ask you to "confirm" credit card information or bank account numbers in unsolicited phone calls, faxes, or e-mails

- Plans that quote discounts in a variety of ways, making price comparisons difficult

- Plans that ask for credit card or bank account numbers before even supplying enrollment information

- Plans that offer you certain services for free, such as "call to see if you are eligible for our free prescription drug offer"

- Plan solicitations with hard-to-locate contact information and a hard-to-locate business address (Legitimate programs and insurers will readily display the location of their headquarters and how to contact them.)

- Plans that are not affiliated with a licensed health insurance carrier or offered by a legitimate known business

Medical Discount Plans: They're Not Health Insurance

Medical discount plans can be useful for some consumers looking to save money on health care. But they are not the same as health insurance. Medical discount plans do not pay any of your health care costs; instead, they require you to pay a fee for a list of health care providers and sellers of health-related products who are willing to offer discounts to members of the plan.

According to the Federal Trade Commission (FTC), the nation's consumer protection agency, some medical discount plans claim to provide big discounts from hundreds of providers for a wide range of services, from doctor visits and dental exams to hospital stays and prescription drugs. But many plans fail to make good on those claims. The FTC and many states have found that although some medical discount plans provide legitimate discounts that benefit their members, many take consumers' money and offer very little in return.

Check It Out

When considering your options, know what you are getting—medical insurance or a medical discount plan. If you are not sure, check with your state insurance commissioner to see if the company offering the plan is registered to sell insurance in your state. If the company is not registered to sell health insurance and you want to buy health insurance, consider shopping elsewhere. Remember that if you buy a health insurance plan, it generally covers a broad array of services, and pays you or your health care provider for your medical bills. If you buy a medical discount plan, you generally are paying for a list of providers and sellers who may be willing to offer discounts on some of their services, products, or procedures. If you're interested in buying a medical discount plan, you should investigate the details before you pay any money.

- Look for a telephone number or website of the company you are considering doing business with so you can get more information.

- Before you pay any money, ask the company for a list of providers who participate in its plan. Call the providers and ask about the services and discounts they are offering.

- If the plan does not provide a list of providers promptly, consider taking your business elsewhere.

- Investigate the details of any plan carefully. Read the fine print, paying special attention to the refund policy. If a plan does not readily provide information and answers before you buy, it is not likely to be responsive once they have your money.

- If your usual medical or dental providers do not participate, see whether other doctors in your area accept the plan and will give you the discount the plan promoter promised. Some legitimate plans offer a get acquainted or initial consultation visit so you can meet a practitioner who participates in the plan before you commit to becoming a member.

- Do the math. Try to calculate what your total payment for a discount plan will be for a given amount of time. You could be responsible for paying a substantial amount up front, in addition to monthly fees and other costs. The costs of the program may total more than the savings you anticipate. Indeed, you may be able to negotiate a similar discount directly with your provider, without having to join a medical discount program.

- Call your local consumer protection office, state Attorney General, or Better Business Bureau to find out whether there are complaints about the business offering the discount plan.

Additional Information

Federal Trade Commission
Consumer Response Center
600 Pennsylvania Ave., N.W.
Washington, DC 20580
Toll-Free: 877-FTC-HELP (877-382-4357)
Toll-Free TDD/TTY: 866-653-4261
Website: http://www.ftc.gov

Chapter 70

Low-Cost or Free Health Insurance for Children

Insure Kids Now! is a national campaign to link the nation's uninsured children—from birth to age 18—to free and low-cost health insurance. Many families simply don't know their children are eligible.

I need health insurance for my children. What are my options?

When you call the free and confidential hotline 877-543-7669, you will be directly connected to your state's program that provides either free or low-cost health insurance for children. The states have different eligibility rules, but in most states, uninsured children 18 years old and younger whose families earn up to $34,100 a year (for a family of four) are eligible. When you call, you will speak with someone from the children's health insurance program in your state. They can send you an application and help you apply.

Is there a limit on the amount of time my child can remain enrolled?

Your child can stay on the program as long as he or she qualifies. Although there is no limit on the amount of time your child can remain

---

"Insure Kids Now! Questions and Answers," an undated document produced by Health Resources and Services Administration (HRSA); available online at http://www.insurekidsnow.gov/questions.htm. Accessed March 15, 2007.

on the program, you will need to renew their coverage periodically, generally every 6–12 months. As long as your children continue to meet the eligibility criteria established by your state, they can remain on the program.

What services does the insurance cover?

For little or no cost, this insurance pays for doctor visits, prescription medicines, hospitalizations, and much more. Most states also cover the cost of dental care, eye care, and medical equipment.

Is this program new?

In 1997 Congress passed legislation that allows states to provide health insurance to more children in working families. These programs build on the Medicaid program that started covering children and adults in the mid-1960s.

Why is health insurance for children and teens important?

Children who have health insurance generally have better health throughout their childhood and into their teens. They are more likely to:

- receive needed shots that prevent disease;
- get treatment for recurring illnesses such as ear infections and asthma;
- get preventative care to keep them well;
- get sick less often; and
- get the treatment they need when they are sick.

How does having health insurance affect my child's ability to learn?

Children who have health insurance have a better chance of being healthy. Having health insurance will allow you to give them the medical care necessary for them to stay healthy and focus on their studies. Children with health insurance are less likely to miss school because they are sick. By helping them go to school every day ready to learn, you can help boost your child's performance in school today and in the future.

How will having insurance help my child stay healthy?

You will be able to pick a doctor for your child and see that doctor every time your child gets sick, without having to worry about how you are going to pay for it. Your child can get immunizations and well-child visits required to attend school and play sports. If your child gets sick, you can get prescription medicines to help him or her get better fast. Finally, you will not have to sit for hours in the emergency room when your child has an illness that could be easily treated in your doctor's office.

How much does it cost?

Health insurance provided to children through these programs is free or low-cost. The costs are different depending on the state and your family's income, but when there are charges, they are minimal.

Who pays for these health insurance programs?

Your tax dollars fund these state and federally sponsored programs. The state and federal governments want to help working families protect their children's health and future. In some states you may need to pay a premium or co-payment for your children's health insurance.

I have teenagers. Are they eligible, too?

Yes, in most states, children from birth until their nineteenth birthday can receive free or low-cost health insurance. Remember each state has its own program.

I have a job. Can my children still qualify?

The majority of children covered by this health insurance come from working families. Many working families who cannot afford or whose children are not covered by employer-sponsored health insurance or other private health insurance, may be eligible.

Who can apply for health insurance for my child?

In addition to parents, in many states, grandparents and legal guardians can also enroll children in their care for free or low-cost health insurance.

What if my children are covered by Medicaid already?

If your children are currently on Medicaid, they already have comprehensive health insurance. If you are having trouble seeing a doctor or getting a needed service, please contact your caseworker or your state Medicaid program.

What if my state tells me that my children are eligible for Medicaid but I don't want to enroll them in Medicaid? Can I qualify for another insurance program?

Children eligible for Medicaid are not eligible to enroll in their state's children's health insurance program (CHIP). Medicaid provides comprehensive health benefits for children.

How do I apply?

In most states, you can complete a short application and send it through the mail.

Is it hard to apply?

Most states have made it very easy to apply for health insurance for your children, often the application is very short. In most states you can complete the application through the mail or over the phone without having to take time off of work. If you have trouble filling out the application, you can ask for help by calling 877-543-7669.

Additional Information

Insure Kids Now
Toll-Free: 877-543-7669
Website: http://www.insurekidsnow.gov

Chapter 71

High-Risk Health Insurance

What are high-risk pools?

High-risk pools are nonprofit associations that are created by states to provide health insurance for residents with preexisting health conditions. Generally, a board of directors oversees the high-risk pool and contracts with a health insurance company to administer benefits and pay enrollees' claims. Individuals enroll in the high-risk pool by purchasing insurance through the association. By law, premiums are capped: They are somewhat higher than premiums charged to healthy people, but they are not as high as premiums for unhealthy individuals on the open market. The high-risk pool is subsidized in order to keep the premiums within the state's cap. The difference between the money collected from premiums and the cost of enrollees' actual claims (plus administrative expenses) is called the high-risk pool's "loss." The amount of this loss is subsidized, often through assessments charged to insurers, and sometimes from other state or federal funds.

Who do high-risk pools help?

High-risk pools are a way to guarantee access to insurance coverage for a small but important segment of the population—people who are deemed uninsurable. Uninsurable people do not have coverage

Excerpted from "High-Risk Health Insurance Pools," © 2006 Families USA (www.familiesusa.org). Reprinted with permission.

through their employers and cannot get coverage in the individual market, either because insurance companies offer them only policies with prohibitively high premiums or because insurers simply refuse to sell them policies due to their poor health. Minnesota, which operates the oldest high-risk pool in the nation, insures about 6 percent of its individually insured population through its high-risk pool. A few other states that have been effective in reaching their uninsurable populations cover 2–3 percent of their states' individually insured populations through their high-risk pools.

In most states, high-risk pools provide coverage for middle class people who may be able to afford insurance but who are unhealthy and therefore cannot find insurers willing to sell them policies. In a few states (Colorado, Connecticut, Montana, New Mexico, Oregon, Washington, and Wisconsin), lower-income people receive additional premium subsidies to help them participate in the high-risk pools.

What alternatives do states use to guarantee access to individual insurance?

Under the federal Health Insurance Portability and Accountability Act (HIPAA), states must guarantee access to insurance for certain individuals who are leaving the group market. People who qualify for this federal guarantee are called "HIPAA-eligible," and they must meet the following criteria:

- they were previously insured for 18 months, the last day of which was through a group plan (usually a plan offered by an employer);

- they have used up any rights to continue their health coverage under the federal COBRA law (Consolidated Omnibus Budget Reconciliation Act of 1985) or under similar state laws;

- they are not eligible for Medicare or Medicaid; and

- they have maintained coverage without a gap of more than 63 days.

For people previously insured through individual policies or for people who were previously uninsured, there is no federal law that guarantees access to insurance.

Thirty-three states use high-risk pools to guarantee access either to all individuals or to HIPAA-eligible individuals. Other states meet federal HIPAA obligations or provide broader guarantees that insurance policies will be issued to all interested individuals by doing the following:

- requiring all insurers in the individual market to accept HIPAA-eligible applicants

- requiring all insurers in the individual market to sell policies to all applicants, regardless of their health (called guaranteed issuance)

- requiring one particular insurer (such as Blue Cross) to accept HIPAA-eligible individuals or to more generally provide an open enrollment period during which it will accept all individuals

- requiring one particular type of insurer (for example, all large insurers or all nonprofit insurers or HMOs that sell individual policies) to guarantee issuance to individuals at any time or during an open enrollment period

- allowing uninsurable individuals to participate in a public program by paying premiums on a sliding fee scale (Tennessee used this approach for several years but has since stopped)

To be effective, public policies that guarantee access to individual insurance must also address the cost of insurance for people with serious health conditions. In states with high-risk pools, capping premiums helps address this issue. Some states also use rate regulation to address costs, either by prohibiting price variation based on health status altogether or by setting limits on how much an insurer can vary premiums based on health status. Since high-risk pool premiums are based on the average costs of premiums for equivalent coverage in the individual market, regulating the rates of all individual insurers can help lower the premiums for high-risk pools.

How are high-risk pools financed?

States use several different mechanisms to subsidize the operating costs of their high-risk pools so that premiums will stay within the caps set by law. One challenge that states face is establishing a fair and broad-based funding system that will grow at the same rate as health expenditures. To do this, some states assess all insurance carriers and HMOs. Because this source of revenue is tied to health care costs, it grows along with health expenditures. However, this kind of assessment is not considered broad-based because it reaches only fully funded health insurance and does not cover the many employers that self-fund health care for their workers.

Large companies often use self-funded insurance. To indirectly reach those employers who self-fund their plans, some states include assessments on stop-loss insurers and reinsurance carriers based on the number of covered lives (that is, the number of people they cover), rather than based on a percentage of premiums collected. (Stop-loss insurance and reinsurance carriers do not collect as many premium dollars as carriers that provide comprehensive coverage because they are only at risk for high-cost claims.) Some states also assess third-party administrators—that is, companies that administer health benefits for an employer who self-funds health insurance. In some states, insurers receive a tax credit for the assessment that they pay, meaning that, in the end, public dollars actually pay for all or part of the high-risk pool subsidy.

Hospital or health care provider surcharges are another source of revenue used by some state high-risk pools. This is another source of broad-based funding that may indirectly spread financing among both self-funded and fully funded plans.

Lastly, a number of states use either a special funding source (such as a tobacco tax) or general appropriations to finance high-risk pools. However, these sources may not grow at the same rate as health inflation, so, over time, they may fall short of the amount needed to subsidize premiums.

In addition to state financing mechanisms, high-risk pools may receive federal grants. Federal grants can be used for the following purposes:

- as seed money to start a high-risk pool in a state that does not have one

- for losses a state incurs by operating a high-risk pool

- to provide additional consumer benefits, such as a premium subsidy for low-income enrollees, an overall reduction in premium costs, reduction or elimination of a waiting list for enrollment, reduction of the waiting period before preexisting conditions are covered, an increase in covered benefits, or establishment of a disease management program

The Centers for Medicare and Medicaid Services (CMS) administers the grant program and announced available funds on May 1, 2006. Information is posted on its website. Bear in mind that while you may want to encourage states to take advantage of these grants now, there is no guarantee that federal grant money will be available to your state in future years.

Fully-Funded Health Coverage Versus Self-Funded Health Coverage

Employers that fully fund health insurance contract with a health insurance company to handle health benefits for their workers. These employers pay premiums to an insurer, and in exchange, the insurer pays health care claims and bears the risk for claims. In contrast, employers who self-fund health insurance directly pay health care claims for their employees, although they may pay a third party administrator to administer health benefits and/or pay a stop-loss insurer to cover a portion of claims that exceed a certain dollar threshold.

States regulate fully-funded insurance and can impose taxes or assessments on such health insurers. However, under the federal Employee Retirement Income Security Act (ERISA), states cannot regulate or directly assess employers' self-funded health benefit programs. Self-funded plans cover about 50 percent of people with employer-based coverage and comprise an even higher percentage of the insurance market in some states. So, without a broad base of assessment funding that reaches this portion of the market, the burden of paying for high-risk pool losses falls only on the fully-funded insurance plans, which are primarily used by small businesses and individuals.

How much do premiums typically cost?

Various state laws set premium caps at different levels. Laws in California, Minnesota, and Oregon cap premiums at 125 percent of average premium rates for comparable plans sold to individuals who are not in the high-risk pool. In practice, some of these states have kept premiums even lower than their state laws require. For example, in 2006, high-risk pool premiums in Oregon are set at 111 percent of the average premium rates for individuals not in the high-risk pool. In some years, Oregon's high-risk pool premiums have been as low as 102 percent of average premiums. Further, for people previously covered through an employer (HIPAA-eligibles), Oregon's high-risk pool premiums are just 100 percent of average premiums.

Most states cap their high-risk pool premiums at no more than 150 percent of average premiums. To be eligible for federal grants, high-risk pools must set premium caps below 200 percent of average premium costs. Since high-risk pool premium costs are based on average premium costs for health insurance policies sold to individuals in a state, states with strong rate regulation will also have lower premium charges in their high-risk pools.

To get an idea of what premiums cost in various states, we looked at premiums that would be charged to a 50-year-old woman purchasing a plan with a $500 deductible (the lowest deductible charged) in the states that have enrolled at least 10,000 people in their high-risk pools. For example, in 2006, a 50-year-old woman seeking a policy with a $500 deductible would pay monthly premiums of $448 in Minnesota (where premiums are set at between 101–125 percent of the average rate for comparable policies), $506 in Oregon (where premiums are capped at 125 percent), $737 in Texas (where premiums are capped at 200 percent), and $865 in Illinois (where premiums are set at between 125–150 percent). Differences between states may reflect differences in benefit levels among state high-risk pools, as well as differences in overall insurance costs that result both from market forces and from rate regulation and enforcement. In some of these states, low-income people receive additional premium subsidies.

What are typical deductibles?

High-risk pools generally offer policies with a range of deductibles. Typically, the lowest deductible is $500, meaning that consumers pay $500 for medical costs before the insurance policy begins to cover their claims. In high-risk pools around the country, deductibles range from as low as $500 to as high as $10,000 a year. Deductibles often deter low-income people from obtaining routine care—they rely on their insurance only for serious health problems when they require hospital care. Some consumers may choose to establish a tax-free Health Savings Account (HAS) in hopes of saving enough money to pay for the deductible, co-insurance, and other medical expenses not covered by their plan. However, not surprisingly, few consumers with high-risk health conditions possess the disposable income needed to establish such a savings account. Nationally, about 90 percent of high-deductible plan enrollees do not have money saved in a Health Savings Account.

Have states done anything to make high-risk pools affordable to low-income consumers?

As noted earlier, a few states (Colorado, Connecticut, Montana, New Mexico, Oregon, Washington, and Wisconsin) provide additional premium subsidies to lower-income people who participate in high-risk pools. These states use a variety of mechanisms to subsidize low-income enrollees.

Oregon: Subsidies are administered through a separate program called Family Health Insurance Assistance, which helps low-income Oregon residents pay for private insurance premiums if they are former Medicaid beneficiaries or have been uninsured for at least six months. Families with incomes below 185 percent of poverty are eligible. High-risk pool policies are among the policies for which they can use their subsidies. Subsidies pay between 50 and 95 percent of premium costs, depending on the person's income, but they cannot be used to cover deductibles or co-insurance.

About 60 percent of the enrollees in Oregon's high-risk pool earn less than $35,000 per year. This group includes, for example, people who work for small businesses that do not offer coverage, people with disabilities, people near retirement age, and divorced women who formerly were covered through their spouses. Currently, about 4,600 of the high-risk pool's 15,000 enrollees receive subsidies.

Oregon's Family Health Insurance Assistance Program is funded in part through a Medicaid waiver, so it uses both state and federal dollars.

In other states, reductions in premium costs for low-income people are offered directly through the high-risk pool.

Colorado: Effective July 2006, premium discounts of 50 percent are provided to people with annual incomes of less than $40,000, and discounts of 40 percent are provided to people with annual incomes between $40,000 and $50,000. The high-risk pool is funded through assessments on insurers and through the unclaimed property trust fund.

Connecticut: One particular plan within the high-risk pool—the Special Health Care Plan—provides lower premiums to low-income members and also offers lower deductibles. Providers in that plan are reimbursed at lower rates than in other plans: They agree to accept 75 percent of Medicare payment rates. The lower premiums are funded by a combination of provider discounts and the assessments on insurers that fund the high-risk pool generally.

Montana: Federal grant money and a state appropriation have subsidized premiums for low-income people by 45 percent. However, enrollment in the premium assistance program is capped due to funding limitations, so the program is sometimes closed to new members.

New Mexico: Premium reductions based on income are provided by the high-risk pool itself. Premiums are reduced by 75 percent for people with incomes below 200 percent of poverty and by 50 percent for people with incomes between 200 and 400 percent of poverty. Assessments and premiums fund the high-risk pool.

Washington: State law requires that enrollees be charged a minimum of 110 percent of the average rate for individual commercial coverage. However, enrollees ages 50–64 with incomes below 300 percent of poverty receive lower rates than other enrollees. (Other enrollees can be charged up to 150 percent of average rates, depending on the policy they purchase.) State funds help to support premium discounts.

Wisconsin: Households with incomes below $25,000 pay 133 percent of standard premium rates, and households with incomes below $10,000 pay 100 percent of standard premium rates.

Assessments on health insurers and provider payment adjustments fund the subsidy.

What questions should consumers ask when they are considering joining a high-risk pool?

- **Am I able to get insurance on the individual market, through an employer, or through a public program such as Medicaid?** If not, high-risk pools may provide an opportunity to purchase coverage. The website of the National Association of State Comprehensive Health Insurance Plans, www.naschip.org, provides contact information for state high-risk pools.

- **What are the residency requirements for coverage through a high-risk pool in my state?** Some state pools will allow people to join immediately upon moving into the state if they intend to stay. Other pools require people to be residents for a period of time before joining. Even in states that require a period of residency for most high-risk pool enrollees, under federal rules, HIPAA-eligibles may be immediately eligible once they demonstrate that they are residents.

- **What do I need to do to prove my eligibility for the high-risk pool?** Am I automatically eligible if I have a certain medical condition, or do I need to apply for individual insurance and show that I have been denied coverage or charged a high rate based on my condition?

- **Is there a waiting period for coverage of preexisting conditions?** If so, what care can I get now, and what treatments will be subject to the waiting period? Most state high-risk pools immediately provide some health coverage to new enrollees, but for new enrollees who were previously uninsured for more than 63 days, high-risk pools commonly exclude coverage of a preexisting health condition for a period of time. These waiting periods for coverage of preexisting conditions are designed to encourage people to sign up for coverage and pay premiums before an illness strikes. It is quite common for high-risk pools to use a six-month waiting period for coverage of a preexisting condition, but some states require waits of as much as 12 months, and other states have shorter waits of three months or no wait at all. States often reduce or eliminate waiting periods for people who had previous health insurance coverage, depending on the length of time they had creditable coverage. (Creditable coverage includes coverage under a group health plan, an individual health insurance policy, COBRA, Medicaid, Medicare, CHAMPUS [Civilian Health and Medical Program of the Uniformed Services], the Indian Health Service, a state high-risk pool, the Federal Employees Health Benefits Program [FEHBP], the Peace Corps Act, or a public health plan, as long as there was not a break in coverage of more than 63 days.)

- **What will happen if I move?** Be aware that if you are covered by a high-risk pool in one state and then move to another state, you may not automatically have the right to enter the new state's high-risk pool. Some state high-risk pools provide reciprocity and guarantee coverage to people who had coverage from a high-risk pool in another state without imposing new waiting periods for coverage of preexisting conditions, while other state high-risk pools do not provide these guarantees.

- **What plan in the high-risk pool is best for me,** considering the deductibles, my savings, and the costs that I can and cannot afford to pay out-of-pocket?

Chapter 72

Communicating Effectively with Insurance Company Personnel

The following excerpt from the take-home guide of the Communicating Effectively with Healthcare Professionals workshop developed by the National Family Caregivers Association with assistance from the National Alliance for Caregiving provides you with practical information for interacting with insurance company personnel, one of the categories of healthcare professionals we all encounter as family caregivers.

Talking with Insurance Personnel

Before you pick up the phone to speak to a claims representative, you need to gather some information. Be prepared to give the person you talk with:

- your name and your relationship to your care recipient;
- the care recipient's birth date;
- the insurance policy number;
- the name and address of the organization that sent the bill;
- the total amount of the bill;
- the diagnosis code on the bill; and

- the Explanation of Benefits (if you are questioning an insurance payment).

When you start the conversation, ask for the name and telephone extension of the individual who is handling your phone call. If you need to call again, you will want to try to speak with the same person.

Keep in mind that billing office personnel and insurance claims representatives are there to serve you. You are the customer. Be assertive. You should expect to:

- be treated with respect and consideration;

- have your concerns clarified;

- have your questions answered with accurate and timely information; and

- be informed of any steps you need to take to move things along.

Communication Tips

Here are some tips for communicating effectively with people who work in the health insurance system.

Be prepared: Before you call an insurance company, write down a list of the questions you have so you can handle everything in one phone call.

Take good notes: Take notes about your phone conversations, including the date of the call and the information you were given as well as with whom you spoke.

Be clear and concise: State clearly and briefly what your question or concern is, what you need, and what you expect.

Be patient: Health insurance issues are frustrating and time-consuming. Accept that you will spend a certain amount of time navigating through automated telephone menus, waiting on hold, and waiting for the claims process to be completed.

Be considerate: Most insurance personnel want to do their jobs well, and they have a tough job to do. Thank them when they have been helpful. Speak to them kindly. Assume that they are trying to help you, not that they are "the enemy."

Chapter 73

Filing a Claim for Your Health or Disability Benefits

If you participate in a health plan or a plan that provides disability benefits, you will want to know how to file a claim for your benefits. The steps outlined in this chapter describe some of your plan's obligations and briefly explain the procedures and timelines for filing a health or disability benefits claim.

Before you file, however, be aware of the Employee Income Retirement Security Act of 1974 (ERISA), a law that protects your health and disability benefits and sets standards for those who administer your plan. Among other things, the law and rules issued by the Department of Labor include requirements for the processing of benefit claims, the timeline for a decision when you file a claim, and your rights when a claim is denied.

You should know that ERISA does not cover some employee benefit plans (such as those sponsored by government entities and most churches). If, however, you are one of the millions of participants and beneficiaries who depend on health or disability benefits from a private-sector employment-based plan, take a few minutes and read on to learn more.

Reviewing the Summary Plan Description

A key document related to your plan is the summary plan description (SPD). The SPD provides a detailed overview of the plan—how

U.S. Department of Labor, September 2006.

it works, what benefits it provides, and how to file a claim for benefits. It also describes your rights as well as your responsibilities under ERISA and your plan. For some single-employer collectively bargained plans, you should also check the collective bargaining agreement's claim filing, grievance, and appeal procedures as they may apply to claims for health and disability benefits.

Before you apply for health or disability benefits, review the SPD to make sure you meet the plan's requirements and understand the procedures for filing a claim. Sometimes claims procedures are contained in a separate booklet that is handed out with your SPD. If you do not have a copy of your plan's SPD or claims procedures, make a written request for one or both to your plan's administrator. Your plan administrator is required to provide you with a copy.

Filing a Claim

An important first step is to check your SPD to make sure you meet your plan's requirements to receive benefits. Your plan might say, for example, that a waiting period must pass before you can enroll and receive benefits or that a dependent is not covered after a certain age. Also, be aware of what your plan requires to file a claim. The SPD or claims procedure booklet must include information on where to file, what to file, and whom to contact if you have questions about your plan, such as the process for providing a required pre-approval for health benefits. Plans cannot charge any filing fees or costs for filing claims and appeals.

If, for any reason, that information is not in the SPD or claims procedure booklet, write your plan administrator, your employer's human resource department (or the office that normally handles claims), or your employer to notify them that you have a claim. Keep a copy of the letter for your records. You may also want to send the letter by certified mail with return receipt requested, so you will have a record that the letter was received and by whom.

If it is not you, but an authorized representative who is filing the claim, that person should refer to the SPD and follow your plan's claims procedure. Your plan may require you to complete a form to name the representative. If it is an emergency situation, the treating physician can automatically become your authorized representative without you having to complete a form.

Remember: When a claim is filed, be sure to keep a copy for your records.

Types of Claims

All health and disability benefit claims must be decided within a specific time limit, depending on the type of claim filed.

Group health claims are divided into three types: *urgent care, pre-service and post-service claims*, with the type of claim determining how quickly a decision must be made. The plan must decide what type of claim it is except when a physician determines that the urgent care is needed.

Urgent care claims are a special kind of pre-service claim that requires a quicker decision because your health would be threatened if the plan took the normal time permitted to decide a pre-service claim. If a physician with knowledge of your medical condition tells the plan that a pre-service claim is urgent, the plan must treat it as an urgent care claim.

Pre-service claims are requests for approval that the plan requires you to obtain before you get medical care, such as preauthorization or a decision on whether a treatment or procedure is medically necessary.

Post-service claims are all other claims for benefits under your group health plan, including claims after medical services have been provided, such as requests for reimbursement or payment of the costs of the services provided. Most claims for group health benefits are post-service claims.

Disability claims are requests for benefits where the plan must make a determination of disability to decide the claim.

Waiting for a Decision on Your Claim

As noted, ERISA sets specific periods of time for plans to evaluate your claim and inform you of the decision. The time limits are counted in calendar days, so weekends and holidays are included. These limits do not govern when the benefits must be paid or provided. If you are entitled to benefits, check your SPD for how and when benefits are paid. Plans are required to pay or provide benefits within a reasonable time after a claim is approved.

Urgent care claims must be decided as soon as possible, taking into account the medical needs of the patient, but no later than 72 hours after the plan receives the claim. The plan must tell you within 24 hours if more information is needed; you will have no less than 48 hours to respond. Then the plan must decide the claim within 48 hours after the missing information is supplied or the time to supply it has elapsed. The plan cannot extend the time to make the initial decision without your consent. The plan must give you notice that your claim has been granted or denied before the end of the time allotted for the decision. The plan can notify you orally of the benefit determination so long as a written notification is furnished to you no later than three days after the oral notification.

Pre-service claims must be decided within a reasonable period of time appropriate to the medical circumstances, but no later than 15 days after the plan has received the claim. The plan may extend the time period up to an additional 15 days if, for reasons beyond the plan's control, the decision cannot be made within the first 15 days. The plan administrator must notify you prior to the expiration of the first 15-day period, explaining the reason for the delay, requesting any additional information, and advising you when the plan expects to make the decision. If more information is requested, you have at least 45 days to supply it. The plan then must decide the claim no later than 15 days after you supply the additional information or after the period of time allowed to supply it ends, whichever comes first. If the plan wants more time, the plan needs your consent. The plan must give you written notice that your claim has been granted or denied before the end of the time allotted for the decision.

Post-service health claims must be decided within a reasonable period of time, but not later than 30 days after the plan has received the claim. If, because of reasons beyond the plan's control, more time is needed to review your request, the plan may extend the time period up to an additional 15 days. However, the plan administrator has to let you know before the end of the first 30-day period, explaining the reason for the delay, requesting any additional information needed, and advising you when a final decision is expected. If more information is requested, you have at least 45 days to supply it. The claim then must be decided no later than 15 days after you supply the additional information or the period of time given by the plan to do so ends, whichever comes first. The plan needs your consent if it wants more time after its first extension. The plan must give you notice that your claim has been denied in whole or in part (paying less than 100% of the claim) before the end of the time allotted for the decision.

Disability claims must be decided within a reasonable period of time, but not later than 45 days after the plan has received the claim. If, because of reasons beyond the plan's control, more time is needed to review your request, the plan can extend the timeframe up to 30 days. The plan must tell you prior to the end of the first 45-day period that additional time is needed, explaining why, any unresolved issues and additional information needed, and when the plan expects to render a final decision. If more information is requested during either extension period, you will have at least 45 days to supply it. The claim then must be decided no later than 30 days after you supply the additional information or the period of time given by the plan to do so ends, whichever comes first. The plan administrator may extend the time period for up to another 30 days as long as it notifies you before the first extension expires. For any additional extensions, the plan needs your consent. The plan must give you notice whether your claim has been denied before the end of the time allotted for the decision.

If your claim is denied, the plan administrator must send you a notice, either in writing or electronically, with a detailed explanation of why your claim was denied and a description of the appeal process. In addition, the plan must include the plan rules, guidelines, protocols, or exclusions (such as medical necessity or experimental treatment) used in the decision or provide you with instructions on how you can request a copy from the plan. The notice may also include a specific request for you to provide the plan with additional information in case you wish to appeal your denial.

Appealing a Denied Claim

Claims are denied for various reasons. Perhaps the services you received are not covered by your plan. Or, perhaps the plan simply needs more information about your claim. Whatever the reason, you have at least 180 days to file an appeal (check your SPD or claims procedure to see if your plan provides a longer period).

Use the information in your claim denial notice in preparing your appeal. You should also be aware that the plan must provide claimants, on request and free of charge, copies of documents, records, and other information relevant to the claim for benefits. The plan also must identify, on your request, any medical or vocational expert whose advice was obtained by the plan. Be sure to include in your appeal all information related to your claim, particularly any additional information or evidence that you want the plan to consider, and get it to the person specified in the denial notice before the end of the 180-day period.

Reviewing an Appeal

On appeal, your claim must be reviewed by someone new who looks at all of the information submitted and consults with qualified medical professionals if a medical judgment is involved. This reviewer cannot be a subordinate of the person who made the initial decision and must give no consideration to that decision.

Plans have specific periods of time within which to review your appeal, depending on the type of claim.

Urgent care claims must be reviewed as soon as possible, taking into account the medical needs of the patient, but not later than 72 hours after the plan receives your request to review a denied claim.

Pre-service claims must be reviewed within a reasonable period of time appropriate to the medical circumstances, but not later than 30 days after the plan receives your request to review a denied claim.

Post-service claims must be reviewed within a reasonable period of time, but not later than 60 days after the plan receives your request to review a denied claim.

Note: If a group health plan needs more time, the plan must get your consent. If you do not agree to more time, the plan must complete the review within the permitted time limit.

Disability claims must be reviewed within a reasonable period of time, but not later than 45 days after the plan receives your request to review a denied claim. If the plan determines special circumstances exist and an extension is needed, the plan may take up to an additional 45 days to decide the appeal. However, before taking the extension, the plan must notify you in writing during the first 45-day period explaining the special circumstances, and the date by which the plan expects to make the decision.

Time Limit Exceptions

There are two exceptions to these time limits. In general, single-employer collectively bargained plans may use a collectively bargained grievance process for their claims appeal procedure if it has provisions on filing, determination, and review of benefit claims. Multi-employer collectively bargained plans are given special timeframes to allow them to schedule reviews on appeal of post-service claims and disability claims for the regular quarterly meetings of their boards of trustees. If you are a participant in one of those plans and you have questions about your plan's procedures, you can consult your plan's SPD or contact the Department of Labor's Employee Benefits Security Administration (EBSA).

Plans can require you to go through two levels of review of a denied health or disability claim to finish the plan's claims process. If two levels of review are required, the maximum time for each review generally is half of the time limit permitted for one review. For example, in the case of a group health plan with one appeal level, as noted, the review of a pre-service claim must be completed within a reasonable period of time appropriate to the medical circumstances but no later than 30 days after the plan gets your appeal. If the plan requires two appeals, each review must be completed within 15 days for pre-service claims. If your claim on appeal is still denied after the first review, the plan has to allow you a reasonable period of time (but not a full 180 days) to file for the second review.

Once the final decision on your claim is made, the plan must send you a written explanation of the decision. The notice must be in plain language that can be understood by participants in the plan. It must include all the specific reasons for the denial of your claim on appeal, refer you to the plan provisions on which the decision is based, tell you if the plan has any additional voluntary levels of appeal, explain your right to receive documents that are relevant to your benefit claim free of charge, and describe your rights to seek judicial review of the plan's decision.

If Your Appeal Is Denied

If the plan's final decision denies your claim, you may want to seek legal advice regarding your rights to bring an action in court to challenge the denial. Normally, you must complete your plan's claim process before filing an action in court to challenge the denial of a claim for benefits. However, if you believe your plan failed to establish or follow a claims procedure consistent with the Department's rules described in this chapter, you may want to seek legal advice regarding your right to ask a court to review your benefit claim without waiting for a decision from the plan. You also may want to contact the nearest EBSA office about your rights if you believe the plan failed to follow any of ERISA's requirements in handling your benefit claim.

Filing a Claim—Summary

- Check your plan's benefits and claims procedure before filing a claim. Read your SPD and contact your plan administrator if you have questions.

- Once your claim is filed, the maximum allowable waiting period for a decision varies by the type of claim, ranging from 72 hours to 45 days. However, your plan can extend certain time periods but must notify you before doing so. Usually, you will receive a decision within this timeframe.

- If your claim is denied, you must receive a written notice, including specific information about why your claim was denied and how to file an appeal.

- You have at least 180 days to request a full and fair review of your denied claim. Use your plan's appeals procedure and be aware that you may need to gather and submit new evidence or information to help the plan in reviewing the claim.

- Reviewing your appeal can take between 72 hours and 60 days depending on the type of claim. The law and the Department's rules allow a disability plan additional time if the plan's administrator has notified you beforehand of the need for an extension. For an appeal of a health claim, the plan needs your permission for an extension. The plan must send you a written notice, telling you whether the appeal was granted or denied.

- If the appeal is denied, the written notice must tell you the reason it was denied, describe any additional appeal levels or voluntary appeal procedures offered by the plan, and contain a statement regarding your rights to seek judicial review of the plan's decision.

- You may decide to seek legal advice if your claim's appeal is denied or if the plan failed to establish or follow reasonable claims procedures. If you believe the plan failed to follow ERISA requirements, you also may want to contact the nearest EBSA office concerning your rights under ERISA.

Additional Information

U.S. Department of Labor
Frances Perkins Building
200 Constitution Ave., N.W.
Washington, DC 20210
Toll-Free: 866-444-3272
Toll-Free TTY: 877-889-5627
Website: http://www.dol.gov/ebsa

Part Eight

Additional Help and Information

Chapter 74

Glossary of Terms Related to Disease Management

activities of daily living (ADL): The tasks of everyday life. These activities include eating, dressing, getting into or out of a bed or chair, taking a bath or shower, and using the toilet. Instrumental activities of daily living are activities related to independent living and include preparing meals, managing money, shopping, doing housework, and using a telephone.

advance directive: A legal document that states the treatment or care a person wishes to receive or not receive if he or she becomes unable to make medical decisions (for example, due to being unconscious or in a coma). Some types of advance directives are living wills and do-not-resuscitate (DNR) orders.

antibiotic: A drug used to treat infections caused by bacteria and other microorganisms.

anxiety: Feelings of fear, dread, and uneasiness that may occur as a reaction to stress. A person with anxiety may sweat, feel restless and tense, and have a rapid heart beat. Extreme anxiety that happens often over time may be a sign of an anxiety disorder.

Unmarked definitions in this chapter are excerpted from PDQ® Cancer Information Summary. National Cancer Institute; Bethesda, MD. Transitional Care Planning (PDQ®): Treatment - Patient. Updated 10/2007. Available at: http:// cancer.gov. Accessed November 9, 2007. Terms marked [1] are excerpted from "Your Health Plan and HIPAA—Making the Law Work for You," U.S. Department of Labor, September 2006.

assessment: In health care, a process used to learn about a patient's condition. This may include a complete medical history, medical tests, a physical exam, a test of learning skills, tests to find out if the patient is able to carry out the tasks of daily living, a mental health evaluation, and a review of social support and community resources available to the patient.

assistive device: A tool that helps a person with a disability to do a certain task. Examples are a cane, wheelchair, scooter, walker, hearing aid, or special bed.

assistive technology: Any device or technology that helps a disabled person. Examples are special grips for holding utensils, computer screen monitors to help a person with low vision read more easily, computers controlled by talking, telephones that make the sound louder, and lifters to help a person rise out of a chair.

bereavement: A state of sadness, grief, and mourning after the loss of a loved one.

blood: A tissue with red blood cells, white blood cells, platelets, and other substances suspended in fluid called plasma. Blood takes oxygen and nutrients to the tissues, and carries away wastes.

blood transfusion: The administration of blood or blood products into a blood vessel.

cancer: A term for diseases in which abnormal cells divide without control. Cancer cells can invade nearby tissues and can spread to other parts of the body through the blood and lymph systems. There are several main types of cancer. Carcinoma is cancer that begins in the skin or in tissues that line or cover internal organs. Sarcoma is cancer that begins in bone, cartilage, fat, muscle, blood vessels, or other connective or supportive tissue. Leukemia is cancer that starts in blood-forming tissue such as the bone marrow, and causes large numbers of abnormal blood cells to be produced and enter the blood. Lymphoma and multiple myeloma are cancers that begin in the cells of the immune system. Central nervous system cancers are cancers that begin in the tissues of the brain and spinal cord.

cardiopulmonary: Having to do with the heart and lungs.

catheter: A flexible tube used to deliver fluids into or withdraw fluids from the body.

cell: The individual unit that makes up the tissues of the body. All living things are made up of one or more cells.

certificate of creditable coverage: A document prepared by a group health plan, health maintenance organization (HMO), or insurance company that shows prior periods of creditable coverage, used to reduce or eliminate the length of a preexisting condition exclusion period.[1]

chaplain: A member of the clergy in charge of a chapel or who works with the military or with an institution, such as a hospital.

chemotherapy: Treatment with drugs that kill cancer cells.

clinical trial: A type of research study that tests how well new medical approaches work in people. These studies test new methods of screening, prevention, diagnosis, or treatment of a disease; also called a clinical study.

COBRA: An abbreviation for the Consolidated Omnibus Budget Reconciliation Act of 1986, a law that provides for a temporary extension of health plan coverage from a prior group health plan.[1]

colostomy: An opening into the colon from the outside of the body. A colostomy provides a new path for waste material to leave the body after part of the colon has been removed.

counseling: The process by which a professional counselor helps a person cope with mental or emotional distress, and understand and solve personal problems.

creditable coverage: A period of prior health coverage, which may be used to offset the length of a preexisting condition exclusion period. This includes coverage under a group health plan, COBRA, Medicare, and Medicaid, or a health maintenance organization (HMO) or individual health insurance policy.[1]

cure: To heal or restore health; a treatment to restore health.

depression: A mental condition marked by ongoing feelings of sadness, despair, loss of energy, and difficulty dealing with normal daily life. Other symptoms of depression include feelings of worthlessness and hopelessness, loss of pleasure in activities, changes in eating or sleeping habits, and thoughts of death or suicide. Depression can affect anyone, and can be successfully treated. Depression affects 15–25%

of cancer patients and up to one-third of the people who have a chronic illness.

diagnosis: The process of identifying a disease by the signs and symptoms.

dietitian: A health professional with special training in nutrition who can help with dietary choices, also called a nutritionist.

DNR order (do not resuscitate order): A type of advance directive in which a person states that health care providers should not perform cardiopulmonary resuscitation (restarting the heart) if his or her heart or breathing stops.

drug: Any substance, other than food, that is used to prevent, diagnose, treat, or relieve symptoms of a disease or abnormal condition. Also refers to a substance that alters mood or body function, or that can be habit-forming or addictive, especially a narcotic.

durable power of attorney (DPA): A type of power of attorney. A power of attorney is a legal document that gives one person (such as a relative, lawyer, or friend) the authority to make legal, medical, or financial decisions for another person. It may go into effect right away, or when that person is no longer able to make decisions for himself or herself. A durable power of attorney remains in effect until the person who grants it dies or cancels it. It does not need to be renewed over time.

enrollment date: The first day of health insurance coverage or the first day of the waiting period (if applicable).[1]

health care proxy (HCP): A type of advance directive that gives a person (such as a relative, lawyer, or friend) the authority to make health care decisions for another person. It becomes active when that person loses the ability to make decisions for himself or herself.

hospice: A program that provides special care for people who are near the end of life and for their families, either at home, in freestanding facilities, or within hospitals.

hygiene: The science of health, and the practice of cleanliness that promotes good health and well-being.

infection: Invasion and multiplication of germs in the body. Infections can occur in any part of the body and can spread throughout the body. The germs may be bacteria, viruses, yeast, or fungi. They can cause a fever and other problems, depending on where the infection occurs. When the body's natural defense system is strong, it can often fight the germs and prevent infection. Some cancer treatments can weaken the natural defense system.

infusion: A method of putting fluids, including drugs, into the bloodstream; also called intravenous infusion.

insured plan: A plan which provides benefits through an insurance company or HMO. Check your summary plan description (SPD) to see if your plan is insured.[1]

late enrollee: An individual who enrolls in the plan at some time other than when first eligible or a special enrollment opportunity.[1]

living will: A type of legal advance directive in which a person describes specific treatment guidelines that are to be followed by health care providers if he or she becomes terminally ill and cannot communicate. A living will usually has instructions about whether to use aggressive medical treatment to keep a person alive, such as cardiopulmonary resuscitation (CPR), artificial nutrition, or use of a respirator.

lung: One of a pair of organs in the chest that supplies the body with oxygen and removes carbon dioxide from the body.

mental health: A person's overall psychological and emotional condition. Good mental health is a state of well-being in which a person is able to cope with everyday events, think clearly, be responsible, meet challenges, and have good relationships with others.

mental health counselor: A specialist who can talk with patients and their families about emotional and personal matters, and can help them make decisions.

nurse: A health professional trained to care for people who are ill or disabled.

nursing home: A place that gives care to people who have physical or mental disabilities and need help with activities of daily living (such as taking a bath, getting dressed, and going to the bathroom) but do not need to be in the hospital.

nutrition: The taking in and use of food and other nourishing material by the body. Nutrition is a three-part process. First, food or drink is consumed. Second, the body breaks down the food or drink into nutrients. Third, the nutrients travel through the bloodstream to different parts of the body where they are used as fuel and for many other purposes. To give the body proper nutrition, a person has to eat and drink enough of the foods that contain key nutrients.

occupational therapist: A health professional trained to help people who are ill or disabled learn to manage their daily activities.

outpatient: A patient who visits a health care facility for diagnosis or treatment without spending the night, sometimes called a day patient.

palliative care: Care given to improve the quality of life of patients who have a serious or life-threatening disease. The goal of palliative care is to prevent or treat as early as possible the symptoms of the disease, side effects caused by treatment of the disease, and psychological, social, and spiritual problems related to the disease or its treatment, also called comfort care, supportive care, and symptom management.

palliative therapy: Treatment given to relieve the symptoms and reduce the suffering caused by cancer and other life-threatening diseases. Palliative cancer therapies are given together with other cancer treatments, from the time of diagnosis, through treatment, survivorship, recurrent or advanced disease, and at the end of life.

physical examination: An exam of the body to check for general signs of disease.

physical therapist: A health professional who teaches exercises and physical activities that help condition muscles and restore strength and movement.

preexisting condition exclusion: A limitation or exclusion of health insurance benefits relating to a condition because that condition was present before the effective date of your health coverage.[1]

preexisting condition exclusion period: The amount of time that you are excluded from health insurance coverage of benefits for a preexisting condition (the maximum is 12 months, or 18 months for late enrollees).[1]

psychological: Having to do with how the mind works and how thoughts and feelings affect behavior.

psychologist: A specialist who can talk with patients and their families about emotional and personal matters and can help them make decisions.

pump: A device that is used to give a controlled amount of a liquid at a specific rate. For example, pumps are used to give drugs (such as chemotherapy or pain medicine) or nutrients.

quality of life: The overall enjoyment of life. Many clinical trials assess the effects of cancer and its treatment on the quality of life. These studies measure aspects of an individual's sense of well-being and ability to carry out various activities.

rehabilitation: In medicine, a process to restore mental or physical abilities lost to injury or disease, in order to function in a normal or near-normal way.

relapse: The return of signs and symptoms of cancer after a period of improvement.

remission: A decrease in or disappearance of signs and symptoms of illness such as cancer. In partial remission, some, but not all, signs and symptoms of disease have disappeared. In complete remission, all signs and symptoms of disease have disappeared, although disease still may be in the body.

respirator: In medicine, a machine used to help a patient breathe, also called ventilator.

screening: Checking for disease when there are no symptoms.

self-insured plan: A group health plan where the employer assumes the risk of paying the benefits itself. An insurance company may provide administration services to a self-insured plan, such as claims administration, but does not assume any risk to pay claims for benefits.[1]

side effect: A problem that occurs when treatment affects healthy tissues or organs. Some common side effects of cancer treatment are fatigue, pain, nausea, vomiting, decreased blood cell counts, hair loss, and mouth sores.

significant break: A break in health insurance coverage for 63 days or more.[1]

similarly situated individuals: Permitted distinctions health insurance plans may make among individuals, such as groups of employees, if based on bona fide employment-based classifications consistent with the employer's usual business practice. For example, part-time and full-time employees can be treated as different groups of similarly situated individuals. In addition, a plan may draw a distinction between employees and their dependents. Plans can also make distinctions between dependents themselves if the distinction is not based on a health factor. For example, a plan can distinguish between spouses and dependent children, or between dependent children based on their age or student status.[1]

social service: A community resource that helps people in need. Services may include help getting to and from medical appointments, home delivery of medication and meals, in-home nursing care, help paying medical costs not covered by insurance, loaning medical equipment, and housekeeping help.

social support: A network of family, friends, neighbors, and community members that is available in times of need to give psychological, physical, and financial help.

social worker: A professional trained to talk with people and their families about emotional or physical needs and to find them support services.

special enrollment: An opportunity for certain individuals to enroll in a group health plan, regardless of the plan's regular enrollment dates. These opportunities occur when you lose eligibility for other coverage or experience certain life events (marriage, birth, adoption, or placement for adoption).[1]

spirituality: Having to do with deep, often religious, feelings and beliefs, including a person's sense of peace, purpose, connection to others, and beliefs about the meaning of life.

stage: The extent of a cancer in the body. Staging is usually based on the size of the tumor, whether lymph nodes contain cancer, and whether the cancer has spread from the original site to other parts of the body.

summary plan description (SPD): A document outlining your plan, usually provided when you enroll in the plan.[1]

supplemental nutrition: A substance or product that is added to a person's diet to make sure they get all the nutrients they need. It may include vitamins, minerals, protein, or fat, and may be given by mouth, by tube feeding, or into a vein.

support group: A group of people with similar disease who meet to discuss how better to cope with their disease and treatment.

supportive care: Care given to improve the quality of life of patients who have a serious or life-threatening disease. The goal of supportive care is to prevent or treat as early as possible the symptoms of the disease, side effects caused by treatment of the disease, and psychological, social, and spiritual problems related to the disease or its treatment; also called palliative care, comfort care, and symptom management.

symptom: An indication that a person has a condition or disease. Some examples of symptoms are headache, fever, fatigue, nausea, vomiting, and pain.

symptom management: Care given to improve the quality of life of patients who have a serious or life-threatening disease. The goal of symptom management is to prevent or treat as early as possible the symptoms of the disease, side effects caused by treatment of the disease, and psychological, social, and spiritual problems related to the disease or its treatment; also called palliative care, comfort care, and supportive care.

tube feeding: A type of enteral nutrition (nutrition that is delivered into the digestive system in a liquid form). For tube feeding, a small tube may be placed through the nose into the stomach or the small intestine. Sometimes it is surgically placed into the stomach or the intestinal tract through an opening made on the outside of the abdomen, depending on how long it will be used. People who are unable to meet their needs with food and beverages alone, and who do not have vomiting or uncontrollable diarrhea may be given tube feedings. Tube feeding can be used to add to what a person is able to eat or can be the only source of nutrition.

waiting period: The time that must pass before coverage can become effective under the terms of a group health plan.[1]

Chapter 75

Additional Resources for Information about Disease Management

Government Organizations

Administration on Aging
National Aging Information
Center
330 Independence Ave., S.W.
Washington, DC 20201
Toll-Free: 800-677-1116
(Eldercare Locator)
Phone: 202-619-7501
Website: http://www.aoa.dhhs.gov
E-mail: AoAInfo@aoa.gov

Agency for Healthcare Research and Quality (AHRQ)
U.S. Dept. of Health and Human
Services (HHS)
P.O. Box 8547
Silver Spring, MD 20907-8547
Toll-Free: 800-358-9295
Website: http://www.ahrq.gov
E-mail: info@ahrq.gov

Centers for Medicare and Medicaid Services (CMS)
500 Security Blvd.
Baltimore, MD 21244-1850
Toll-Free: 800-633-4227
Toll-Free TTY: 877-486-2048
Phone: 410-786-3000
Website: http://cms.hhs.gov

Centers for Disease Control and Prevention (CDC)
1600 Clifton Rd.
Atlanta, GA 30333
Toll-Free: 800-311-3435
Phone: 404-639-3534
Website: http://www.cdc.gov
E-mail: cdcinfo@cdc.gov

Resources in this chapter were compiled from several sources deemed reliable; all contact information was verified and updated in November 2007.

Equal Employment Opportunity Commission (EEOC)
1801 L Street, N.W.
Washington, DC 20507
Toll-Free: 800-669-4000
Toll-Free TDD: 800-669-6820
Phone: 202-663-4900
Website: http://www.eeoc.gov

Federal Trade Commission (FTC)
Consumer Response Center
600 Pennsylvania Ave., N.W.
Washington, DC 20580
Toll-Free: 877-FTC-HELP
(877-382-4357)
Toll-Free TDD/TTY: 866-653-4261
Website: http://www.ftc.gov

Health Resources and Services Administration (HRSA)
Information Center
P.O. Box 2910
Merrifield, VA 22116
Toll-Free: 888-275-4772
Toll-Free TTY: 877-489-4772
Fax: 703-821-2098
Website: http://www.hrsa.gov
E-mail: ask@hrsa.gov

Healthfinder®
National Health Information
Center
P.O. Box 1133
Washington, DC 20013-1133
Toll-Free: 800-336-4797
Phone: 301-565-4167
Fax: 301-984-4256
Website: http://
www.healthfinder.gov
E-mail: healthfinder@nhic.org

National Cancer Institute (NCI)
NCI Public Inquiries Office
6116 Executive Blvd.
Suite 3036A, MSC8322
Bethesda, MD 20892-8322
Toll-Free: 800-4-CANCER
(422-6237)
Toll-Free TTY: 800-332-8615
Website: http://www.cancer.gov
E-mail:
cancergovstaff@mail.nih.gov

National Diabetes Information Clearinghouse
1 Information Way
Bethesda, MD 20892-3560
Toll-Free: 800-860-8747
Phone: 301-654-3327
Fax: 703-738-4929
Website: http://
diabetes.niddk.nih.gov
E-mail: ndic@info.niddk.nih.gov

National Center for Chronic Disease Prevention and Health Promotion
4770 Buford Hwy., N.E.
MS K-40
Atlanta, GA 30341
Toll-Free: 800-311-3435
Phone: 404-639-3534
Website: http://www.cdc.gov/
nccdphp
E-mail: ccdinfo@cdc.gov

National Center for Complementary and Alternative Medicine (NCCAM) Clearinghouse
P.O. Box 7923
Gaithersburg, MD 20898
Bethesda, MD 20892-2182
Toll-Free: 888-644-6226
Toll-Free TTY: 866-464-3615
Phone: 301-519-3153
Fax: 866-464-3616
Website: http://nccam.nih.gov
E-mail: info@nccam.nih.gov

National Health Information Center
P.O. Box 1133
Washington, DC 20013-1133
Toll-Free: 800-336-4797
Phone: 301-565-4167
Fax: 301-984-4256
Website: http://www.health.gov/NHIC
E-mail: nhicinfo@health.org

National Heart, Lung, and Blood Institute (NHLBI)
P.O. Box 30105
Bethesda, MD 20824-0105
Phone: 301-592-8573
TTY: 240-629-3255
Fax: 240-629-3246
Website: http://www.nhlbi.nih.gov
E-mail: nhlbiinfo@nhlbi.nih.gov

National Human Genome Research Institute (NHGRI)
National Institutes of Health
31 Center Drive
Bethesda, MD 20892-2152
Phone: 301-402-0911
Fax: 301-402-4831
Website: http://www.genome.gov

National Institute of Arthritis and Musculoskeletal and Skin Diseases (NIAMS)
1 AMS Circle
Bethesda, MD 20892-3675
Toll-Free: 877-226-4267
Phone: 301-495-4484
TTY: 301-565-2966
Fax: 301-718-6366
Website: http://www.niams.nih.gov
E-mail: niamsinfo@mail.nih.gov

National Institute of Child Health and Human Development (NICHD)
Information Resource Center
P.O. Box 3006
Rockville, MD 20847
Toll-Free: 800-370-2943
Toll-Free TTY: 888-320-6942
Fax: 301-984-1473
Website: http://www.nichd.nih.gov
E-mail: nichdinformationResourceCenter@mail.nih.gov

National Institute of Diabetes and Digestive and Kidney Diseases (NIDDK)
Office of Communications and Public Liaison
Building 31, Room 9A06
31 Center Drive, MSC 2560
Bethesda, MD 20892-2560
NIDDK Information Clearing-house Toll-Free: 800-891-5390
Phone: 301-496-3583
Website: http://www2.niddk.nih.gov
E-mail: dwebmaster@extra.niddk.nih.gov

National Institute of Mental Health (NIMH)
Office of Communications and Public Liaison
6001 Executive Blvd.
Rm. 8184, MSC 9663
Bethesda, MD 20892-9663
Phone: 301-443-4513
TTY: 301-443-8431
Fax: 301-443-4279
Website: http://www.nimh.nih.gov
E-mail: nimhinfo@nih.gov

National Institute of Neurological Disorders and Stroke (NINDS)
P.O. Box 5801
Bethesda, MD 20824
Toll-Free: 800-352-9424
Phone: 301-496-5751
TTY: 301-496-5981
Website: http://www.ninds.nih.gov
E-mail: braininfo@ninds.nih.gov

National Institute on Aging (NIA)
P.O. Box 8057
Gaithersburg, MD 20898
Toll-Free: 800-222-2225
Toll-Free TTY: 800-222-4225
Phone: 301-496-1752
Fax: 301-496-1072
Website: http://www.nia.nih.gov

National Institutes of Health (NIH)
9000 Rockville Pike
Bethesda, MD 20892
Phone: 301-496-4000
TTY: 301-402-9612
Website: http://www.nih.gov
E-mail: NIHinfo@od.nih.gov

National Women's Health Information Center (NWHIC)
8270 Willow Oaks Corporate Dr.
Fairfax, VA 22031
Toll-Free: 800-994-9662
Toll-Free TDD: 888-220-5446
Website: http://www.womenshealth.gov, or http://www.4woman.gov

Office of Minority Health Resource Center (OMH-RC)
P.O. Box 37337
Washington, DC 20013-7337
Toll-Free: 800-444-6472
TTY: 301-230-7199
Fax: 301-230-7198
Website: http://www.omhrc.gov
E-mail: info@omhrc.gov

Substance Abuse and Mental Health Services Administration (SAMHSA)
1 Choke Cherry Rd.
Rockville, MD 20857
Toll-Free: 877-726-4727
Website: http://www.samhsa.gov

U.S. Food and Drug Administration (FDA)
Office of Consumer Affairs
5600 Fishers Lane
HFE-50
Rockville, MD 20857
Toll-Free: 888-463-6332
Phone: 301-827-4420
Fax: 301-443-9767
Website: http://www.fda.gov

U.S. National Library of Medicine
8600 Rockville Pike
Bethesda, MD 20894
Toll-Free: 888-346-3656
Toll-Free TDD: 800-735-2258
Phone: 301-594-5983
Fax: 301-402-1384
Website: http://www.nlm.nih.gov
E-mail: custserv@nlm.nih.gov

Private Organizations

ABLEDATA
8630 Fenton St., Suite 930
Silver Spring, MD 20910
Toll-Free: 800-227-0216
TTY: 301-608-8912
Fax: 301-608-8958
Website: http://www.abledata.com
E-mail: abledata@verizon.net

Alzheimer's Association
225 N. Michigan Ave., Floor 17
Chicago, IL 60601-7633
Toll-Free: 800-272-3900
Phone: 312-335-8700
Fax: 312-335-1110
Website: http://www.alz.org
E-mail: info@alz.org

American Academy of Family Physicians
P.O. Box 11210
Shawnee Mission, KS 66207-1210
Toll-Free: 800-274-2237
Phone: 913-906-6000
Website: http://www.aafp.org
E-mail: fp@aafp.org

American Cancer Society (ACS)
13599 Clifton Rd., N.E.
Atlanta, GA 30329
Toll-Free: 800-227-2345
Toll-Free TTY: 866-228-4327
Website: http://www.cancer.org

American Health Information Management Association (AHIMA)
233 N. Michigan Ave., 21st Floor
Chicago, IL 60601-5800
Phone: 312-233-1100
Fax: 312-233-1090
Website: http://www.myphr.com
E-mail: info@ahima.org

American Heart Association (AHA)
National Center
7272 Greenville Ave.
Dallas, TX 75231
Toll-Free: 800-242-8721
Website: http://
www.americanheart.org

American Lung Association (ALA)
61 Broadway, 6th Fl.
New York, NY 10006
Toll-Free: 800-586-4872 (for location of nearest ALA group)
Toll-Free: 800-548-8252 (to speak with a lung health professional)
Phone: 212-315-8700
Website: http://www.lungusa.org

American Medical Association (AMA)
515 N. State St.
Chicago, IL 60610
Toll-Free: 800-621-8335
Phone: 312-464-5000
Fax: 312-464-5600
Website: http://www.ama-assn.org

Cleveland Clinic
9500 Euclid Ave.
Cleveland, OH 44195
Toll-Free: 800-223-2273
Phone: 216-444-2200
TTY: 216-444-0261
Website: http://
www.clevelandclinic.org

National Family Caregivers Association (NFCA)
10400 Connecticut Ave.
Suite 500
Kensington, MD 20895-3944
Toll-Free: 800-896-3650
Phone: 301-942-6430
Fax: 301 942 2302
Website: http://www.nfcacares.org
E-mail:
info@thefamilycaregiver.org

National Health Care Anti-Fraud Association
1201 New York Ave., N.W.
Suite 1120
Washington, DC 20005
Phone: 202-659-5955
Fax: 202-785-6764
Website: http://www.nhcaa.org
E-mail: nhcaa@nhcaa.org

National Patient Advocate Foundation
725 15th St. N.W., 10th Fl.
Washington, DC 20005
Phone: 202-347-8009
Fax: 202-347-5579
Website: http://www.npaf.org

National Patient Safety Foundation
132 MASS MoCA Way
North Adams, MA 01247
Phone: 413-663-8900
Fax: 413-663-8905
Website: http://www.npsf.org
E-mail: info@npsf.org

National Rehabilitation Information Center
4200 Forbes Blvd., Suite 202
Lanham, MD 20706-4829
Toll-Free: 800-346-2742
Phone: 301-459-5900
Fax: 301-459-4263
TTY: 301-459-5984
Website: http://www.naric.com
E-mail:
naricinfo@heitechservices.com

Nemours Foundation Center for Children's Health Media
1600 Rockland Rd.
Wilmington, DE 19803
Phone: 302-651-4000
Website: http://
www.kidshealth.org, or
http://www.teenshealth.org
E-mail: info@kidshealth.org

Chapter 76

Directory of Health Insurance Information

The organizations listed are offered as a place to begin when seeking further information about health insurance. They are listed in alphabetical order. Readers should consult qualified experts before making decisions about health insurance.

Agency for Healthcare Research and Quality (AHRQ)
U.S. Department of Health and Human Services
P.O. Box 8547
Silver Spring MD 20907-8547
Toll-Free: 800-358-9295
Website: http://www.ahrq.gov
E-mail: info@ahrq.gov

AHRQ offers a publication titled "Questions and Answers about Health Insurance," available at http://www.ahrq.gov/consumer/insuranceqa/insuranceqa.pdf.

AARP
601 E Street, N.W.
Washington, DC 20049
Toll-Free: 800-424-3410
Phone: 202-434-2277
Website: http://www.aarp.org

Resources in this chapter were compiled from several sources deemed reliable; all contact information was verified and updated in November 2007.

AARP provides publications and online information on a variety of topics including health insurance.

America's Health Insurance Plans
601 Pennsylvania Ave., N.W.
South Bldg., Suite 500
Washington, DC 20004
Phone: 202-778-3200
Fax: 202-331-7487
Website: http://hiaa.org
E-mail: ahip@ahip.org

The AHIP website offers a national directory of health insurance plans where visitors have access to a variety of insurance products designed to help manage healthcare coverage decisions.

Centers for Medicare and Medicaid Services (CMS)
7500 Security Blvd.
Baltimore, MD 21244-1850
Toll-Free: 877-267-2323
Toll Free TTY: 866-226-1819
Phone: 410-786-3000
TTY: 410-786-0727
Website: http://cms.hhs.gov, or http://www.medicare.gov

Coalition against Insurance Fraud
1012 14th St. N.W., Suite 200
Washington, DC 20005
Phone: 202-393-7330
Fax: 202-393-7329
Website: http://www.InsuranceFraud.org
E-mail: info@insurancefraud.org

Families USA
201 New York Ave. N.W., Suite 1100
Washington, DC 20005
Phone: 202-628-3030
Fax: 202-347-2417
Website: http://www.familiesusa.org
E-mail: info@familiesusa.org

Federal Trade Commission
Consumer Response Center
600 Pennsylvania Ave., N.W.
Washington, DC 20580
Toll-Free: 877-FTC-HELP (877-382-4357)
Toll-Free TDD/TTY: 866-653-4261
Website: http:www.ftc.gov

healthinsuranceinfo.net
Georgetown University Health Policy Institute
Website: http://www.healthinsuranceinfo.net/

This website has online consumer guides for getting and keeping health insurance according to each state's guidelines and offers current news information about health insurance.

Insurance Information Institute
Consumer Affairs
110 William St., 24th Floor
New York, NY 10038
Toll-Free: 800-331-9146
Phone: 212-346-5500
Website: http://www.iii.org

Kaiser Family Foundation
Website: http://www.kff.org

The Kaiser Family Foundation offers "A Consumer Guide to Handling Disputes with Your Employer or Private Health Plan, 2005 Update," on their website at http://kff.org/consumerguide/7350.cfm.

MedlinePlus Encyclopedia
Website: http://www.nlm.nih.gov/medlineplus/healthinsurance.html

MedlinePlus, a service of the National Institutes of Health (NIH) National Library of Medicine, lists many sources for information about health insurance.

National Association of Insurance Commissioners
Executive Headquarters
2301 McGee St., Suite 800
Kansas City, MO 64108-2662
Toll-Free: 866-470-NAIC (6242)
Phone: 816-842-3600
Fax: 816-783-8175
Website: http://naic.org

Patient Advocate Foundation
700 Thimble Shoals Blvd.
Suite 200
Newport News, VA 23606
Toll-Free: 800-532-5274
Fax: 757-873-8999
Website: http://www.patientadvocate.org
E-mail: help@patientadvocate.org

U.S. Department of Labor
Frances Perkins Building
200 Constitution Ave., N.W.
Washington, DC 20210
Toll-Free: 866-444-3272
Toll-Free TTY: 877-889-5627
Website: http://www.dol.gov/ebsa

The DOL website includes information to help consumers in filing claims health or disability benefits.

U.S. Department of the Treasury
Internal Revenue Service
Toll-Free for Individuals: 800-829-1040
Toll-Free for Businesses: 800-829-4933
Website: http://www.treas.gov

Offers information about health savings accounts (HSA).

Chapter 77

Directory of Organizations that Provide Financial Assistance for Medical Treatments

Cancer and chronic illness impose heavy economic burdens on both patients and their families. For many people, a portion of medical expenses is paid by their health insurance plan. For individuals who do not have health insurance or who need financial assistance to cover health care costs, resources are available, including government-sponsored programs and services supported by nonprofit organizations. Patients and their families should discuss any concerns they may have about health care costs with their physician, medical social worker, or the business office of their hospital or clinic.

This chapter includes an alphabetical listing of some of the government agencies, organizations, and programs that are designed to provide assistance for patients and their families. However, resources provided by individual organizations vary, and it is important to check with a specific group to determine if financial aid is currently available.

Government Programs

Bureau of Primary Health Care
Website: http://ask.hrsa.gov/pc (to locate a health center)

The Health Resources and Services Administration's (HRSA) Bureau of Primary Health Care offers health centers that provide health

Excerpted from "Financial Assistance and Other Resources for People with Cancer," National Cancer Institute (NCI), February 2007. All contact information was verified and updated in November 2007.

care to low-income and other vulnerable populations. Health centers care for people regardless of their ability to pay. They provide primary and preventive health care, as well as services such as transportation and translation.

Centers for Medicare and Medicaid Services (CMS)
7500 Security Blvd.
Baltimore, MD 21244-1850
Toll-Free: 877-267-2323, Toll Free TTY: 866-226-1819
Phone: 410-786-3000, TTY: 410-786-0727
Website: http://cms.hhs.gov

Hill-Burton Free and Reduced Cost Health Care
Toll-Free: 800-638-0742 (Maryland residents call 800-492-0359)
Website: http://www.hrsa.gov/hillburton/default.htm

Hill-Burton is a program through which hospitals receive construction and modernization funds from the federal government. Hospitals that receive Hill-Burton funds are required by law to provide a reasonable volume of services to people who cannot afford to pay for their hospitalization and make their services available to all residents in the facility's area. To find a Hill-Burton program in your area, visit http://www.hrsa.gov/hillburton/hillburtonfacilities.htm, or call their toll-free number.

Internal Revenue Service (IRS)
Toll-Free: 800-829-1040
Website: http://www.irs.gov

The Internal Revenue Service (IRS) can provide information about tax deductions for medical costs that are not covered by insurance policies. For example, tax deductible expenses might include mileage for trips to and from medical appointments, out-of-pocket costs for treatment, prescription drugs or equipment, and the cost of meals during lengthy medical visits. Deductible-qualified medical expenses include those incurred by the patient, spouse, and dependents. Medical expenses may also be deducted for someone who would have qualified as a dependent for the purpose of taking personal exemptions except that the person did not meet the gross income or joint return test. Nursing home expenses are allowable as medical expenses in certain instances. If the patient, a spouse, or dependent is in a nursing home, and the primary reason for being there is for medical care, the entire cost, including meals and lodging, is a medical expense. The local IRS office, tax consultants, or certified public accountants can determine whether medical costs are tax deductible.

Medicaid (Medical Assistance)

Toll-Free: 877-267-2323
Website: http://www.cms.hhs.gov/home/medicaid.asp?

Medicaid (Medical Assistance), a jointly funded, federal-state health insurance program for people who need financial assistance for medical expenses, is coordinated by the Centers for Medicare and Medicaid Services (CMS). At a minimum, states must provide home care services to people who receive federal income assistance such as social security income (SSI) and aid to families with dependent children (AFDC). Medicaid coverage includes part-time nursing, home care aide services, and medical supplies and equipment. Information about coverage is available from local state welfare offices, state health departments, state social services agencies, or the state Medicaid office. Check the local telephone directory for the number to call. Information about specific state contacts is also available on the Medicaid website.

Medicare

Toll-Free: 800-333-4227
Toll-Free TTY: 877-486-2048
Website: http://www.medicare.gov

Medicare is a federal health insurance program also administered by the CMS. Eligible individuals include those who are 65 or older, people of any age with permanent kidney failure, and disabled people under age 65. Medicare is divided into two parts, part A and part B. Part A pays for hospital care, home health care, hospice care, and care in Medicare-certified nursing facilities. Part B covers medically necessary services, including diagnostic studies, physicians' services, durable home medical equipment, and ambulance transportation; Part B also covers screening exams for several types of cancer. To receive information on eligibility, explanations of coverage, and related publications, call Medicare or visit their website.

State and Local Government-Funded Programs

Some nonprofit community hospitals are able to provide care for patients in need of financial assistance. Other hospitals have indigent or charity care programs funded by state and local governments. For information about these programs, contact a hospital social worker, who will be able to explain these types of programs. Another type of assistance may be offered through your local health department.

State and local social services agencies can provide help with food, housing, prescription drugs, transportation, and other medical expenses for those who are not eligible for other programs. Information can be obtained by contacting your state or local agency; this number is found in the local telephone directory.

State Children's Health Insurance Programs (SCHIP)
Toll-Free: 877-543-7669
Website: http://www.insurekidsnow.gov

The State Children's Health Insurance Program (SCHIP) is a federal-state partnership that offers low-cost or free health insurance coverage to uninsured infants, children, and teens. Callers will be referred to the program in their state for further information about what the program covers, who is eligible, and the minimum qualifications. In most states, uninsured children age 18 and younger whose families earn up to $34,100 a year (for a family of four) are eligible. For a list of health insurance coverage and eligibility by state, go to http://www.insurekidsnow.gov/states.htm on the internet.

U.S. Department of Veterans Affairs (VA)
Toll-Free: 877-222-8387
Website: http://www1.va.gov/health

The Department of Veterans Affairs (VA) provides eligible veterans with treatment for service-connected injuries and other medical conditions. The VA offers limited medical benefits to family members of eligible veterans.

Nonprofit Organizations

American Cancer Society (ACS)
13599 Clifton Rd., N.E.
Atlanta, GA 30329
Toll-Free: 800-227-2345
Toll-Free TTY: 866-228-4327
Website: http://www.cancer.org

ACS Hope Lodge
Website: http://www.cancer.org/docroot/SHR/content/SHR_2.1_x
_Hope_Lodge.asp?sitearea=SHR

Hope Lodge is a temporary housing program supported by ACS. It provides free, temporary housing facilities for cancer patients who are undergoing treatment. For more information about this program, or to find locations of Hope Lodges, call the ACS's toll-free number or visit the Hope Lodge website.

ACS Road to Recovery

The Road to Recovery is an ACS service program that provides transportation for cancer patients to their treatments and home again. Transportation is provided according to the needs and available resources in the community and can be arranged by calling the toll-free number or by contacting your local ACS office.

Brain Tumor Society
124 Watertown St., Suite 3-H
Watertown, MA 02472
Toll-Free: 800-770-8287
Phone: 617-924-9997, Fax: 617-924-9998
Website: http://www.tbts.org
E-mail: info@tbts.org

The Brain Tumor Society is a national nonprofit agency that provides information about brain tumors and related conditions for patients and their families. Financial assistance is given through the agency's BTS CARES financial assistance program. This program provides supplementary financial assistance to individuals experiencing financial need. This program covers specific nonmedical costs related to a primary brain tumor diagnosis. Direct medical expenses are not covered.

CancerCare, Inc.
National Office
275 Seventh Ave., Floor 22
New York, NY 10001
Toll-Free: 800-813-4673
Phone: 212-712-8400, Fax: 212-712-8495
Website: http://www.cancercare.org
E-mail: info@cancercare.org

CancerCare is a national nonprofit agency that offers free support, information, financial assistance, and practical help to people with cancer and their loved ones. Financial assistance is given in the form of limited grants for certain treatment expenses. Services are provided by oncology social workers and are available in person, over the telephone, and through the agency's website. Information about financial assistance for all cancers is available at http://www.cancercare.org/get_help/assistance/cc_financial.php.

CancerCare has also partnered with Susan G. Komen to create the Linking A.R.M.S. program, which provides limited financial assistance for hormonal and oral chemotherapy, pain and antinausea medication, lymphedema supplies, and durable medical equipment for women with breast cancer.

CancerCare operates the AVONCares program for medically underserved women, in partnership with the Avon Foundation. This program provides financial assistance to low-income, under- and uninsured, underserved women throughout the country who need supportive services (transportation, child care, and home care) related to the treatment of breast and cervical cancers.

Candlelighters® Childhood Cancer Foundation (CCCF)
National Office
P.O. Box 498
Kensington, MD 20895-0498
Toll-Free: 800-366-2223, Phone: 301-962-3520, Fax: 301-062-3521
Website: http://www.candlelighters.org

CCCF is a nonprofit organization that provides information, peer support, and advocacy through publications, an information clearinghouse, and a network of local support groups to families of chronically and terminally ill children. The CCCF website contains a list of organizations to which eligible families can apply for financial assistance. This list is available at http://www.candlelighters.org/financialassistance.stm. In addition, some local CCCF affiliates offer financial assistance.

Leukemia and Lymphoma Society (LLS)
1311 Mamaroneck Ave.
White Plains, NY 10605-5221
Toll-Free: 800-955-4572, Phone: 914-949-5213
Website: http://www.leukemia-lymphoma.org
E-mail: infocenter@leukemia-lymphoma.org

LLS offers information and financial aid to patients in significant financial need who have leukemia, non-Hodgkin lymphoma, Hodgkin lymphoma, or multiple myeloma. The LLS's "Patient Financial Aid" web page provides more information about the types of service available, application forms, and eligibility requirements at http://www.leukemia-lymphoma.org/all_page?item_id=4603.

LIVESTRONG ™

P.O. Box 161150
Austin, TX 78716-1150
Toll-Free: 866-235-7205
Phone: 512-236-8820
Website: http://www.livestrong.org

The LIVESTRONG™ Survivor Care partnership between CancerCare and the Lance Armstrong Foundation provides financial assistance to cancer survivors. For patients who are six months post-treatment with no evidence of disease, limited financial assistance is available for transportation to follow-up appointments, medical co-pays, cancer-related medications, and neuropsychological evaluation.

National Patient Travel Center

4620 Haygood Rd., Ste. 1
Virginia Beach, VA 23455
Toll-Free: 800-296-1217
Fax: 800-550-1767
Website: http://www.patienttravel.org
E-mail: info@nationalpatienttravelcenter.org

The National Patient Travel Center provides information about all forms of charitable, long-distance medical air transportation and provides referrals to all appropriate sources of help available in the national charitable medical air transportation network.

NeedyMeds

P.O. Box 219
Gloucester, MA 01931
Website: http://www.needymeds.com

NeedyMeds is a 501(3)(c) nonprofit organization with the mission of helping people who cannot afford medicine or health care costs. The information at NeedyMeds can be obtained anonymously and is free of charge. NeedyMeds is an information source similar to the Yellow Pages; it does not supply medications or financial assistance, but helps people find assistance programs and other available resources.

Patient Advocate Foundation (PAF)

700 Thimble Shoals Boulevard, Suite 200
Newport News, VA 23606
Toll-Free: 800-532-5274
Website: http://www.patientadvocate.org

PAF provides education, legal counseling, and referrals to patients and survivors concerning managed care, insurance, financial issues, job discrimination, and debt crisis matters. The PAF's Co-Pay Relief program provides limited payment assistance for medicine to insured patients who financially and medically qualify. For more information about the Co-Pay Relief program, visit http://www.copays.org, or call toll-free 866-512-3861.

Patient Assistant Programs for Medications

Patient assistance programs are offered by some pharmaceutical manufacturers to help pay for medications. To learn whether a specific drug might be available at reduced cost through such a program, talk with a physician or a medical social worker, or visit the drug manufacturer's website. Most pharmaceutical companies' websites will have a section titled "patient assistance programs."

Ronald McDonald House Charities
One Kroc Drive
Oak Brook, IL 60523
Phone: 630-623-7048
Fax: 630-623-7488
Website: http://www.rmhc.com
E-mail: info@rmhc.org

Ronald McDonald Houses, supported by Ronald McDonald House Charities, provide a "home away from home" for families of seriously ill children receiving treatment at nearby hospitals. Ronald McDonald Houses are temporary residences near the medical facility, where family members can sleep, eat, relax, and find support from other families in similar situations. In return, families are asked to make a donation ranging on average from $5 to $20 per day, but if that isn't possible, their stay is free.

Voluntary Agencies and Service Organizations

Community voluntary agencies and service organizations such as the United Way of America , Salvation Army, Lutheran Social Services, Jewish Social Services, and Catholic Charities may offer help. These organizations are listed in your local phone directory. Some churches and synagogues may provide financial help or services to their members.

Index

Index

Page numbers followed by 'n' indicate a footnote. Page numbers in *italics* indicate a table or illustration.

599

613

Health Reference Series

COMPLETE CATALOG

List price $87 per volume. **School and library price $78 per volume.**

Adolescent Health Sourcebook, 2nd Edition

Basic Consumer Health Information about the Physical, Mental, and Emotional Growth and Development of Adolescents, Including Medical Care, Nutritional and Physical Activity Requirements, Puberty, Sexual Activity, Acne, Tanning, Body Piercing, Common Physical Illnesses and Disorders, Eating Disorders, Attention Deficit Hyperactivity Disorder, Depression, Bullying, Hazing, and Adolescent Injuries Related to Sports, Driving, and Work

Along with Substance Abuse Information about Nicotine, Alcohol, and Drug Use, a Glossary, and Directory of Additional Resources

Edited by Joyce Brennfleck Shannon. 683 pages. 2006. 978-0-7808-0943-7.

"It is written in clear, nontechnical language aimed at general readers. . . . Recommended for public libraries, community colleges, and other agencies serving health care consumers."
— *American Reference Books Annual, 2003*

"Recommended for school and public libraries. Parents and professionals dealing with teens will appreciate the easy-to-follow format and the clearly written text. This could become a 'must have' for every high school teacher." — *E-Streams, Jan '03*

"A good starting point for information related to common medical, mental, and emotional concerns of adolescents." — *School Library Journal, Nov '02*

"This book provides accurate information in an easy to access format. It addresses topics that parents and caregivers might not be aware of and provides practical, useable information."
— *Doody's Health Sciences Book Review Journal, Sep-Oct '02*

"Recommended reference source."
— *Booklist, American Library Association, Sep '02*

AIDS Sourcebook, 3rd Edition

Basic Consumer Health Information about Acquired Immune Deficiency Syndrome (AIDS) and Human Immunodeficiency Virus (HIV) Infection, Including Facts about Transmission, Prevention, Diagnosis, Treatment, Opportunistic Infections, and Other Complications, with a Section for Women and Children, Including Details about Associated Gynecological Concerns, Pregnancy, and Pediatric Care

Along with Updated Statistical Information, Reports on Current Research Initiatives, a Glossary, and Directories of Internet, Hotline, and Other Resources

Edited by Dawn D. Matthews. 664 pages. 2003. 978-0-7808-0631-3.

"The 3rd edition of the *AIDS Sourcebook*, part of Omnigraphics' *Health Reference Series*, is a welcome update. . . . This resource is highly recommended for academic and public libraries."
— *American Reference Books Annual, 2004*

"Excellent sourcebook. This continues to be a highly recommended book. There is no other book that provides as much information as this book provides."
— *AIDS Book Review Journal, Dec-Jan '00*

"Recommended reference source."
— *Booklist, American Library Association, Dec '99*

Alcoholism Sourcebook, 2nd Edition

Basic Consumer Health Information about Alcohol Use, Abuse, and Dependence, Featuring Facts about the Physical, Mental, and Social Health Effects of Alcohol Addiction, Including Alcoholic Liver Disease, Pancreatic Disease, Cardiovascular Disease, Neurological Disorders, and the Effects of Drinking during Pregnancy

Along with Information about Alcohol Treatment, Medications, and Recovery Programs, in Addition to Tips for Reducing the Prevalence of Underage Drinking, Statistics about Alcohol Use, a Glossary of Related Terms, and Directories of Resources for More Help and Information

Edited by Amy L. Sutton. 653 pages. 2006. 978-0-7808-0942-0.

"This title is one of the few reference works on alcoholism for general readers. For some readers this will be a welcome complement to the many self-help books on the market. Recommended for collections serving general readers and consumer health collections."
— *E-Streams, Mar '01*

"This book is an excellent choice for public and academic libraries."
— *American Reference Books Annual, 2001*

"Recommended reference source."
— *Booklist, American Library Association, Dec '00*

"Presents a wealth of information on alcohol use and abuse and its effects on the body and mind, treatment, and prevention." — *SciTech Book News, Dec '00*

"Important new health guide which packs in the latest consumer information about the problems of alcoholism." — *Reviewer's Bookwatch, Nov '00*

SEE ALSO *Drug Abuse Sourcebook*

Allergies Sourcebook, 3rd Edition

Basic Consumer Health Information about Allergic Disorders, Such as Anaphylaxis, Hives, Eczema, Rhinitis, Sinusitis, and Conjunctivitis, and Their Triggers, Including Pollen, Mold, Dust Mites, Animal Dander, Insects, Chemicals, Food, Food Additives, and Medications;

Along with Advice about the Diagnosis and Treatment of Allergy Symptoms, a Glossary of Related Terms, a Directory of Resources for Help and Information, and Suggestions for Additional Reading

Edited by Amy L. Sutton. 598 pages. 2007. 978-0-7808-0950-5.

"This book brings a great deal of useful material together. . . . This is an excellent addition to public and consumer health library collections."
— *American Reference Books Annual, 2003*

"This second edition would be useful to laypersons with little or advanced knowledge of the subject matter. This book would also serve as a resource for nursing and other health care professions students. It would be useful in public, academic, and hospital libraries with consumer health collections." — *E-Streams, Jul '02*

∎

Alternative Medicine Sourcebook

SEE *Complementary & Alternative Medicine Sourcebook*

∎

Alzheimer's Disease Sourcebook, 3rd Edition

Basic Consumer Health Information about Alzheimer's Disease, Other Dementias, and Related Disorders, Including Multi-Infarct Dementia, AIDS Dementia Complex, Dementia with Lewy Bodies, Huntington's Disease, Wernicke-Korsakoff Syndrome (Alcohol-Related Dementia), Delirium, and Confusional States

Along with Information for People Newly Diagnosed with Alzheimer's Disease and Caregivers, Reports Detailing Current Research Efforts in Prevention, Diagnosis, and Treatment, Facts about Long-Term Care Issues, and Listings of Sources for Additional Information

Edited by Karen Bellenir. 645 pages. 2003. 978-0-7808-0666-5.

"This very informative and valuable tool will be a great addition to any library serving consumers, students and health care workers."
— *American Reference Books Annual, 2004*

"This is a valuable resource for people affected by dementias such as Alzheimer's. It is easy to navigate and includes important information and resources."
— *Doody's Review Service, Feb '04*

"Recommended reference source."
— *Booklist, American Library Association, Oct '99*

SEE ALSO *Brain Disorders Sourcebook*

Arthritis Sourcebook, 2nd Edition

Basic Consumer Health Information about Osteoarthritis, Rheumatoid Arthritis, Other Rheumatic Disorders, Infectious Forms of Arthritis, and Diseases with Symptoms Linked to Arthritis, Featuring Facts about Diagnosis, Pain Management, and Surgical Therapies

Along with Coping Strategies, Research Updates, a Glossary, and Resources for Additional Help and Information

Edited by Amy L. Sutton. 593 pages. 2004. 978-0-7808-0667-2.

"This easy-to-read volume is recommended for consumer health collections within public or academic libraries." — *E-Streams, May '05*

"As expected, this updated edition continues the excellent reputation of this series in providing sound, usable health information. . . . Highly recommended."
— *American Reference Books Annual, 2005*

"Excellent reference." — *The Bookwatch, Jan '05*

∎

Asthma Sourcebook, 2nd Edition

Basic Consumer Health Information about the Causes, Symptoms, Diagnosis, and Treatment of Asthma in Infants, Children, Teenagers, and Adults, Including Facts about Different Types of Asthma, Common Co-Occurring Conditions, Asthma Management Plans, Triggers, Medications, and Medication Delivery Devices

Along with Asthma Statistics, Research Updates, a Glossary, a Directory of Asthma-Related Resources, and More

Edited by Karen Bellenir. 609 pages. 2006. 978-0-7808-0866-9.

"A worthwhile reference acquisition for public libraries and academic medical libraries whose readers desire a quick introduction to the wide range of asthma information." — *Choice, Association of College & Research Libraries, Jun '01*

"Recommended reference source."
— *Booklist, American Library Association, Feb '01*

"Highly recommended." — *The Bookwatch, Jan '01*

"There is much good information for patients and their families who deal with asthma daily."
— *American Medical Writers Association Journal, Winter '01*

"This informative text is recommended for consumer health collections in public, secondary school, and community college libraries and the libraries of universities with a large undergraduate population."
— *American Reference Books Annual, 2001*

∎

Attention Deficit Disorder Sourcebook

Basic Consumer Health Information about Attention Deficit/Hyperactivity Disorder in Children and Adults,

Including Facts about Causes, Symptoms, Diagnostic Criteria, and Treatment Options Such as Medications, Behavior Therapy, Coaching, and Homeopathy

Along with Reports on Current Research Initiatives, Legal Issues, and Government Regulations, and Featuring a Glossary of Related Terms, Internet Resources, and a List of Additional Reading Material

Edited by Dawn D. Matthews. 470 pages. 2002. 978-0-7808-0624-5.

"Recommended reference source."
— Booklist, American Library Association, Jan '03

"This book is recommended for all school libraries and the reference or consumer health sections of public libraries." — American Reference Books Annual, 2003

■

Back & Neck Sourcebook, 2nd Edition

Basic Consumer Health Information about Spinal Pain, Spinal Cord Injuries, and Related Disorders, Such as Degenerative Disk Disease, Osteoarthritis, Scoliosis, Sciatica, Spina Bifida, and Spinal Stenosis, and Featuring Facts about Maintaining Spinal Health, Self-Care, Pain Management, Rehabilitative Care, Chiropractic Care, Spinal Surgeries, and Complementary Therapies

Along with Suggestions for Preventing Back and Neck Pain, a Glossary of Related Terms, and a Directory of Resources

Edited by Amy L. Sutton. 633 pages. 2004. 978-0-7808-0738-9.

"Recommended . . . an easy to use, comprehensive medical reference book." — E-Streams, Sep '05

"The strength of this work is its basic, easy-to-read format. Recommended." — Reference and User Services Quarterly, American Library Association, Winter '97

■

Blood & Circulatory Disorders Sourcebook, 2nd Edition

Basic Consumer Health Information about the Blood and Circulatory System and Related Disorders, Such as Anemia and Other Hemoglobin Diseases, Cancer of the Blood and Associated Bone Marrow Disorders, Clotting and Bleeding Problems, and Conditions That Affect the Veins, Blood Vessels, and Arteries, Including Facts about the Donation and Transplantation of Bone Marrow, Stem Cells, and Blood and Tips for Keeping the Blood and Circulatory System Healthy

Along with a Glossary of Related Terms and Resources for Additional Help and Information

Edited by Amy L. Sutton. 659 pages. 2005. 978-0-7808-0746-4.

"Highly recommended pick for basic consumer health reference holdings at all levels."
— The Bookwatch, Aug '05

"Recommended reference source."
— Booklist, American Library Association, Feb '99

"An important reference sourcebook written in simple language for everyday, non-technical users. "
— Reviewer's Bookwatch, Jan '99

■

Brain Disorders Sourcebook, 2nd Edition

Basic Consumer Health Information about Acquired and Traumatic Brain Injuries, Infections of the Brain, Epilepsy and Seizure Disorders, Cerebral Palsy, and Degenerative Neurological Disorders, Including Amyotrophic Lateral Sclerosis (ALS), Dementias, Multiple Sclerosis, and More

Along with Information on the Brain's Structure and Function, Treatment and Rehabilitation Options, Reports on Current Research Initiatives, a Glossary of Terms Related to Brain Disorders and Injuries, and a Directory of Sources for Further Help and Information

Edited by Sandra J. Judd. 625 pages. 2005. 978-0-7808-0744-0.

"Highly recommended pick for basic consumer health reference holdings at all levels."
— The Bookwatch, Aug '05

"Belongs on the shelves of any library with a consumer health collection." — E-Streams, Mar '00

"Recommended reference source."
— Booklist, American Library Association, Oct '99

SEE ALSO Alzheimer's Disease Sourcebook

■

Breast Cancer Sourcebook, 2nd Edition

Basic Consumer Health Information about Breast Cancer, Including Facts about Risk Factors, Prevention, Screening and Diagnostic Methods, Treatment Options, Complementary and Alternative Therapies, Post-Treatment Concerns, Clinical Trials, Special Risk Populations, and New Developments in Breast Cancer Research

Along with Breast Cancer Statistics, a Glossary of Related Terms, and a Directory of Resources for Additional Help and Information

Edited by Sandra J. Judd. 595 pages. 2004. 978-0-7808-0668-9.

"This book will be an excellent addition to public, community college, medical, and academic libraries."
— American Reference Books Annual, 2006

"It would be a useful reference book in a library or on loan to women in a support group."
— Cancer Forum, Mar '03

"Recommended reference source."
— Booklist, American Library Association, Jan '02

"This reference source is highly recommended. It is quite informative, comprehensive and detailed in nature, and yet it offers practical advice in easy-to-read language. It could be thought of as the 'bible' of breast cancer for the consumer." — *E-Streams, Jan '02*

"From the pros and cons of different screening methods and results to treatment options, *Breast Cancer Sourcebook* provides the latest information on the subject." — *Library Bookwatch, Dec '01*

"This thoroughgoing, very readable reference covers all aspects of breast health and cancer.... Readers will find much to consider here. Recommended for all public and patient health collections." — *Library Journal, Sep '01*

SEE ALSO *Cancer Sourcebook for Women, Women's Health Concerns Sourcebook*

Breastfeeding Sourcebook

Basic Consumer Health Information about the Benefits of Breastmilk, Preparing to Breastfeed, Breastfeeding as a Baby Grows, Nutrition, and More, Including Information on Special Situations and Concerns Such as Mastitis, Illness, Medications, Allergies, Multiple Births, Prematurity, Special Needs, and Adoption

Along with a Glossary and Resources for Additional Help and Information

Edited by Jenni Lynn Colson. 388 pages. 2002. 978-0-7808-0332-9.

"Particularly useful is the information about professional lactation services and chapters on breastfeeding when returning to work.... *Breastfeeding Sourcebook* will be useful for public libraries, consumer health libraries, and technical schools offering nurse assistant training, especially in areas where Internet access is problematic." — *American Reference Books Annual, 2003*

SEE ALSO *Pregnancy & Birth Sourcebook*

Burns Sourcebook

Basic Consumer Health Information about Various Types of Burns and Scalds, Including Flame, Heat, Cold, Electrical, Chemical, and Sun Burns

Along with Information on Short-Term and Long-Term Treatments, Tissue Reconstruction, Plastic Surgery, Prevention Suggestions, and First Aid

Edited by Allan R. Cook. 604 pages. 1999. 978-0-7808-0204-9.

"This is an exceptional addition to the series and is highly recommended for all consumer health collections, hospital libraries, and academic medical centers." — *E-Streams, Mar '00*

"This key reference guide is an invaluable addition to all health care and public libraries in confronting this ongoing health issue." —*American Reference Books Annual, 2000*

"Recommended reference source." —*Booklist, American Library Association, Dec '99*

SEE ALSO *Dermatological Disorders Sourcebook*

Cancer Sourcebook, 5th Edition

Basic Consumer Health Information about Major Forms and Stages of Cancer, Featuring Facts about Head and Neck Cancers, Lung Cancers, Gastrointestinal Cancers, Genitourinary Cancers, Lymphomas, Blood Cell Cancers, Endocrine Cancers, Skin Cancers, Bone Cancers, Metastatic Cancers, and More

Along with Facts about Cancer Treatments, Cancer Risks and Prevention, a Glossary of Related Terms, Statistical Data, and a Directory of Resources for Additional Information

Edited by Karen Bellenir. 1,133 pages. 2007. 978-0-7808-0947-5.

"With cancer being the second leading cause of death for Americans, a prodigious work such as this one, which locates centrally so much cancer-related information, is clearly an asset to this nation's citizens and others." —*Journal of the National Medical Association, 2004*

"This title is recommended for health sciences and public libraries with consumer health collections." —*E-Streams, Feb '01*

"... can be effectively used by cancer patients and their families who are looking for answers in a language they can understand. Public and hospital libraries should have it on their shelves." —*American Reference Books Annual, 2001*

"Recommended reference source." —*Booklist, American Library Association, Dec '00*

SEE ALSO *Breast Cancer Sourcebook, Cancer Sourcebook for Women, Pediatric Cancer Sourcebook, Prostate Cancer Sourcebook*

Cancer Sourcebook for Women, 3rd Edition

Basic Consumer Health Information about Leading Causes of Cancer in Women, Featuring Facts about Gynecologic Cancers and Related Concerns, Such as Breast Cancer, Cervical Cancer, Endometrial Cancer, Uterine Sarcoma, Vaginal Cancer, Vulvar Cancer, and Common Non-Cancerous Gynecologic Conditions, in Addition to Facts about Lung Cancer, Colorectal Cancer, and Thyroid Cancer in Women

Along with Information about Cancer Risk Factors, Screening and Prevention, Treatment Options, and Tips on Coping with Life after Cancer Treatment, a Glossary of Cancer Terms, and a Directory of Resources for Additional Help and Information

Edited by Amy L. Sutton. 715 pages. 2006. 978-0-7808-0867-6.

"An excellent addition to collections in public, consumer health, and women's health libraries." —*American Reference Books Annual, 2003*

"Overall, the information is excellent, and complex topics are clearly explained. As a reference book for the consumer it is a valuable resource to assist them to make informed decisions about cancer and its treatments." — *Cancer Forum, Nov '02*

■

Cancer Survivorship Sourcebook

Basic Consumer Health Information about the Physical, Educational, Emotional, Social, and Financial Needs of Cancer Patients from Diagnosis, through Cancer Treatment, and Beyond, Including Facts about Researching Specific Types of Cancer and Learning about Clinical Trials and Treatment Options, and Featuring Tips for Coping with the Side Effects of Cancer Treatments and Adjusting to Life after Cancer Treatment Concludes

Along with Suggestions for Caregivers, Friends, and Family Members of Cancer Patients, a Glossary of Cancer Care Terms, and Directories of Related Resources

Edited by Karen Bellenir. 6561 pages. 2007. 978-0-7808-0985-7.

■

Cardiovascular Diseases & Disorders Sourcebook, 3rd Edition

Basic Consumer Health Information about Heart and Vascular Diseases and Disorders, Such as Angina, Heart Attacks, Arrhythmias, Cardiomyopathy, Valve Disease, Atherosclerosis, and Aneurysms, with Information about Managing Cardiovascular Risk Factors and Maintaining Heart Health, Medications and Procedures Used to Treat Cardiovascular Disorders, and Concerns of Special Significance to Women

Along with Reports on Current Research Initiatives, a Glossary of Related Medical Terms, and a Directory of Sources for Further Help and Information

Edited by Sandra J. Judd. 713 pages. 2005. 978-0-7808-0739-6.

■

Caregiving Sourcebook

Basic Consumer Health Information for Caregivers, Including a Profile of Caregivers, Caregiving Responsibilities and Concerns, Tips for Specific Conditions, Care Environments, and the Effects of Caregiving

Along with Facts about Legal Issues, Financial Information, and Future Planning, a Glossary, and a Listing of Additional Resources

Edited by Joyce Brennfleck Shannon. 600 pages. 2001. 978-0-7808-0331-2.

■

Child Abuse Sourcebook

Basic Consumer Health Information about the Physical, Sexual, and Emotional Abuse of Children, with Additional Facts about Neglect, Munchausen Syndrome by Proxy (MSBP), Shaken Baby Syndrome, and Controversial Issues Related to Child Abuse, Such as Withholding Medical Care, Corporal Punishment, and Child Maltreatment in Youth Sports, and Featuring Facts about Child Protective Services, Foster Care, Adoption, Parenting Challenges, and Other Abuse Prevention Efforts

Along with a Glossary of Related Terms and Resources for Additional Help and Information

Edited by Dawn D. Matthews. 620 pages. 2004. 978-0-7808-0705-1.

Childhood Diseases & Disorders Sourcebook

Basic Consumer Health Information about Medical Problems Often Encountered in Pre-Adolescent Children, Including Respiratory Tract Ailments, Ear Infections, Sore Throats, Disorders of the Skin and Scalp, Digestive and Genitourinary Diseases, Infectious Diseases, Inflammatory Disorders, Chronic Physical and Developmental Disorders, Allergies, and More

Along with Information about Diagnostic Tests, Common Childhood Surgeries, and Frequently Used Medications, with a Glossary of Important Terms and Resource Directory

Edited by Chad T. Kimball. 662 pages. 2003. 978-0-7808-0458-6.

"This is an excellent book for new parents and should be included in all health care and public libraries."
— *American Reference Books Annual, 2004*

SEE ALSO: *Healthy Children Sourcebook*

■

Colds, Flu & Other Common Ailments Sourcebook

Basic Consumer Health Information about Common Ailments and Injuries, Including Colds, Coughs, the Flu, Sinus Problems, Headaches, Fever, Nausea and Vomiting, Menstrual Cramps, Diarrhea, Constipation, Hemorrhoids, Back Pain, Dandruff, Dry and Itchy Skin, Cuts, Scrapes, Sprains, Bruises, and More

Along with Information about Prevention, Self-Care, Choosing a Doctor, Over-the-Counter Medications, Folk Remedies, and Alternative Therapies, and Including a Glossary of Important Terms and a Directory of Resources for Further Help and Information

Edited by Chad T. Kimball. 638 pages. 2001. 978-0-7808-0435-7.

"A good starting point for research on common illnesses. It will be a useful addition to public and consumer health library collections."
— *American Reference Books Annual, 2002*

"Will prove valuable to any library seeking to maintain a current, comprehensive reference collection of health resources. . . . Excellent reference."
— *The Bookwatch, Aug '01*

"Recommended reference source."
— *Booklist, American Library Association, Jul '01*

■

Communication Disorders Sourcebook

Basic Information about Deafness and Hearing Loss, Speech and Language Disorders, Voice Disorders, Balance and Vestibular Disorders, and Disorders of Smell, Taste, and Touch

Edited by Linda M. Ross. 533 pages. 1996. 978-0-7808-0077-9.

"This is skillfully edited and is a welcome resource for the layperson. It should be found in every public and medical library." — *Booklist Health Sciences Supplement, American Library Association, Oct '97*

■

Complementary & Alternative Medicine Sourcebook, 3rd Edition

Basic Consumer Health Information about Complementary and Alternative Medical Therapies, Including Acupuncture, Ayurveda, Traditional Chinese Medicine, Herbal Medicine, Homeopathy, Naturopathy, Biofeedback, Hypnotherapy, Yoga, Art Therapy, Aromatherapy, Clinical Nutrition, Vitamin and Mineral Supplements, Chiropractic, Massage, Reflexology, Crystal Therapy, Therapeutic Touch, and More

Along with Facts about Alternative and Complementary Treatments for Specific Conditions Such as Cancer, Diabetes, Osteoarthritis, Chronic Pain, Menopause, Gastrointestinal Disorders, Headaches, and Mental Illness, a Glossary, and a Resource List for Additional Help and Information

Edited by Sandra J. Judd. 657 pages. 2006. 978-0-7808-0864-5.

"Recommended for public, high school, and academic libraries that have consumer health collections. Hospital libraries that also serve the public will find this to be a useful resource." — *E-Streams, Feb '03*

"Recommended reference source."
— *Booklist, American Library Association, Jan '03*

"An important alternate health reference."
— *MBR Bookwatch, Oct '02*

"A great addition to the reference collection of every type of library." — *American Reference Books Annual, 2000*

■

Congenital Disorders Sourcebook, 2nd Edition

Basic Consumer Health Information about Non-hereditary Birth Defects and Disorders Related to Prematurity, Gestational Injuries, Congenital Infections, and Birth Complications, Including Heart Defects, Hydrocephalus, Spina Bifida, Cleft Lip and Palate, Cerebral Palsy, and More

Along with Facts about the Prevention of Birth Defects, Fetal Surgery and Other Treatment Options, Research Initiatives, a Glossary of Related Terms, and Resources for Additional Information and Support

Edited by Sandra J. Judd. 647 pages. 2006. 978-0-7808-0945-1.

"Recommended reference source."
— *Booklist, American Library Association, Oct '97*

SEE ALSO *Pregnancy & Birth Sourcebook*

■

Contagious Diseases Sourcebook

Basic Consumer Health Information about Infectious Diseases Spread by Person-to-Person Contact through

Direct Touch, Airborne Transmission, Sexual Contact, or Contact with Blood or Other Body Fluids, Including Hepatitis, Herpes, Influenza, Lice, Measles, Mumps, Pinworm, Ringworm, Severe Acute Respiratory Syndrome (SARS), Streptococcal Infections, Tuberculosis, and Others

Along with Facts about Disease Transmission, Antimicrobial Resistance, and Vaccines, with a Glossary and Directories of Resources for More Information

Edited by Karen Bellenir. 643 pages. 2004. 978-0-7808-0736-5.

"This easy-to-read volume is recommended for consumer health collections within public or academic libraries." —E-Streams, May '05

"This informative book is highly recommended for public libraries, consumer health collections, and secondary schools and undergraduate libraries."
—American Reference Books Annual, 2005

"Excellent reference." —The Bookwatch, Jan '05

Death & Dying Sourcebook, 2nd Edition

Basic Consumer Health Information about End-of-Life Care and Related Perspectives and Ethical Issues, Including End-of-Life Symptoms and Treatments, Pain Management, Quality-of-Life Concerns, the Use of Life Support, Patients' Rights and Privacy Issues, Advance Directives, Physician-Assisted Suicide, Caregiving, Organ and Tissue Donation, Autopsies, Funeral Arrangements, and Grief

Along with Statistical Data, Information about the Leading Causes of Death, a Glossary, and Directories of Support Groups and Other Resources

Edited by Joyce Brennfleck Shannon. 653 pages. 2006. 978-0-7808-0871-3.

"Public libraries, medical libraries, and academic libraries will all find this sourcebook a useful addition to their collections."
—American Reference Books Annual, 2001

"An extremely useful resource for those concerned with death and dying in the United States."
—Respiratory Care, Nov '00

"Recommended reference source."
—Booklist, American Library Association, Aug '00

"This book is a definite must for all those involved in end-of-life care." —Doody's Review Service, 2000

Dental Care & Oral Health Sourcebook, 2nd Edition

Basic Consumer Health Information about Dental Care, Including Oral Hygiene, Dental Visits, Pain Management, Cavities, Crowns, Bridges, Dental Implants, and Fillings, and Other Oral Health Concerns, Such as Gum Disease, Bad Breath, Dry Mouth, Genetic and Developmental Abnormalities, Oral Cancers, Orthodontics, and Temporomandibular Disorders

Along with Updates on Current Research in Oral Health, a Glossary, a Directory of Dental and Oral Health Organizations, and Resources for People with Dental and Oral Health Disorders

Edited by Amy L. Sutton. 609 pages. 2003. 978-0-7808-0634-4.

"This book could serve as a turning point in the battle to educate consumers in issues concerning oral health."
—American Reference Books Annual, 2004

"Unique source which will fill a gap in dental sources for patients and the lay public. A valuable reference tool even in a library with thousands of books on dentistry. Comprehensive, clear, inexpensive, and easy to read and use. It fills an enormous gap in the health care literature." —Reference & User Services Quarterly, American Library Association, Summer '98

"Recommended reference source."
—Booklist, American Library Association, Dec '97

Depression Sourcebook

Basic Consumer Health Information about Unipolar Depression, Bipolar Disorder, Postpartum Depression, Seasonal Affective Disorder, and Other Types of Depression in Children, Adolescents, Women, Men, the Elderly, and Other Selected Populations

Along with Facts about Causes, Risk Factors, Diagnostic Criteria, Treatment Options, Coping Strategies, Suicide Prevention, a Glossary, and a Directory of Sources for Additional Help and Information

Edited by Karen Bellenir. 602 pages. 2002. 978-0-7808-0611-5.

"*Depression Sourcebook* is of a very high standard. Its purpose, which is to serve as a reference source to the lay reader, is very well served."
—Journal of the National Medical Association, 2004

"Invaluable reference for public and school library collections alike." —Library Bookwatch, Apr '03

"Recommended for purchase."
—American Reference Books Annual, 2003

Dermatological Disorders Sourcebook, 2nd Edition

Basic Consumer Health Information about Conditions and Disorders Affecting the Skin, Hair, and Nails, Such as Acne, Rosacea, Rashes, Dermatitis, Pigmentation Disorders, Birthmarks, Skin Cancer, Skin Injuries, Psoriasis, Scleroderma, and Hair Loss, Including Facts about Medications and Treatments for Dermatological Disorders and Tips for Maintaining Healthy Skin, Hair, and Nails

Along with Information about How Aging Affects the Skin, a Glossary of Related Terms, and a Directory of Resources for Additional Help and Information

Edited by Amy L. Sutton. 645 pages. 2005. 978-0-7808-0795-2.

629

"... comprehensive, easily read reference book."
—*Doody's Health Sciences Book Reviews, Oct '97*

SEE ALSO *Burns Sourcebook*

■

Diabetes Sourcebook, 3rd Edition

Basic Consumer Health Information about Type 1 Diabetes (Insulin-Dependent or Juvenile-Onset Diabetes), Type 2 Diabetes (Noninsulin-Dependent or Adult-Onset Diabetes), Gestational Diabetes, Impaired Glucose Tolerance (IGT), and Related Complications, Such as Amputation, Eye Disease, Gum Disease, Nerve Damage, and End-Stage Renal Disease, Including Facts about Insulin, Oral Diabetes Medications, Blood Sugar Testing, and the Role of Exercise and Nutrition in the Control of Diabetes

Along with a Glossary and Resources for Further Help and Information

Edited by Dawn D. Matthews. 622 pages. 2003. 978-0-7808-0629-0.

"This edition is even more helpful than earlier versions. . . . It is a truly valuable tool for anyone seeking readable and authoritative information on diabetes."
—*American Reference Books Annual, 2004*

"An invaluable reference." —*Library Journal, May '00*

Selected as one of the 250 "Best Health Sciences Books of 1999." —*Doody's Rating Service, Mar-Apr '00*

"Provides useful information for the general public."
—*Healthlines, University of Michigan Health Management Research Center, Sep/Oct '99*

"... provides reliable mainstream medical information . . . belongs on the shelves of any library with a consumer health collection." —*E-Streams, Sep '99*

"Recommended reference source."
—*Booklist, American Library Association, Feb '99*

■

Diet & Nutrition Sourcebook, 3rd Edition

Basic Consumer Health Information about Dietary Guidelines and the Food Guidance System, Recommended Daily Nutrient Intakes, Serving Proportions, Weight Control, Vitamins and Supplements, Nutrition Issues for Different Life Stages and Lifestyles, and the Needs of People with Specific Medical Concerns, Including Cancer, Celiac Disease, Diabetes, Eating Disorders, Food Allergies, and Cardiovascular Disease

Along with Facts about Federal Nutrition Support Programs, a Glossary of Nutrition and Dietary Terms, and Directories of Additional Resources for More Information about Nutrition

Edited by Joyce Brennfleck Shannon. 633 pages. 2006. 978-0-7808-0800-3.

"This book is an excellent source of basic diet and nutrition information." —*Booklist Health Sciences Supplement, American Library Association, Dec '00*

"This reference document should be in any public library, but it would be a very good guide for beginning students in the health sciences. If the other books in this publisher's series are as good as this, they should all be in the health sciences collections."
—*American Reference Books Annual, 2000*

"This book is an excellent general nutrition reference for consumers who desire to take an active role in their health care for prevention. Consumers of all ages who select this book can feel confident they are receiving current and accurate information." —*Journal of Nutrition for the Elderly, Vol. 19, No. 4, 2000*

SEE ALSO *Digestive Diseases & Disorders Sourcebook, Eating Disorders Sourcebook, Gastrointestinal Diseases & Disorders Sourcebook, Vegetarian Sourcebook*

■

Digestive Diseases & Disorders Sourcebook

Basic Consumer Health Information about Diseases and Disorders that Impact the Upper and Lower Digestive System, Including Celiac Disease, Constipation, Crohn's Disease, Cyclic Vomiting Syndrome, Diarrhea, Diverticulosis and Diverticulitis, Gallstones, Heartburn, Hemorrhoids, Hernias, Indigestion (Dyspepsia), Irritable Bowel Syndrome, Lactose Intolerance, Ulcers, and More

Along with Information about Medications and Other Treatments, Tips for Maintaining a Healthy Digestive Tract, a Glossary, and Directory of Digestive Diseases Organizations

Edited by Karen Bellenir. 335 pages. 2000. 978-0-7808-0327-5.

"This title would be an excellent addition to all public or patient-research libraries."
—*American Reference Books Annual, 2001*

"This title is recommended for public, hospital, and health sciences libraries with consumer health collections." —*E-Streams, Jul-Aug '00*

"Recommended reference source."
—*Booklist, American Library Association, May '00*

SEE ALSO *Eating Disorders Sourcebook, Gastrointestinal Diseases & Disorders Sourcebook*

■

Disabilities Sourcebook

Basic Consumer Health Information about Physical and Psychiatric Disabilities, Including Descriptions of Major Causes of Disability, Assistive and Adaptive Aids, Workplace Issues, and Accessibility Concerns

Along with Information about the Americans with Disabilities Act, a Glossary, and Resources for Additional Help and Information

Edited by Dawn D. Matthews. 616 pages. 2000. 978-0-7808-0389-3.

"It is a must for libraries with a consumer health section." —*American Reference Books Annual, 2002*

"A much needed addition to the Omnigraphics *Health Reference Series*. A current reference work to provide people with disabilities, their families, caregivers or those who work with them, a broad range of information in one volume, has not been available until now. . . . It is recommended for all public and academic library reference collections." —*E-Streams, May '01*

"An excellent source book in easy-to-read format covering many current topics; highly recommended for all libraries." —*Choice, Association of College & Research Libraries, Jan '01*

"Recommended reference source." —*Booklist, American Library Association, Jul '00*

■

Domestic Violence Sourcebook, 2nd Edition

Basic Consumer Health Information about the Causes and Consequences of Abusive Relationships, Including Physical Violence, Sexual Assault, Battery, Stalking, and Emotional Abuse, and Facts about the Effects of Violence on Women, Men, Young Adults, and the Elderly, with Reports about Domestic Violence in Selected Populations, and Featuring Facts about Medical Care, Victim Assistance and Protection, Prevention Strategies, Mental Health Services, and Legal Issues

Along with a Glossary of Related Terms and Resources for Additional Help and Information

Edited by Dawn D. Matthews. 628 pages. 2004. 978-0-7808-0669-6.

"Educators, clergy, medical professionals, police, and victims and their families will benefit from this realistic and easy-to-understand resource." —*American Reference Books Annual, 2005*

"Recommended for all collections supporting consumer health information. It should also be considered for any collection needing general, readable information on domestic violence." —*E-Streams, Jan '05*

"This sourcebook complements other books in its field, providing a one-stop resource . . . Recommended." —*Choice, Association of College & Research Libraries, Jan '05*

"Interested lay persons should find the book extremely beneficial. . . . A copy of *Domestic Violence and Child Abuse Sourcebook* should be in every public library in the United States." —*Social Science & Medicine, No. 56, 2003*

"This is important information. The Web has many resources but this sourcebook fills an important societal need. I am not aware of any other resources of this type." —*Doody's Review Service, Sep '01*

"Recommended reference source." —*Booklist, American Library Association, Apr '01*

"Important pick for college-level health reference libraries." —*The Bookwatch, Mar '01*

"Because this problem is so widespread and because this book includes a lot of issues within one volume, this work is recommended for all public libraries." —*American Reference Books Annual, 2001*

SEE ALSO Child Abuse Sourcebook

■

Drug Abuse Sourcebook, 2nd Edition

Basic Consumer Health Information about Illicit Substances of Abuse and the Misuse of Prescription and Over-the-Counter Medications, Including Depressants, Hallucinogens, Inhalants, Marijuana, Stimulants, and Anabolic Steroids

Along with Facts about Related Health Risks, Treatment Programs, Prevention Programs, a Glossary of Abuse and Addiction Terms, a Glossary of Drug-Related Street Terms, and a Directory of Resources for More Information

Edited by Catherine Ginther. 607 pages. 2004. 978-0-7808-0740-2.

"Commendable for organizing useful, normally scattered government and association-produced data into a logical sequence." —*American Reference Books Annual, 2006*

"This easy-to-read volume is recommended for consumer health collections within public or academic libraries." —*E-Streams, Sep '05*

"An excellent library reference." —*The Bookwatch, May '05*

"Containing a wealth of information, this book will be useful to the college student just beginning to explore the topic of substance abuse. This resource belongs in libraries that serve a lower-division undergraduate or community college clientele as well as the general public." —*Choice, Association of College & Research Libraries, Jun '01*

"Recommended reference source." —*Booklist, American Library Association, Feb '01*

SEE ALSO Alcoholism Sourcebook

■

Ear, Nose & Throat Disorders Sourcebook, 2nd Edition

Basic Consumer Health Information about Disorders of the Ears, Hearing Loss, Vestibular Disorders, Nasal and Sinus Problems, Throat and Vocal Cord Disorders, and Otolaryngologic Cancers, Including Facts about Ear Infections and Injuries, Genetic and Congenital Deafness, Sensorineural Hearing Disorders, Tinnitus, Vertigo, Ménière Disease, Rhinitis, Sinusitis, Snoring, Sore Throats, Hoarseness, and More

Along with Reports on Current Research Initiatives, a Glossary of Related Medical Terms, and a Directory of Sources for Further Help and Information

Edited by Sandra J. Judd. 659 pages. 2006. 978-0-7808-0872-0.

"Overall, this sourcebook is helpful for the consumer seeking information on ENT issues. It is recommended for public libraries."
— *American Reference Books Annual, 1999*

"Recommended reference source."
— *Booklist, American Library Association, Dec '98*

Eating Disorders Sourcebook, 2nd Edition

Basic Consumer Health Information about Anorexia Nervosa, Bulimia Nervosa, Binge Eating, Compulsive Exercise, Female Athlete Triad, and Other Eating Disorders, Including Facts about Body Image and Other Cultural and Age-Related Risk Factors, Prevention Efforts, Adverse Health Effects, Treatment Options, and the Recovery Process

Along with Guidelines for Healthy Weight Control, a Glossary, and Directories of Additional Resources

Edited by Joyce Brennfleck Shannon. 585 pages. 2007. 978-0-7808-0948-2.

"Recommended for health science libraries that are open to the public, as well as hospital libraries. This book is a good resource for the consumer who is concerned about eating disorders." — *E-Streams, Mar '02*

"This volume is another convenient collection of excerpted articles. Recommended for school and public library patrons; lower-division undergraduates; and two-year technical program students."
— *Choice, Association of College & Research Libraries, Jan '02*

"Recommended reference source."
— *Booklist, American Library Association, Oct '01*

SEE ALSO *Diet & Nutrition Sourcebook, Digestive Diseases & Disorders Sourcebook, Gastrointestinal Diseases & Disorders Sourcebook*

Emergency Medical Services Sourcebook

Basic Consumer Health Information about Preventing, Preparing for, and Managing Emergency Situations, When and Who to Call for Help, What to Expect in the Emergency Room, the Emergency Medical Team, Patient Issues, and Current Topics in Emergency Medicine

Along with Statistical Data, a Glossary, and Sources of Additional Help and Information

Edited by Jenni Lynn Colson. 494 pages. 2002. 978-0-7808-0420-3.

"Handy and convenient for home, public, school, and college libraries. Recommended."
— *Choice, Association of College & Research Libraries, Apr '03*

"This reference can provide the consumer with answers to most questions about emergency care in the United States, or it will direct them to a resource where the answer can be found."
— *American Reference Books Annual, 2003*

"Recommended reference source."
— *Booklist, American Library Association, Feb '03*

Endocrine & Metabolic Disorders Sourcebook

Basic Information for the Layperson about Pancreatic and Insulin-Related Disorders Such as Pancreatitis, Diabetes, and Hypoglycemia; Adrenal Gland Disorders Such as Cushing's Syndrome, Addison's Disease, and Congenital Adrenal Hyperplasia; Pituitary Gland Disorders Such as Growth Hormone Deficiency, Acromegaly, and Pituitary Tumors; Thyroid Disorders Such as Hypothyroidism, Graves' Disease, Hashimoto's Disease, and Goiter; Hyperparathyroidism; and Other Diseases and Syndromes of Hormone Imbalance or Metabolic Dysfunction

Along with Reports on Current Research Initiatives

Edited by Linda M. Shin. 574 pages. 1998. 978-0-7808-0207-0.

"Omnigraphics has produced another needed resource for health information consumers."
— *American Reference Books Annual, 2000*

"Recommended reference source."
— *Booklist, American Library Association, Dec '98*

Environmental Health Sourcebook, 2nd Edition

Basic Consumer Health Information about the Environment and Its Effect on Human Health, Including the Effects of Air Pollution, Water Pollution, Hazardous Chemicals, Food Hazards, Radiation Hazards, Biological Agents, Household Hazards, Such as Radon, Asbestos, Carbon Monoxide, and Mold, and Information about Associated Diseases and Disorders, Including Cancer, Allergies, Respiratory Problems, and Skin Disorders

Along with Information about Environmental Concerns for Specific Populations, a Glossary of Related Terms, and Resources for Further Help and Information

Edited by Dawn D. Matthews. 673 pages. 2003. 978-0-7808-0632-0.

"This recently updated edition continues the level of quality and the reputation of the numerous other volumes in Omnigraphics' *Health Reference Series*."
— *American Reference Books Annual, 2004*

"An excellent updated edition."
— *The Bookwatch, Oct '03*

"Recommended reference source."
— *Booklist, American Library Association, Sep '98*

"This book will be a useful addition to anyone's library." — *Choice Health Sciences Supplement, Association of College & Research Libraries, May '98*

". . . a good survey of numerous environmentally induced physical disorders . . . a useful addition to anyone's library."
— *Doody's Health Sciences Book Reviews, Jan '98*

Ethnic Diseases Sourcebook

Basic Consumer Health Information for Ethnic and Racial Minority Groups in the United States, Including General Health Indicators and Behaviors, Ethnic Diseases, Genetic Testing, the Impact of Chronic Diseases, Women's Health, Mental Health Issues, and Preventive Health Care Services

Along with a Glossary and a Listing of Additional Resources

Edited by Joyce Brennfleck Shannon. 664 pages. 2001. 978-0-7808-0336-7.

"Recommended for health sciences libraries where public health programs are a priority."
— E-Streams, Jan '02

"Not many books have been written on this topic to date, and the *Ethnic Diseases Sourcebook* is a strong addition to the list. It will be an important introductory resource for health consumers, students, health care personnel, and social scientists. It is recommended for public, academic, and large hospital libraries."
— American Reference Books Annual, 2002

"Recommended reference source."
— Booklist, American Library Association, Oct '01

"Will prove valuable to any library seeking to maintain a current, comprehensive reference collection of health resources. . . . An excellent source of health information about genetic disorders which affect particular ethnic and racial minorities in the U.S."
— The Bookwatch, Aug '01

Eye Care Sourcebook, 2nd Edition

Basic Consumer Health Information about Eye Care and Eye Disorders, Including Facts about the Diagnosis, Prevention, and Treatment of Common Refractive Problems Such as Myopia, Hyperopia, Astigmatism, and Presbyopia, and Eye Diseases, Including Glaucoma, Cataract, Age-Related Macular Degeneration, and Diabetic Retinopathy

Along with a Section on Vision Correction and Refractive Surgeries, Including LASIK and LASEK, a Glossary, and Directories of Resources for Additional Help and Information

Edited by Amy L. Sutton. 543 pages. 2003. 978-0-7808-0635-1.

". . . a solid reference tool for eye care and a valuable addition to a collection."
— American Reference Books Annual, 2004

Family Planning Sourcebook

Basic Consumer Health Information about Planning for Pregnancy and Contraception, Including Traditional Methods, Barrier Methods, Hormonal Methods, Permanent Methods, Future Methods, Emergency Contraception, and Birth Control Choices for Women at Each Stage of Life

Along with Statistics, a Glossary, and Sources of Additional Information

Edited by Amy Marcaccio Keyzer. 520 pages. 2001. 978-0-7808-0379-4.

"Recommended for public, health, and undergraduate libraries as part of the circulating collection."
— E-Streams, Mar '02

"Information is presented in an unbiased, readable manner, and the sourcebook will certainly be a necessary addition to those public and high school libraries where Internet access is restricted or otherwise problematic." — American Reference Books Annual, 2002

"Recommended reference source."
— Booklist, American Library Association, Oct '01

"Will prove valuable to any library seeking to maintain a current, comprehensive reference collection of health resources. . . . Excellent reference."
— The Bookwatch, Aug '01

SEE ALSO Pregnancy & Birth Sourcebook

Fitness & Exercise Sourcebook, 3rd Edition

Basic Consumer Health Information about the Physical and Mental Benefits of Fitness, Including Cardiorespiratory Endurance, Muscular Strength, Muscular Endurance, and Flexibility, with Facts about Sports Nutrition and Exercise-Related Injuries and Tips about Physical Activity and Exercises for People of All Ages and for People with Health Concerns

Along with Advice on Selecting and Using Exercise Equipment, Maintaining Exercise Motivation, a Glossary of Related Terms, and a Directory of Resources for More Help and Information

Edited by Amy L. Sutton. 663 pages. 2007. 978-0-7808-0946-8.

"This work is recommended for all general reference collections."
— American Reference Books Annual, 2002

"Highly recommended for public, consumer, and school grades fourth through college." — E-Streams, Nov '01

"Recommended reference source."
— Booklist, American Library Association, Oct '01

"The information appears quite comprehensive and is considered reliable. . . . This second edition is a welcomed addition to the series."
— Doody's Review Service, Sep '01

Food Safety Sourcebook

Basic Consumer Health Information about the Safe Handling of Meat, Poultry, Seafood, Eggs, Fruit Juices, and Other Food Items, and Facts about Pesticides, Drinking Water, Food Safety Overseas, and the Onset, Duration, and Symptoms of Foodborne Illnesses, Including Types of Pathogenic Bacteria, Parasitic Protozoa, Worms, Viruses, and Natural Toxins

Along with the Role of the Consumer, the Food Handler, and the Government in Food Safety; a Glossary, and Resources for Additional Help and Information

Edited by Dawn D. Matthews. 339 pages. 1999. 978-0-7808-0326-8.

"This book is recommended for public libraries and universities with home economic and food science programs."
— E-Streams, Nov '00

"Recommended reference source."
— Booklist, American Library Association, May '00

"This book takes the complex issues of food safety and foodborne pathogens and presents them in an easily understood manner. [It does] an excellent job of covering a large and often confusing topic."
— American Reference Books Annual, 2000

Forensic Medicine Sourcebook

Basic Consumer Information for the Layperson about Forensic Medicine, Including Crime Scene Investigation, Evidence Collection and Analysis, Expert Testimony, Computer-Aided Criminal Identification, Digital Imaging in the Courtroom, DNA Profiling, Accident Reconstruction, Autopsies, Ballistics, Drugs and Explosives Detection, Latent Fingerprints, Product Tampering, and Questioned Document Examination

Along with Statistical Data, a Glossary of Forensics Terminology, and Listings of Sources for Further Help and Information

Edited by Annemarie S. Muth. 574 pages. 1999. 978-0-7808-0232-2.

"Given the expected widespread interest in its content and its easy to read style, this book is recommended for most public and all college and university libraries."
— E-Streams, Feb '01

"Recommended for public libraries."
— Reference & User Services Quarterly, American Library Association, Spring 2000

"Recommended reference source."
— Booklist, American Library Association, Feb '00

"A wealth of information, useful statistics, references are up-to-date and extremely complete. This wonderful collection of data will help students who are interested in a career in any type of forensic field. It is a great resource for attorneys who need information about types of expert witnesses needed in a particular case. It also offers useful information for fiction and nonfiction writers whose work involves a crime. A fascinating compilation. All levels."
— Choice, Association of College & Research Libraries, Jan '00

"There are several items that make this book attractive to consumers who are seeking certain forensic data.... This is a useful current source for those seeking general forensic medical answers."
— American Reference Books Annual, 2000

Gastrointestinal Diseases & Disorders Sourcebook, 2nd Edition

Basic Consumer Health Information about the Upper and Lower Gastrointestinal (GI) Tract, Including the Esophagus, Stomach, Intestines, Rectum, Liver, and Pancreas, with Facts about Gastroesophageal Reflux Disease, Gastritis, Hernias, Ulcers, Celiac Disease, Diverticulitis, Irritable Bowel Syndrome, Hemorrhoids, Gastrointestinal Cancers, and Other Diseases and Disorders Related to the Digestive Process

Along with Information about Commonly Used Diagnostic and Surgical Procedures, Statistics, Reports on Current Research Initiatives and Clinical Trials, a Glossary, and Resources for Additional Help and Information

Edited by Sandra J. Judd. 681 pages. 2006. 978-0-7808-0798-3.

"... very readable form. The successful editorial work that brought this material together into a useful and understandable reference makes accessible to all readers information that can help them more effectively understand and obtain help for digestive tract problems."
— Choice, Association of College & Research Libraries, Feb '97

SEE ALSO Diet & Nutrition Sourcebook, Digestive Diseases & Disorders Sourcebook, Eating Disorders Sourcebook

Genetic Disorders Sourcebook, 3rd Edition

Basic Consumer Health Information about Hereditary Diseases and Disorders, Including Facts about the Human Genome, Genetic Inheritance Patterns, Disorders Associated with Specific Genes, Such as Sickle Cell Disease, Hemophilia, and Cystic Fibrosis, Chromosome Disorders, Such as Down Syndrome, Fragile X Syndrome, and Turner Syndrome, and Complex Diseases and Disorders Resulting from the Interaction of Environmental and Genetic Factors, Such as Allergies, Cancer, and Obesity

Along with Facts about Genetic Testing, Suggestions for Parents of Children with Special Needs, Reports on Current Research Initiatives, a Glossary of Genetic Terminology, and Resources for Additional Help and Information

Edited by Karen Bellenir. 777 pages. 2004. 978-0-7808-0742-6.

"This text is recommended for any library with an interest in providing consumer health resources."
— E-Streams, Aug '05

"This is a valuable resource for anyone wishing to have an understandable description of any of the topics or disorders included. The editor succeeds in making complex genetic issues understandable."
— Doody's Book Review Service, May '05

"A good acquisition for public libraries."
— American Reference Books Annual, 2005

Head Trauma Sourcebook

Basic Information for the Layperson about Open-Head and Closed-Head Injuries, Treatment Advances, Recovery, and Rehabilitation

Along with Reports on Current Research Initiatives

Edited by Karen Bellenir. 414 pages. 1997. 978-0-7808-0208-7.

Headache Sourcebook

Basic Consumer Health Information about Migraine, Tension, Cluster, Rebound and Other Types of Headaches, with Facts about the Cause and Prevention of Headaches, the Effects of Stress and the Environment, Headaches during Pregnancy and Menopause, and Childhood Headaches

Along with a Glossary and Other Resources for Additional Help and Information

Edited by Dawn D. Matthews. 362 pages. 2002. 978-0-7808-0337-4.

Healthy Aging Sourcebook

Basic Consumer Health Information about Maintaining Health through the Aging Process, Including Advice on Nutrition, Exercise, and Sleep, Help in Making Decisions about Midlife Issues and Retirement, and Guidance Concerning Practical and Informed Choices in Health Consumerism

Along with Data Concerning the Theories of Aging, Different Experiences in Aging by Minority Groups, and Facts about Aging Now and Aging in the Future; and Featuring a Glossary, a Guide to Consumer Help, Additional Suggested Reading, and Practical Resource Directory

Edited by Jenifer Swanson. 536 pages. 1999. 978-0-7808-0390-9.

SEE ALSO *Physical & Mental Issues in Aging Sourcebook*

Healthy Children Sourcebook

Basic Consumer Health Information about the Physical and Mental Development of Children between the Ages of 3 and 12, Including Routine Health Care, Preventative Health Services, Safety and First Aid,

Healthy Sleep, Dental Care, Nutrition, and Fitness, and Featuring Parenting Tips on Such Topics as Bedwetting, Choosing Day Care, Monitoring TV and Other Media, and Establishing a Foundation for Substance Abuse Prevention

Along with a Glossary of Commonly Used Pediatric Terms and Resources for Additional Help and Information

Edited by Chad T. Kimball. 647 pages. 2003. 978-0-7808-0247-6.

SEE ALSO *Childhood Diseases & Disorders Sourcebook*

Healthy Heart Sourcebook for Women

Basic Consumer Health Information about Cardiac Issues Specific to Women, Including Facts about Major Risk Factors and Prevention, Treatment and Control Strategies, and Important Dietary Issues

Along with a Special Section Regarding the Pros and Cons of Hormone Replacement Therapy and Its Impact on Heart Health, and Additional Help, Including Recipes, a Glossary, and a Directory of Resources

Edited by Dawn D. Matthews. 336 pages. 2000. 978-0-7808-0329-9.

SEE ALSO *Cardiovascular Diseases & Disorders Sourcebook, Women's Health Concerns Sourcebook*

Hepatitis Sourcebook

Basic Consumer Health Information about Hepatitis A, Hepatitis B, Hepatitis C, and Other Forms of Hepatitis, Including Autoimmune Hepatitis, Alcoholic Hepatitis, Nonalcoholic Steatohepatitis, and Toxic Hepatitis, with

Facts about Risk Factors, Screening Methods, Diagnostic Tests, and Treatment Options

Along with Information on Liver Health, Tips for People Living with Chronic Hepatitis, Reports on Current Research Initiatives, a Glossary of Terms Related to Hepatitis, and a Directory of Sources for Further Help and Information

Edited by Sandra J. Judd. 597 pages. 2005. 978-0-7808-0749-5.

"Highly recommended."
— American Reference Books Annual, 2006

■

Household Safety Sourcebook

Basic Consumer Health Information about Household Safety, Including Information about Poisons, Chemicals, Fire, and Water Hazards in the Home

Along with Advice about the Safe Use of Home Maintenance Equipment, Choosing Toys and Nursery Furniture, Holiday and Recreation Safety, a Glossary, and Resources for Further Help and Information

Edited by Dawn D. Matthews. 606 pages. 2002. 978-0-7808-0338-1.

"This work will be useful in public libraries with large consumer health and wellness departments."
— American Reference Books Annual, 2003

"As a sourcebook on household safety this book meets its mark. It is encyclopedic in scope and covers a wide range of safety issues that are commonly seen in the home." — E-Streams, Jul '02

■

Hypertension Sourcebook

Basic Consumer Health Information about the Causes, Diagnosis, and Treatment of High Blood Pressure, with Facts about Consequences, Complications, and Co-Occurring Disorders, Such as Coronary Heart Disease, Diabetes, Stroke, Kidney Disease, and Hypertensive Retinopathy, and Issues in Blood Pressure Control, Including Dietary Choices, Stress Management, and Medications

Along with Reports on Current Research Initiatives and Clinical Trials, a Glossary, and Resources for Additional Help and Information

Edited by Dawn D. Matthews and Karen Bellenir. 613 pages. 2004. 978-0-7808-0674-0.

"Academic, public, and medical libraries will want to add the Hypertension Sourcebook to their collections."
— E-Streams, Aug '05

"The strength of this source is the wide range of information given about hypertension."
— American Reference Books Annual, 2005

■

Immune System Disorders Sourcebook, 2nd Edition

Basic Consumer Health Information about Disorders of the Immune System, Including Immune System Function and Response, Diagnosis of Immune Disorders, Information about Inherited Immune Disease, Acquired Immune Disease, and Autoimmune Diseases, Including Primary Immune Deficiency, Acquired Immunodeficiency Syndrome (AIDS), Lupus, Multiple Sclerosis, Type 1 Diabetes, Rheumatoid Arthritis, and Graves' Disease

Along with Treatments, Tips for Coping with Immune Disorders, a Glossary, and a Directory of Additional Resources

Edited by Joyce Brennfleck Shannon. 671 pages. 2005. 978-0-7808-0748-8.

"Highly recommended for academic and public libraries." — American Reference Books Annual, 2006

"The updated second edition is a 'must' for any consumer health library seeking a solid resource covering the treatments, symptoms, and options for immune disorder sufferers. . . . An excellent guide."
— MBR Bookwatch, Jan '06

■

Infant & Toddler Health Sourcebook

Basic Consumer Health Information about the Physical and Mental Development of Newborns, Infants, and Toddlers, Including Neonatal Concerns, Nutrition Recommendations, Immunization Schedules, Common Pediatric Disorders, Assessments and Milestones, Safety Tips, and Advice for Parents and Other Caregivers

Along with a Glossary of Terms and Resource Listings for Additional Help

Edited by Jenifer Swanson. 585 pages. 2000. 978-0-7808-0246-9.

"As a reference for the general public, this would be useful in any library." — E-Streams, May '01

"Recommended reference source."
— Booklist, American Library Association, Feb '01

"This is a good source for general use."
— American Reference Books Annual, 2001

■

Infectious Diseases Sourcebook

Basic Consumer Health Information about Non-Contagious Bacterial, Viral, Prion, Fungal, and Parasitic Diseases Spread by Food and Water, Insects and Animals, or Environmental Contact, Including Botulism, E. Coli, Encephalitis, Legionnaires' Disease, Lyme Disease, Malaria, Plague, Rabies, Salmonella, Tetanus, and Others, and Facts about Newly Emerging Diseases, Such as Hantavirus, Mad Cow Disease, Monkeypox, and West Nile Virus

Along with Information about Preventing Disease Transmission, the Threat of Bioterrorism, and Current Research Initiatives, with a Glossary and Directory of Resources for More Information

Edited by Karen Bellenir. 634 pages. 2004. 978-0-7808-0675-7.

"This reference continues the excellent tradition of the *Health Reference Series* in consolidating a wealth of information on a selected topic into a format that is easy to use and accessible to the general public."
— *American Reference Books Annual, 2005*

"Recommended for public and academic libraries."
— *E-Streams, Jan '05*

■

Injury & Trauma Sourcebook

Basic Consumer Health Information about the Impact of Injury, the Diagnosis and Treatment of Common and Traumatic Injuries, Emergency Care, and Specific Injuries Related to Home, Community, Workplace, Transportation, and Recreation

Along with Guidelines for Injury Prevention, a Glossary, and a Directory of Additional Resources

Edited by Joyce Brennfleck Shannon. 696 pages. 2002. 978-0-7808-0421-0.

"This publication is the most comprehensive work of its kind about injury and trauma."
— *American Reference Books Annual, 2003*

"This sourcebook provides concise, easily readable, basic health information about injuries. . . . This book is well organized and an easy to use reference resource suitable for hospital, health sciences and public libraries with consumer health collections."
— *E-Streams, Nov '02*

"Practitioners should be aware of guides such as this in order to facilitate their use by patients and their families."
— *Doody's Health Sciences Book Review Journal, Sep-Oct '02*

"Recommended reference source."
— *Booklist, American Library Association, Sep '02*

"Highly recommended for academic and medical reference collections."
— *Library Bookwatch, Sep '02*

■

Kidney & Urinary Tract Diseases & Disorders Sourcebook

SEE Urinary Tract & Kidney Diseases & Disorders Sourcebook

■

Learning Disabilities Sourcebook, 2nd Edition

Basic Consumer Health Information about Learning Disabilities, Including Dyslexia, Developmental Speech and Language Disabilities, Non-Verbal Learning Disorders, Developmental Arithmetic Disorder, Developmental Writing Disorder, and Other Conditions That Impede Learning Such as Attention Deficit/Hyperactivity Disorder, Brain Injury, Hearing Impairment, Klinefelter Syndrome, Dyspraxia, and Tourette's Syndrome

Along with Facts about Educational Issues and Assistive Technology, Coping Strategies, a Glossary of Re-

lated Terms, and Resources for Further Help and Information

Edited by Dawn D. Matthews. 621 pages. 2003. 978-0-7808-0626-9.

"The second edition of Learning Disabilities Sourcebook far surpasses the earlier edition in that it is more focused on information that will be useful as a consumer health resource."
— *American Reference Books Annual, 2004*

"Teachers as well as consumers will find this an essential guide to understanding various syndromes and their latest treatments. [An] invaluable reference for public and school library collections alike."
— *Library Bookwatch, Apr '03*

Named "Outstanding Reference Book of 1999."
— *New York Public Library, Feb '00*

"An excellent candidate for inclusion in a public library reference section. It's a great source of information. Teachers will also find the book useful. Definitely worth reading."
— *Journal of Adolescent & Adult Literacy, Feb 2000*

"Readable . . . provides a solid base of information regarding successful techniques used with individuals who have learning disabilities, as well as practical suggestions for educators and family members. Clear language, concise descriptions, and pertinent information for contacting multiple resources add to the strength of this book as a useful tool."
— *Choice, Association of College & Research Libraries, Feb '99*

"Recommended reference source."
— *Booklist, American Library Association, Sep '98*

"A useful resource for libraries and for those who don't have the time to identify and locate the individual publications."
— *Disability Resources Monthly, Sep '98*

■

Leukemia Sourcebook

Basic Consumer Health Information about Adult and Childhood Leukemias, Including Acute Lymphocytic Leukemia (ALL), Chronic Lymphocytic Leukemia (CLL), Acute Myelogenous Leukemia (AML), Chronic Myelogenous Leukemia (CML), and Hairy Cell Leukemia, and Treatments Such as Chemotherapy, Radiation Therapy, Peripheral Blood Stem Cell and Marrow Transplantation, and Immunotherapy

Along with Tips for Life During and After Treatment, a Glossary, and Directories of Additional Resources

Edited by Joyce Brennfleck Shannon. 587 pages. 2003. 978-0-7808-0627-6.

"Unlike other medical books for the layperson, . . . the language does not talk down to the reader. . . . This volume is highly recommended for all libraries."
— *American Reference Books Annual, 2004*

". . . a fine title which ranges from diagnosis to alternative treatments, staging, and tips for life during and after diagnosis."
— *The Bookwatch, Dec '03*

Liver Disorders Sourcebook

Basic Consumer Health Information about the Liver and How It Works; Liver Diseases, Including Cancer, Cirrhosis, Hepatitis, and Toxic and Drug Related Diseases; Tips for Maintaining a Healthy Liver; Laboratory Tests, Radiology Tests, and Facts about Liver Transplantation

Along with a Section on Support Groups, a Glossary, and Resource Listings

Edited by Joyce Brennfleck Shannon. 591 pages. 2000. 978-0-7808-0383-1.

"A valuable resource."
—*American Reference Books Annual, 2001*

"This title is recommended for health sciences and public libraries with consumer health collections."
— *E-Streams, Oct '00*

"Recommended reference source."
—*Booklist, American Library Association, Jun '00*

Lung Disorders Sourcebook

Basic Consumer Health Information about Emphysema, Pneumonia, Tuberculosis, Asthma, Cystic Fibrosis, and Other Lung Disorders, Including Facts about Diagnostic Procedures, Treatment Strategies, Disease Prevention Efforts, and Such Risk Factors as Smoking, Air Pollution, and Exposure to Asbestos, Radon, and Other Agents

Along with a Glossary and Resources for Additional Help and Information

Edited by Dawn D. Matthews. 678 pages. 2002. 978-0-7808-0339-8.

"This title is a great addition for public and school libraries because it provides concise health information on the lungs."
— *American Reference Books Annual, 2003*

"Highly recommended for academic and medical reference collections." — *Library Bookwatch, Sep '02*

SEE ALSO *Respiratory Diseases & Disorders Sourcebook*

Medical Tests Sourcebook, 2nd Edition

Basic Consumer Health Information about Medical Tests, Including Age-Specific Health Tests, Important Health Screenings and Exams, Home-Use Tests, Blood and Specimen Tests, Electrical Tests, Scope Tests, Genetic Testing, and Imaging Tests, Such as X-Rays, Ultrasound, Computed Tomography, Magnetic Resonance Imaging, Angiography, and Nuclear Medicine

Along with a Glossary and Directory of Additional Resources

Edited by Joyce Brennfleck Shannon. 654 pages. 2004. 978-0-7808-0670-2.

"Recommended for hospital and health sciences

libraries with consumer health collections."
— *E-Streams, Mar '00*

"This is an overall excellent reference with a wealth of general knowledge that may aid those who are reluctant to get vital tests performed."
— *Today's Librarian, Jan '00*

"A valuable reference guide."
— *American Reference Books Annual, 2000*

Men's Health Concerns Sourcebook, 2nd Edition

Basic Consumer Health Information about the Medical and Mental Concerns of Men, Including Theories about the Shorter Male Lifespan, the Leading Causes of Death and Disability, Physical Concerns of Special Significance to Men, Reproductive and Sexual Concerns, Sexually Transmitted Diseases, Men's Mental and Emotional Health, and Lifestyle Choices That Affect Wellness, Such as Nutrition, Fitness, and Substance Use

Along with a Glossary of Related Terms and a Directory of Organizational Resources in Men's Health

Edited by Robert Aquinas McNally. 644 pages. 2004. 978-0-7808-0671-9.

"A very accessible reference for non-specialist general readers and consumers." — *The Bookwatch, Jun '04*

"This comprehensive resource and the series are highly recommended."
—*American Reference Books Annual, 2000*

"Recommended reference source."
— *Booklist, American Library Association, Dec '98*

Mental Health Disorders Sourcebook, 3rd Edition

Basic Consumer Health Information about Mental and Emotional Health and Mental Illness, Including Facts about Depression, Bipolar Disorder, and Other Mood Disorders, Phobias, Post-Traumatic Stress Disorder (PTSD), Obsessive-Compulsive Disorder, and Other Anxiety Disorders, Impulse Control Disorders, Eating Disorders, Personality Disorders, and Psychotic Disorders, Including Schizophrenia and Dissociative Disorders

Along with Statistical Information, a Special Section Concerning Mental Health Issues in Children and Adolescents, a Glossary, and Directories of Resources for Additional Help and Information

Edited by Karen Bellenir. 661 pages. 2005. 978-0-7808-0747-1.

"Recommended for public libraries and academic libraries with an undergraduate program in psychology."
— *American Reference Books Annual, 2006*

"Recommended reference source."
—*Booklist, American Library Association, Jun '00*

Mental Retardation Sourcebook

Basic Consumer Health Information about Mental Retardation and Its Causes, Including Down Syndrome, Fetal Alcohol Syndrome, Fragile X Syndrome, Genetic Conditions, Injury, and Environmental Sources

Along with Preventive Strategies, Parenting Issues, Educational Implications, Health Care Needs, Employment and Economic Matters, Legal Issues, a Glossary, and a Resource Listing for Additional Help and Information

Edited by Joyce Brennfleck Shannon. 642 pages. 2000. 978-0-7808-0377-0.

"Public libraries will find the book useful for reference and as a beginning research point for students, parents, and caregivers."
— *American Reference Books Annual, 2001*

"The strength of this work is that it compiles many basic fact sheets and addresses for further information in one volume. It is intended and suitable for the general public. This sourcebook is relevant to any collection providing health information to the general public."
— *E-Streams, Nov '00*

"From preventing retardation to parenting and family challenges, this covers health, social and legal issues and will prove an invaluable overview."
— *Reviewer's Bookwatch, Jul '00*

Movement Disorders Sourcebook

Basic Consumer Health Information about Neurological Movement Disorders, Including Essential Tremor, Parkinson's Disease, Dystonia, Cerebral Palsy, Huntington's Disease, Myasthenia Gravis, Multiple Sclerosis, and Other Early-Onset and Adult-Onset Movement Disorders, Their Symptoms and Causes, Diagnostic Tests, and Treatments

Along with Mobility and Assistive Technology Information, a Glossary, and a Directory of Additional Resources

Edited by Joyce Brennfleck Shannon. 655 pages. 2003. 978-0-7808-0628-3.

". . . a good resource for consumers and recommended for public, community college and undergraduate libraries." — *American Reference Books Annual, 2004*

Muscular Dystrophy Sourcebook

Basic Consumer Health Information about Congenital, Childhood-Onset, and Adult-Onset Forms of Muscular Dystrophy, Such as Duchenne, Becker, Emery-Dreifuss, Distal, Limb-Girdle, Facioscapulohumeral (FSHD), Myotonic, and Ophthalmoplegic Muscular Dystrophies, Including Facts about Diagnostic Tests, Medical and Physical Therapies, Management of Co-Occurring Conditions, and Parenting Guidelines

Along with Practical Tips for Home Care, a Glossary, and Directories of Additional Resources

Edited by Joyce Brennfleck Shannon. 577 pages. 2004. 978-0-7808-0676-4.

"This book is highly recommended for public and academic libraries as well as health care offices that support the information needs of patients and their families."
— *E-Streams, Apr '05*

"Excellent reference."   — *The Bookwatch, Jan '05*

Obesity Sourcebook

Basic Consumer Health Information about Diseases and Other Problems Associated with Obesity, and Including Facts about Risk Factors, Prevention Issues, and Management Approaches

Along with Statistical and Demographic Data, Information about Special Populations, Research Updates, a Glossary, and Source Listings for Further Help and Information

Edited by Wilma Caldwell and Chad T. Kimball. 376 pages. 2001. 978-0-7808-0333-6.

"The book synthesizes the reliable medical literature on obesity into one easy-to-read and useful resource for the general public."
— *American Reference Books Annual, 2002*

"This is a very useful resource book for the lay public."
— *Doody's Review Service, Nov '01*

"Well suited for the health reference collection of a public library or an academic health science library that serves the general population." — *E-Streams, Sep '01*

"Recommended reference source."
— *Booklist, American Library Association, Apr '01*

"Recommended pick both for specialty health library collections and any general consumer health reference collection." — *The Bookwatch, Apr '01*

Oral Health Sourcebook

SEE *Dental Care & Oral Health Sourcebook*

Osteoporosis Sourcebook

Basic Consumer Health Information about Primary and Secondary Osteoporosis and Juvenile Osteoporosis and Related Conditions, Including Fibrous Dysplasia, Gaucher Disease, Hyperthyroidism, Hypophosphatasia, Myeloma, Osteopetrosis, Osteogenesis Imperfecta, and Paget's Disease

Along with Information about Risk Factors, Treatments, Traditional and Non-Traditional Pain Management, a Glossary of Related Terms, and a Directory of Resources

Edited by Allan R. Cook. 584 pages. 2001. 978-0-7808-0239-1.

"This would be a book to be kept in a staff or patient library. The targeted audience is the layperson, but the therapist who needs a quick bit of information on a particular topic will also find the book useful."
— *Physical Therapy, Jan '02*

"This resource is recommended as a great reference source for public, health, and academic libraries, and is another triumph for the editors of Omnigraphics."
— *American Reference Books Annual, 2002*

"Recommended for all public libraries and general health collections, especially those supporting patient education or consumer health programs."
— *E-Streams, Nov '01*

"Will prove valuable to any library seeking to maintain a current, comprehensive reference collection of health resources. . . . From prevention to treatment and associated conditions, this provides an excellent survey."
— *The Bookwatch, Aug '01*

"Recommended reference source."
— *Booklist, American Library Association, Jul '01*

SEE ALSO *Healthy Aging Sourcebook, Physical & Mental Issues in Aging Sourcebook, Women's Health Concerns Sourcebook*

Pain Sourcebook, 2nd Edition

Basic Consumer Health Information about Specific Forms of Acute and Chronic Pain, Including Muscle and Skeletal Pain, Nerve Pain, Cancer Pain, and Disorders Characterized by Pain, Such as Fibromyalgia, Shingles, Angina, Arthritis, and Headaches

Along with Information about Pain Medications and Management Techniques, Complementary and Alternative Pain Relief Options, Tips for People Living with Chronic Pain, a Glossary, and a Directory of Sources for Further Information

Edited by Karen Bellenir. 670 pages. 2002. 978-0-7808-0612-2.

"A source of valuable information. . . . This book offers help to nonmedical people who need information about pain and pain management. It is also an excellent reference for those who participate in patient education."
— *Doody's Review Service, Sep '02*

"Highly recommended for academic and medical reference collections."
— *Library Bookwatch, Sep '02*

"The text is readable, easily understood, and well indexed. This excellent volume belongs in all patient education libraries, consumer health sections of public libraries, and many personal collections."
— *American Reference Books Annual, 1999*

"The information is basic in terms of scholarship and is appropriate for general readers. Written in journalistic style . . . intended for non-professionals. Quite thorough in its coverage of different pain conditions and summarizes the latest clinical information regarding pain treatment."
— *Choice, Association of College and Research Libraries, Jun '98*

"Recommended reference source."
— *Booklist, American Library Association, Mar '98*

Pediatric Cancer Sourcebook

Basic Consumer Health Information about Leukemias, Brain Tumors, Sarcomas, Lymphomas, and Other Cancers in Infants, Children, and Adolescents, Including Descriptions of Cancers, Treatments, and Coping Strategies

Along with Suggestions for Parents, Caregivers, and Concerned Relatives, a Glossary of Cancer Terms, and Resource Listings

Edited by Edward J. Prucha. 587 pages. 1999. 978-0-7808-0245-2.

"An excellent source of information. Recommended for public, hospital, and health science libraries with consumer health collections."
— *E-Streams, Jun '00*

"Recommended reference source."
— *Booklist, American Library Association, Feb '00*

"A valuable addition to all libraries specializing in health services and many public libraries."
— *American Reference Books Annual, 2000*

SEE ALSO *Childhood Diseases & Disorders Sourcebook, Healthy Children Sourcebook*

Physical & Mental Issues in Aging Sourcebook

Basic Consumer Health Information on Physical and Mental Disorders Associated with the Aging Process, Including Concerns about Cardiovascular Disease, Pulmonary Disease, Oral Health, Digestive Disorders, Musculoskeletal and Skin Disorders, Metabolic Changes, Sexual and Reproductive Issues, and Changes in Vision, Hearing, and Other Senses

Along with Data about Longevity and Causes of Death, Information on Acute and Chronic Pain, Descriptions of Mental Concerns, a Glossary of Terms, and Resource Listings for Additional Help

Edited by Jenifer Swanson. 660 pages. 1999. 978-0-7808-0233-9.

"This is a treasure of health information for the layperson."
— *Choice Health Sciences Supplement, Association of College & Research Libraries, May '00*

"Recommended for public libraries."
— *American Reference Books Annual, 2000*

"Recommended reference source."
— *Booklist, American Library Association, Oct '99*

SEE ALSO *Healthy Aging Sourcebook*

Podiatry Sourcebook, 2nd Edition

Basic Consumer Health Information about Disorders, Diseases, Deformities, and Injuries that Affect the Foot and Ankle, Including Sprains, Corns, Calluses, Bunions, Plantar Warts, Plantar Fasciitis, Neuromas, Clubfoot, Flat Feet, Achilles Tendonitis, and Much More

Along with Information about Selecting a Foot Care Specialist, Foot Fitness, Shoes and Socks, Diagnostic Tests and Corrective Procedures, Financial Assistance for Corrective Devices, a Glossary of Related Terms, and a Directory of Resources for Additional Help and Information

Edited by Ivy L. Alexander. 543 pages. 2007. 978-0-7808-0944-4.

"Recommended reference source."
— Booklist, American Library Association, Feb '02

"There is a lot of information presented here on a topic that is usually only covered sparingly in most larger comprehensive medical encyclopedias."
— American Reference Books Annual, 2002

■

Pregnancy & Birth Sourcebook, 2nd Edition

Basic Consumer Health Information about Conception and Pregnancy, Including Facts about Fertility, Infertility, Pregnancy Symptoms and Complications, Fetal Growth and Development, Labor, Delivery, and the Postpartum Period, as Well as Information about Maintaining Health and Wellness during Pregnancy and Caring for a Newborn

Along with Information about Public Health Assistance for Low-Income Pregnant Women, a Glossary, and Directories of Agencies and Organizations Providing Help and Support

Edited by Amy L. Sutton. 626 pages. 2004. 978-0-7808-0672-6.

"Will appeal to public and school reference collections strong in medicine and women's health. . . . Deserves a spot on any medical reference shelf."
— The Bookwatch, Jul '04

"A well-organized handbook. Recommended."
— Choice, Association of College & Research Libraries, Apr '98

"Recommended reference source."
— Booklist, American Library Association, Mar '98

"Recommended for public libraries."
— American Reference Books Annual, 1998

SEE ALSO Breastfeeding Sourcebook, Congenital Disorders Sourcebook, Family Planning Sourcebook

■

Prostate & Urological Disorders Sourcebook

Basic Consumer Health Information about Urogenital and Sexual Disorders in Men, Including Prostate and Other Andrological Cancers, Prostatitis, Benign Prostatic Hyperplasia, Testicular and Penile Trauma, Cryptorchidism, Peyronie Disease, Erectile Dysfunction, and Male Factor Infertility, and Facts about Commonly Used Tests and Procedures, Such as Prostatectomy, Vasectomy, Vasectomy Reversal, Penile Implants, and Semen Analysis

Along with a Glossary of Andrological Terms and a Directory of Resources for Additional Information

Edited by Karen Bellenir. 631 pages. 2005. 978-0-7808-0797-6.

Prostate Cancer Sourcebook

Basic Consumer Health Information about Prostate Cancer, Including Information about the Associated Risk Factors, Detection, Diagnosis, and Treatment of Prostate Cancer

Along with Information on Non-Malignant Prostate Conditions, and Featuring a Section Listing Support and Treatment Centers and a Glossary of Related Terms

Edited by Dawn D. Matthews. 358 pages. 2001. 978-0-7808-0324-4.

"Recommended reference source."
— Booklist, American Library Association, Jan '02

"A valuable resource for health care consumers seeking information on the subject. . . . All text is written in a clear, easy-to-understand language that avoids technical jargon. Any library that collects consumer health resources would strengthen their collection with the addition of the Prostate Cancer Sourcebook."
— American Reference Books Annual, 2002

SEE ALSO Men's Health Concerns Sourcebook

■

Reconstructive & Cosmetic Surgery Sourcebook

Basic Consumer Health Information on Cosmetic and Reconstructive Plastic Surgery, Including Statistical Information about Different Surgical Procedures, Things to Consider Prior to Surgery, Plastic Surgery Techniques and Tools, Emotional and Psychological Considerations, and Procedure-Specific Information

Along with a Glossary of Terms and a Listing of Resources for Additional Help and Information

Edited by M. Lisa Weatherford. 374 pages. 2001. 978-0-7808-0214-8.

"An excellent reference that addresses cosmetic and medically necessary reconstructive surgeries. . . . The style of the prose is calm and reassuring, discussing the many positive outcomes now available due to advances in surgical techniques."
— American Reference Books Annual, 2002

"Recommended for health science libraries that are open to the public, as well as hospital libraries that are open to the patients. This book is a good resource for the consumer interested in plastic surgery."
— E-Streams, Dec '01

"Recommended reference source."
— Booklist, American Library Association, Jul '01

■

Rehabilitation Sourcebook

Basic Consumer Health Information about Rehabilitation for People Recovering from Heart Surgery, Spinal Cord Injury, Stroke, Orthopedic Impairments, Amputation, Pulmonary Impairments, Traumatic Injury, and More, Including Physical Therapy, Occupational Therapy, Speech/Language Therapy, Massage Therapy, Dance Therapy, Art Therapy, and Recreational Therapy

Along with Information on Assistive and Adaptive Devices, a Glossary, and Resources for Additional Help and Information

Edited by Dawn D. Matthews. 531 pages. 1999. 978-0-7808-0236-0.

"This is an excellent resource for public library reference and health collections."
— American Reference Books Annual, 2001

"Recommended reference source."
— Booklist, American Library Association, May '00

Respiratory Diseases & Disorders Sourcebook

Basic Information about Respiratory Diseases and Disorders, Including Asthma, Cystic Fibrosis, Pneumonia, the Common Cold, Influenza, and Others, Featuring Facts about the Respiratory System, Statistical and Demographic Data, Treatments, Self-Help Management Suggestions, and Current Research Initiatives

Edited by Allan R. Cook and Peter D. Dresser. 771 pages. 1995. 978-0-7808-0037-3.

"Designed for the layperson and for patients and their families coping with respiratory illness. . . . an extensive array of information on diagnosis, treatment, management, and prevention of respiratory illnesses for the general reader."
— Choice, Association of College & Research Libraries, Jun '96

"A highly recommended text for all collections. It is a comforting reminder of the power of knowledge that good books carry between their covers."
— Academic Library Book Review, Spring '96

"A comprehensive collection of authoritative information presented in a nontechnical, humanitarian style for patients, families, and caregivers."
— Association of Operating Room Nurses, Sep/Oct '95

SEE ALSO Lung Disorders Sourcebook

Sexually Transmitted Diseases Sourcebook, 3rd Edition

Basic Consumer Health Information about Chlamydial Infections, Gonorrhea, Hepatitis, Herpes, HIV/AIDS, Human Papillomavirus, Pubic Lice, Scabies, Syphilis, Trichomoniasis, Vaginal Infections, and Other Sexually Transmitted Diseases, Including Facts about Risk Factors, Symptoms, Diagnosis, Treatment, and the Prevention of Sexually Transmitted Infections

Along with Updates on Current Research Initiatives, a Glossary of Related Terms, and Resources for Additional Help and Information

Edited by Amy L. Sutton. 629 pages. 2006. 978-0-7808-0824-9.

"Recommended for consumer health collections in public libraries, and secondary school and community college libraries."
— American Reference Books Annual, 2002

"Every school and public library should have a copy of this comprehensive and user-friendly reference book."
— Choice, Association of College & Research Libraries, Sep '01

"This is a highly recommended book. This is an especially important book for all school and public libraries."
— AIDS Book Review Journal, Jul-Aug '01

"Recommended reference source."
— Booklist, American Library Association, Apr '01

Sleep Disorders Sourcebook, 2nd Edition

Basic Consumer Health Information about Sleep and Sleep Disorders, Including Insomnia, Sleep Apnea, Restless Legs Syndrome, Narcolepsy, Parasomnias, and Other Health Problems That Affect Sleep, Plus Facts about Diagnostic Procedures, Treatment Strategies, Sleep Medications, and Tips for Improving Sleep Quality

Along with a Glossary of Related Terms and Resources for Additional Help and Information

Edited by Amy L. Sutton. 567 pages. 2005. 978-0-7808-0743-3.

"This book will be useful for just about everybody, especially the 40 million Americans with sleep disorders."
— American Reference Books Annual, 2006

"Recommended for public libraries and libraries supporting health care professionals." — E-Streams, Sep '05

". . . key medical library acquisition."
— The Bookwatch, Jun '05

Smoking Concerns Sourcebook

Basic Consumer Health Information about Nicotine Addiction and Smoking Cessation, Featuring Facts about the Health Effects of Tobacco Use, Including Lung and Other Cancers, Heart Disease, Stroke, and Respiratory Disorders, Such as Emphysema and Chronic Bronchitis

Along with Information about Smoking Prevention Programs, Suggestions for Achieving and Maintaining a Smoke-Free Lifestyle, Statistics about Tobacco Use, Reports on Current Research Initiatives, a Glossary of Related Terms, and Directories of Resources for Additional Help and Information

Edited by Karen Bellenir. 621 pages. 2004. 978-0-7808-0323-7.

"Provides everything needed for the student or general reader seeking practical details on the effects of tobacco use." — The Bookwatch, Mar '05

"Public libraries and consumer health care libraries will find this work useful."
— American Reference Books Annual, 2005

Sports Injuries Sourcebook, 3rd Edition

Basic Consumer Health Information about Sprains and Strains, Fractures, Growth Plate Injuries, Overtraining Injuries, and Injuries to the Head, Face, Shoulders, Elbows, Hands, Spinal Column, Knees, Ankles, and Feet, and with Facts about Heat-Related Illness, Steroids and Sport Supplements, Protective Equipment, Diagnostic Procedures, Treatment Options, and Rehabilitation

Along with a Glossary of Related Terms and a Directory of Resources for Additional Help and Information

Edited by Sandra J. Judd. 651 pages. 2007. 978-0-7808-0949-9.

"This is an excellent reference for consumers and it is recommended for public, community college, and undergraduate libraries."
— *American Reference Books Annual, 2003*

"Recommended reference source."
— *Booklist, American Library Association, Feb '03*

Stress-Related Disorders Sourcebook

Basic Consumer Health Information about Stress and Stress-Related Disorders, Including Stress Origins and Signals, Environmental Stress at Work and Home, Mental and Emotional Stress Associated with Depression, Post-Traumatic Stress Disorder, Panic Disorder, Suicide, and the Physical Effects of Stress on the Cardiovascular, Immune, and Nervous Systems

Along with Stress Management Techniques, a Glossary, and a Listing of Additional Resources

Edited by Joyce Brennfleck Shannon. 610 pages. 2002. 978-0-7808-0560-6.

"Well written for a general readership, the *Stress-Related Disorders Sourcebook* is a useful addition to the health reference literature."
— *American Reference Books Annual, 2003*

"I am impressed by the amount of information. It offers a thorough overview of the causes and consequences of stress for the layperson. . . . A well-done and thorough reference guide for professionals and nonprofessionals alike."
— *Doody's Review Service, Dec '02*

Stroke Sourcebook

Basic Consumer Health Information about Stroke, Including Ischemic, Hemorrhagic, Transient Ischemic Attack (TIA), and Pediatric Stroke, Stroke Triggers and Risks, Diagnostic Tests, Treatments, and Rehabilitation Information

Along with Stroke Prevention Guidelines, Legal and Financial Information, a Glossary, and a Directory of Additional Resources

Edited by Joyce Brennfleck Shannon. 606 pages. 2003. 978-0-7808-0630-6.

"This volume is highly recommended and should be in every medical, hospital, and public library."
— *American Reference Books Annual, 2004*

"Highly recommended for the amount and variety of topics and information covered." — *Choice, Nov '03*

Surgery Sourcebook

Basic Consumer Health Information about Inpatient and Outpatient Surgeries, Including Cardiac, Vascular, Orthopedic, Ocular, Reconstructive, Cosmetic, Gynecologic, and Ear, Nose, and Throat Procedures and More

Along with Information about Operating Room Policies and Instruments, Laser Surgery Techniques, Hospital Errors, Statistical Data, a Glossary, and Listings of Sources for Further Help and Information

Edited by Annemarie S. Muth and Karen Bellenir. 596 pages. 2002. 978-0-7808-0380-0.

"Large public libraries and medical libraries would benefit from this material in their reference collections."
— *American Reference Books Annual, 2004*

"Invaluable reference for public and school library collections alike." — *Library Bookwatch, Apr '03*

Thyroid Disorders Sourcebook

Basic Consumer Health Information about Disorders of the Thyroid and Parathyroid Glands, Including Hypothyroidism, Hyperthyroidism, Graves Disease, Hashimoto Thyroiditis, Thyroid Cancer, and Parathyroid Disorders, Featuring Facts about Symptoms, Risk Factors, Tests, and Treatments

Along with Information about the Effects of Thyroid Imbalance on Other Body Systems, Environmental Factors That Affect the Thyroid Gland, a Glossary, and a Directory of Additional Resources

Edited by Joyce Brennfleck Shannon. 599 pages. 2005. 978-0-7808-0745-7.

"Recommended for consumer health collections."
— *American Reference Books Annual, 2006*

"Highly recommended pick for basic consumer health reference holdings at all levels."
— *The Bookwatch, Aug '05*

Transplantation Sourcebook

Basic Consumer Health Information about Organ and Tissue Transplantation, Including Physical and Financial Preparations, Procedures and Issues Relating to Specific Solid Organ and Tissue Transplants, Rehabilitation, Pediatric Transplant Information, the Future of Transplantation, and Organ and Tissue Donation

Along with a Glossary and Listings of Additional Resources

Edited by Joyce Brennfleck Shannon. 628 pages. 2002. 978-0-7808-0322-0.

"Along with these advances [in transplantation technology] have come a number of daunting questions for potential transplant patients, their families, and their health care providers. This reference text is the best single tool to address many of these questions. . . . It will be a much-needed addition to the reference collections in health care, academic, and large public libraries."
— *American Reference Books Annual, 2003*

"Recommended for libraries with an interest in offering consumer health information." — *E-Streams, Jul '02*

"This is a unique and valuable resource for patients facing transplantation and their families."
— *Doody's Review Service, Jun '02*

Traveler's Health Sourcebook

Basic Consumer Health Information for Travelers, Including Physical and Medical Preparations, Transportation Health and Safety, Essential Information about Food and Water, Sun Exposure, Insect and Snake Bites, Camping and Wilderness Medicine, and Travel with Physical or Medical Disabilities

Along with International Travel Tips, Vaccination Recommendations, Geographical Health Issues, Disease Risks, a Glossary, and a Listing of Additional Resources

Edited by Joyce Brennfleck Shannon. 613 pages. 2000. 978-0-7808-0384-8.

"Recommended reference source."
— *Booklist, American Library Association, Feb '01*

"This book is recommended for any public library, any travel collection, and especially any collection for the physically disabled."
— *American Reference Books Annual, 2001*

SEE ALSO *Worldwide Health Sourcebook*

Urinary Tract & Kidney Diseases & Disorders Sourcebook, 2nd Edition

Basic Consumer Health Information about the Urinary System, Including the Bladder, Urethra, Ureters, and Kidneys, with Facts about Urinary Tract Infections, Incontinence, Congenital Disorders, Kidney Stones, Cancers of the Urinary Tract and Kidneys, Kidney Failure, Dialysis, and Kidney Transplantation

Along with Statistical and Demographic Information, Reports on Current Research in Kidney and Urologic Health, a Summary of Commonly Used Diagnostic Tests, a Glossary of Related Terms, and a Directory of Resources for Additional Help and Information

Edited by Ivy L. Alexander. 649 pages. 2005. 978-0-7808-0750-1.

"A good choice for a consumer health information library or for a medical library needing information to refer to their patients."
— *American Reference Books Annual, 2006*

Vegetarian Sourcebook

Basic Consumer Health Information about Vegetarian Diets, Lifestyle, and Philosophy, Including Definitions of Vegetarianism and Veganism, Tips about Adopting Vegetarianism, Creating a Vegetarian Pantry, and Meeting Nutritional Needs of Vegetarians, with Facts Regarding Vegetarianism's Effect on Pregnant and Lactating Women, Children, Athletes, and Senior Citizens

Along with a Glossary of Commonly Used Vegetarian Terms and Resources for Additional Help and Information

Edited by Chad T. Kimball. 360 pages. 2002. 978-0-7808-0439-5.

"Organizes into one concise volume the answers to the most common questions concerning vegetarian diets and lifestyles. This title is recommended for public and secondary school libraries." — *E-Streams, Apr '03*

"Invaluable reference for public and school library collections alike." — *Library Bookwatch, Apr '03*

"The articles in this volume are easy to read and come from authoritative sources. The book does not necessarily support the vegetarian diet but instead provides the pros and cons of this important decision. The Vegetarian Sourcebook is recommended for public libraries and consumer health libraries."
— *American Reference Books Annual, 2003*

SEE ALSO *Diet & Nutrition Sourcebook*

Women's Health Concerns Sourcebook, 2nd Edition

Basic Consumer Health Information about the Medical and Mental Concerns of Women, Including Maintaining Health and Wellness, Gynecological Concerns, Breast Health, Sexuality and Reproductive Issues, Menopause, Cancer in Women, Leading Causes of Death and Disability among Women, Physical Concerns of Special Significance to Women, and Women's Mental and Emotional Health

Along with a Glossary of Related Terms and Directories of Resources for Additional Help and Information

Edited by Amy L. Sutton. 746 pages. 2004. 978-0-7808-0673-3.

"This is a useful reference book, which makes the reader knowledgeable about several issues that concern women's health. It is recommended for public libraries and home library collections." — *E-Streams, May '05*

"A useful addition to public and consumer health library collections."
— *American Reference Books Annual, 2005*

"A highly recommended title."
— *The Bookwatch, May '04*

"Handy compilation. There is an impressive range of diseases, devices, disorders, procedures, and other physical and emotional issues covered . . . well organized, illustrated, and indexed." — *Choice, Association of College & Research Libraries, Jan '98*

SEE ALSO *Breast Cancer Sourcebook, Cancer Sourcebook for Women, Healthy Heart Sourcebook for Women, Osteoporosis Sourcebook*

Workplace Health & Safety Sourcebook

Basic Consumer Health Information about Workplace Health and Safety, Including the Effect of Workplace Hazards on the Lungs, Skin, Heart, Ears, Eyes, Brain, Reproductive Organs, Musculoskeletal System, and Other Organs and Body Parts

Along with Information about Occupational Cancer, Personal Protective Equipment, Toxic and Hazardous Chemicals, Child Labor, Stress, and Workplace Violence

Edited by Chad T. Kimball. 626 pages. 2000. 978-0-7808-0231-5.

"As a reference for the general public, this would be useful in any library."   —*E-Streams, Jun '01*

"Provides helpful information for primary care physicians and other caregivers interested in occupational medicine. . . . General readers; professionals."
     —*Choice, Association of College & Research Libraries, May '01*

"Recommended reference source."
     —*Booklist, American Library Association, Feb '01*

"Highly recommended."   —*The Bookwatch, Jan '01*

Worldwide Health Sourcebook

Basic Information about Global Health Issues, Including Malnutrition, Reproductive Health, Disease Dispersion and Prevention, Emerging Diseases, Risky Health Behaviors, and the Leading Causes of Death

Along with Global Health Concerns for Children, Women, and the Elderly, Mental Health Issues, Research and Technology Advancements, and Economic, Environmental, and Political Health Implications, a Glossary, and a Resource Listing for Additional Help and Information

Edited by Joyce Brennfleck Shannon. 614 pages. 2001. 978-0-7808-0330-5.

"Named an Outstanding Academic Title."
     —*Choice, Association of College & Research Libraries, Jan '02*

"Yet another handy but also unique compilation in the extensive *Health Reference Series*, this is a useful work because many of the international publications reprinted or excerpted are not readily available. Highly recommended."   —*Choice, Association of College & Research Libraries, Nov '01*

"Recommended reference source."
     —*Booklist, American Library Association, Oct '01*

SEE ALSO *Traveler's Health Sourcebook*

645

Teen Health Series
Helping Young Adults Understand, Manage, and Avoid Serious Illness

List price $65 per volume. **School and library price $58 per volume.**

Alcohol Information for Teens
Health Tips about Alcohol and Alcoholism

Including Facts about Underage Drinking, Preventing Teen Alcohol Use, Alcohol's Effects on the Brain and the Body, Alcohol Abuse Treatment, Help for Children of Alcoholics, and More

Edited by Joyce Brennfleck Shannon. 370 pages. 2005. 978-0-7808-0741-9.

"Boxed facts and tips add visual interest to the well-researched and clearly written text."
— *Curriculum Connection, Apr '06*

Allergy Information for Teens
Health Tips about Allergic Reactions Such as Anaphylaxis, Respiratory Problems, and Rashes

Including Facts about Identifying and Managing Allergies to Food, Pollen, Mold, Animals, Chemicals, Drugs, and Other Substances

Edited by Karen Bellenir. 410 pages. 2006. 978-0-7808-0799-0.

Asthma Information for Teens
Health Tips about Managing Asthma and Related Concerns

Including Facts about Asthma Causes, Triggers, Symptoms, Diagnosis, and Treatment

Edited by Karen Bellenir. 386 pages. 2005. 978-0-7808-0770-9.

"Highly recommended for medical libraries, public school libraries, and public libraries."
— *American Reference Books Annual, 2006*

"It is so clearly written and well organized that even hesitant readers will be able to find the facts they need, whether for reports or personal information. . . . A succinct but complete resource."
— *School Library Journal, Sep '05*

Body Information for Teens
Health Tips about Maintaining Well-Being for a Lifetime

Including Facts about the Development and Functioning of the Body's Systems, Organs, and Structures and the Health Impact of Lifestyle Choices

Edited by Sandra Augustyn Lawton. 458 pages. 2007. 978-0-7808-0443-2.

Cancer Information for Teens
Health Tips about Cancer Awareness, Prevention, Diagnosis, and Treatment

Including Facts about Frequently Occurring Cancers, Cancer Risk Factors, and Coping Strategies for Teens Fighting Cancer or Dealing with Cancer in Friends or Family Members

Edited by Wilma R. Caldwell. 428 pages. 2004. 978-0-7808-0678-8.

"Recommended for school libraries, or consumer libraries that see a lot of use by teens."
— *E-Streams, May '05*

"A valuable educational tool."
— *American Reference Books Annual, 2005*

"Young adults and their parents alike will find this new addition to the *Teen Health Series* an important reference to cancer in teens."
— *Children's Bookwatch, Feb '05*

Complementary and Alternative Medicine Information for Teens
Health Tips about Non-Traditional and Non-Western Medical Practices

Including Information about Acupuncture, Chiropractic Medicine, Dietary and Herbal Supplements, Hypnosis, Massage Therapy, Prayer and Spirituality, Reflexology, Yoga, and More

Edited by Sandra Augustyn Lawton. 405 pages. 2006. 978-0-7808-0966-6.

Diabetes Information for Teens
Health Tips about Managing Diabetes and Preventing Related Complications

Including Information about Insulin, Glucose Control, Healthy Eating, Physical Activity, and Learning to Live with Diabetes

Edited by Sandra Augustyn Lawton. 410 pages. 2006. 978-0-7808-0811-9.

Diet Information for Teens, 2nd Edition

Health Tips about Diet and Nutrition

Including Facts about Dietary Guidelines, Food Groups, Nutrients, Healthy Meals, Snacks, Weight Control, Medical Concerns Related to Diet, and More

Edited by Karen Bellenir. 432 pages. 2006. 978-0-7808-0820-1.

"Full of helpful insights and facts throughout the book. ... An excellent resource to be placed in public libraries or even in personal collections."
— *American Reference Books Annual, 2002*

"Recommended for middle and high school libraries and media centers as well as academic libraries that educate future teachers of teenagers. It is also a suitable addition to health science libraries that serve patrons who are interested in teen health promotion and education."
— *E-Streams, Oct '01*

"This comprehensive book would be beneficial to collections that need information about nutrition, dietary guidelines, meal planning, and weight control. ... This reference is so easy to use that its purchase is recommended."
— *The Book Report, Sep-Oct '01*

"This book is written in an easy to understand format describing issues that many teens face every day, and then provides thoughtful explanations so that teens can make informed decisions. This is an interesting book that provides important facts and information for today's teens."
— *Doody's Health Sciences Book Review Journal, Jul-Aug '01*

"A comprehensive compendium of diet and nutrition. The information is presented in a straightforward, plain-spoken manner. This title will be useful to those working on reports on a variety of topics, as well as to general readers concerned about their dietary health."
— *School Library Journal, Jun '01*

Drug Information for Teens, 2nd Edition

Health Tips about the Physical and Mental Effects of Substance Abuse

Including Information about Marijuana, Inhalants, Club Drugs, Stimulants, Hallucinogens, Opiates, Prescription and Over-the-Counter Drugs, Herbal Products, Tobacco, Alcohol, and More

Edited by Sandra Augustyn Lawton. 468 pages. 2006. 978-0-7808-0862-1.

"A clearly written resource for general readers and researchers alike."
— *School Library Journal*

"This book is well-balanced. ... a must for public and school libraries."
— *VOYA: Voice of Youth Advocates, Dec '03*

"The chapters are quick to make a connection to their teenage reading audience. The prose is straightforward and the book lends itself to spot reading. It should be useful both for practical information and for research, and it is suitable for public and school libraries."
— *American Reference Books Annual, 2003*

"Recommended reference source."
— *Booklist, American Library Association, Feb '03*

"This is an excellent resource for teens and their parents. Education about drugs and substances is key to discouraging teen drug abuse and this book provides this much needed information in a way that is interesting and factual."
— *Doody's Review Service, Dec '02*

Eating Disorders Information for Teens

Health Tips about Anorexia, Bulimia, Binge Eating, and Other Eating Disorders

Including Information on the Causes, Prevention, and Treatment of Eating Disorders, and Such Other Issues as Maintaining Healthy Eating and Exercise Habits

Edited by Sandra Augustyn Lawton. 337 pages. 2005. 978-0-7808-0783-9.

"An excellent resource for teens and those who work with them."
— *VOYA: Voice of Youth Advocates, Apr '06*

"A welcome addition to high school and undergraduate libraries." — *American Reference Books Annual, 2006*

"This book covers the topic in a lucid manner but delves deeper into every aspect of an eating disorder. A solid addition for any nonfiction or reference collection."
— *School Library Journal, Dec '05*

Fitness Information for Teens

Health Tips about Exercise, Physical Well-Being, and Health Maintenance

Including Facts about Aerobic and Anaerobic Conditioning, Stretching, Body Shape and Body Image, Sports Training, Nutrition, and Activities for Non-Athletes

Edited by Karen Bellenir. 425 pages. 2004. 978-0-7808-0679-5.

"Another excellent offering from Omnigraphics in their *Teen Health Series*. ... This book will be a great addition to any public, junior high, senior high, or secondary school library."
— *American Reference Books Annual, 2005*

Learning Disabilities Information for Teens

Health Tips about Academic Skills Disorders and Other Disabilities That Affect Learning

Including Information about Common Signs of Learning Disabilities, School Issues, Learning to Live with a Learning Disability, and Other Related Issues

Edited by Sandra Augustyn Lawton. 337 pages. 2005. 978-0-7808-0796-9.

"This book provides a wealth of information for any reader interested in the signs, causes, and consequences

of learning disabilities, as well as related legal rights and educational interventions.... Public and academic libraries should want this title for both students and general readers."
— *American Reference Books Annual, 2006*

■

Mental Health Information for Teens, 2nd Edition

Health Tips about Mental Wellness and Mental Illness

Including Facts about Mental and Emotional Health, Depression and Other Mood Disorders, Anxiety Disorders, Behavior Disorders, Self-Injury, Psychosis, Schizophrenia, and More

Edited by Karen Bellenir. 400 pages. 2006. 978-0-7808-0863-8.

"In both language and approach, this user-friendly entry in the *Teen Health Series* is on target for teens needing information on mental health concerns."
— *Booklist, American Library Association, Jan '02*

"Readers will find the material accessible and informative, with the shaded notes, facts, and embedded glossary insets adding appropriately to the already interesting and succinct presentation."
— *School Library Journal, Jan '02*

"This title is highly recommended for any library that serves adolescents and parents/caregivers of adolescents."
— *E-Streams, Jan '02*

"Recommended for high school libraries and young adult collections in public libraries. Both health professionals and teenagers will find this book useful."
— *American Reference Books Annual, 2002*

"This is a nice book written to enlighten the society, primarily teenagers, about common teen mental health issues. It is highly recommended to teachers and parents as well as adolescents."
— *Doody's Review Service, Dec '01*

■

Sexual Health Information for Teens

Health Tips about Sexual Development, Human Reproduction, and Sexually Transmitted Diseases

Including Facts about Puberty, Reproductive Health, Chlamydia, Human Papillomavirus, Pelvic Inflammatory Disease, Herpes, AIDS, Contraception, Pregnancy, and More

Edited by Deborah A. Stanley. 391 pages. 2003. 978-0-7808-0445-6.

"This work should be included in all high school libraries and many larger public libraries.... highly recommended."
— *American Reference Books Annual, 2004*

"*Sexual Health* approaches its subject with appropriate seriousness and offers easily accessible advice and information."
— *School Library Journal, Feb '04*

Skin Health Information for Teens

Health Tips about Dermatological Concerns and Skin Cancer Risks

Including Facts about Acne, Warts, Hives, and Other Conditions and Lifestyle Choices, Such as Tanning, Tattooing, and Piercing, That Affect the Skin, Nails, Scalp, and Hair

Edited by Robert Aquinas McNally. 429 pages. 2003. 978-0-7808-0446-3.

"This volume, as with others in the series, will be a useful addition to school and public library collections." — *American Reference Books Annual, 2004*

"There is no doubt that this reference tool is valuable."
— *VOYA: Voice of Youth Advocates, Feb '04*

"This volume serves as a one-stop source and should be a necessity for any health collection."
— *Library Media Connection*

■

Sports Injuries Information for Teens

Health Tips about Sports Injuries and Injury Protection

Including Facts about Specific Injuries, Emergency Treatment, Rehabilitation, Sports Safety, Competition Stress, Fitness, Sports Nutrition, Steroid Risks, and More

Edited by Joyce Brennfleck Shannon. 405 pages. 2003. 978-0-7808-0447-0.

"This work will be useful in the young adult collections of public libraries as well as high school libraries."
— *American Reference Books Annual, 2004*

■

Suicide Information for Teens

Health Tips about Suicide Causes and Prevention

Including Facts about Depression, Risk Factors, Getting Help, Survivor Support, and More

Edited by Joyce Brennfleck Shannon. 368 pages. 2005. 978-0-7808-0737-2.

■

Tobacco Information for Teens

Health Tips about the Hazards of Using Cigarettes, Smokeless Tobacco, and Other Nicotine Products

Including Facts about Nicotine Addiction, Immediate and Long-Term Health Effects of Tobacco Use, Related Cancers, Smoking Cessation, Tobacco Use Prevention, and Tobacco Use Statistics

Edited by Karen Bellenir. 440 pages. 2007. 978-0-7808-0976-5.

Health Reference Series

Adolescent Health Sourcebook,
  2nd Edition
AIDS Sourcebook, 3rd Edition
Alcoholism Sourcebook, 2nd Edition
Allergies Sourcebook, 3rd Edition
Alzheimer's Disease Sourcebook,
  3rd Edition
Arthritis Sourcebook, 2nd Edition
Asthma Sourcebook, 2nd Edition
Attention Deficit Disorder Sourcebook
Back & Neck Sourcebook, 2nd Edition
Blood & Circulatory Disorders
  Sourcebook, 2nd Edition
Brain Disorders Sourcebook, 2nd Edition
Breast Cancer Sourcebook, 2nd Edition
Breastfeeding Sourcebook
Burns Sourcebook
Cancer Sourcebook, 5th Edition
Cancer Sourcebook for Women,
  3rd Edition
Cancer Survivorship Sourcebook
Cardiovascular Diseases & Disorders
  Sourcebook, 3rd Edition
Caregiving Sourcebook
Child Abuse Sourcebook
Childhood Diseases & Disorders
  Sourcebook
Colds, Flu & Other Common Ailments
  Sourcebook
Communication Disorders Sourcebook
Complementary & Alternative Medicine
  Sourcebook, 3rd Edition
Congenital Disorders Sourcebook,
  2nd Edition
Contagious Diseases Sourcebook
Cosmetic & Reconstructive Surgery
  Sourcebook, 2nd
Death & Dying Sourcebook, 2nd Edition
Dental Care & Oral Health Sourcebook,
  2nd Edition
Depression Sourcebook

Dermatological Disorders Sourcebook,
  2nd Edition
Diabetes Sourcebook, 3rd Edition
Diet & Nutrition Sourcebook,
  3rd Edition
Digestive Diseases & Disorder
  Sourcebook
Disabilities Sourcebook
Domestic Violence Sourcebook,
  2nd Edition
Drug Abuse Sourcebook, 2nd Edition
Ear, Nose & Throat Disorders
  Sourcebook, 2nd Edition
Eating Disorders Sourcebook, 2nd Edition
Emergency Medical Services Sourcebook
Endocrine & Metabolic Disorders
  Sourcebook, 2nd Edition
EnvironmentalHealth Sourcebook,
  2nd Edition
Ethnic Diseases Sourcebook
Eye Care Sourcebook, 2nd Edition
Family Planning Sourcebook
Fitness & Exercise Sourcebook,
  3rd Edition
Food Safety Sourcebook
Forensic Medicine Sourcebook
Gastrointestinal Diseases & Disorders
  Sourcebook, 2nd Edition
Genetic Disorders Sourcebook,
  3rd Edition
Head Trauma Sourcebook
Headache Sourcebook
Health Insurance Sourcebook
Healthy Aging Sourcebook
Healthy Children Sourcebook
Healthy Heart Sourcebook for Women
Hepatitis Sourcebook
Household Safety Sourcebook
Hypertension Sourcebook
Immune System Disorders Sourcebook,
  2nd Edition
Infant & Toddler Health Sourcebook
Infectious Diseases Sourcebook